OCULAR IMMUNOLOGY
TODAY

OCULAR IMMUNOLOGY TODAY

Proceedings of the 5th International Symposium on the
Immunology and Immunopathology of the Eye,
Tokyo, 13–15 March 1990

Editors:

MASAHIKO USUI
Department of Ophthalmology
Tokyo Medical College
Tokyo, Japan

SHIGEAKI OHNO
Department of Ophthalmology
Yokohama City University School of Medicine
Yokohama, Japan

KOKI AOKI
Aoki Eye Hospital
Sapporo, Japan

 1990

EXCERPTA MEDICA, AMSTERDAM – NEW YORK – OXFORD

International Congress Series No. 918
ISBN 0 444 81367 5

This book is printed on acid-free paper.

Published by:
Elsevier Science Publishers B.V.
(Biomedical Division)
P.O. Box 211
1000 AE Amsterdam
The Netherlands

Sole distributors for the USA and Canada:
Elsevier Science Publishing Company Inc.
655 Avenue of the Americas
New York, NY 10010
USA

Printed in The Netherlands

*We wish to dedicate this book
to the pioneer of ocular immunology,
Dr. Seiji Sugiura.*

PREFACE

Immunology is one of the most important and rapidly progressing biological sciences, and this is also true in the field of ophthalmology.

The Fifth International Symposium on the Immunology and Immunopathology of the Eye (IIPE) was held at the Tokyo Medical College Hospital (Tokyo, Japan) from 13–15 March 1990, as one of the presymposia of the XXVI International Congress of Ophthalmology (ICO) in Singapore. The 210 participants from 15 countries benefitted from an interesting scientific program, and also had a chance to absorb something of the Japanese culture during the social program.

It is now 16 years since the first Symposium was held at Strasbourg in France, and significant progress has been made in all areas of ocular immunology during that period. The mechanisms that produce many previously mysterious diseases of the eye are now known to be immunological. International cooperation in research fostered by symposia such as this, is vital to maintaining the momentum of endeavors that will perhaps ultimately give us practical methods of immunotherapy for a number of currently intractable diseases, such as Behçet's disease or Vogt-Koyanagi-Harada disease.

The Symposium was organized around 7 main themes. We received many interesting and valuable papers which have been included in this Proceedings. In addition, spirited discussion sessions following each paper were a significant feature of the Symposium. Additionally, this meeting was a great success due to the constant efforts of many people, and unfortunately there is no space to thank them individually. In particular however, the members of the International Advisory Committee, the International Organizing Committee, and the Local Organizing Committee are to be commended for their labors.

Also, we wish to thank our many sponsors, whose assistance helped make the Symposium possible and allowed us to provide scholarships to 19 young scientists and 6 special awards for poster presentations.

In conclusion, we hope that the Sixth Symposium, which will be held in Maryland, USA, proves to be as successful or even more so than was the Tokyo one.

Masahiko Usui, M.D.
Shigeaki Ohno, M.D.
Koki Aoki, M.D.

FOREWORD

The 5th International Symposium on Ocular Immunology was held at the auditorium of the Tokyo Medical College from 13 to 15 March, 1990. The symposium was well attended, and many interesting and important papers were presented with lively discussions. We are proud of the well organized meeting, thanks to our local organizing committee headed by the president, Prof. Masahiko Usui. We look forward to the proceedings of the symposium, to be published within three months after the meeting, and hope that the volume will prove to be a milestone for the progress of ocular immunology.

Immunology and molecular biology are the two most rapidly developing fields in biology, and they are intimately related. The progress in the field of immunology has given us a powerful armamentarium for the battle against such eye diseases as uveitis, allergic conjunctivitis, corneal transplantation, and many other eye conditions for which immunological reaction is among the important factors. The treatment of the immunological conditions is making rapid progress, as is research on the etiological factors causing immune reactions.

I sincerely hope that this book, recording the symposium, will prove to be fruitful in distributing information about the most recent developments in the field, settling the controversy and finding the path of research leading to the discovery of effective treatments for the difficult eye conditions related to immunology. It will also serve all of those who attended the symposium as a token of memory for such a pleasant and useful meeting.

The symposium was followed by the 26th International Congress of Ophthalmology held in Singapore, from 18 to 23 March, 1990. The congress included sessions on ocular immunology, and some of the participants of the IIPE symposium took part in the programme, presenting the recent progress in the field of ocular immunology not only to specialists in this field but also to ophthalmologists in other fields. I sincerely hope that the next symposium will have still better liaison with the main congress, the 27th International Congress of Ophthalmology to be held in Toronto from 26 June to 1 July, 1994.

Akira Nakajima, M.D.
Chairman, Advisory Committee,
Professor Emeritus, Juntendo University,
The President, International Council
of Ophthalmology

CONTENTS

ANIMAL MODELS

MOLECULAR BIOLOGY

INFECTION

GENERAL OCULAR IMMUNOLOGY

IMMUNOTHERAPY

SPECIAL LECTURE

© 1990 Elsevier Science Publishers (Biomedical Division)
Ocular Immunology Today. M. Usui, S. Ohno and K. Aoki, editors.

THE EARLY HISTORY OF OCULAR IMMUNOPATHOLOGY

ARTHUR M. SILVERSTEIN

Institute of the History of Medicine, Johns Hopkins University
School of Medicine, Baltimore, Maryland 21205 (U.S.A.)

The manner in which the young and dynamic field of immunology
affected the clinical field of ophthalmology early in this century
illustrates well how the basic sciences may influence clinical
interests and clinical practice. While many other clinical fields
of medicine attempted to integrate the turn-of-century immunological
excitement into their clinical and research programs, ophthalmology
is perhaps unique in having maintained that interest from that time
up to the present day, even during the half-century or so when
mainstream immunology abandoned its biomedical concerns in favor of
more immunochemical approaches.

CONCEPTUAL TRENDS IN EARLY IMMUNOLOGY

Immunology was born as a laboratory science at the hands of
Louis Pasteur. His demonstrations of the ability to attenuate
pathogens and utilize them for preventive vaccination in the case of
chicken cholera, anthrax, rabies, and other diseases excited the
interest of the world. These successes were further magnified by
the discovery by von Behring and Kitasato that circulating antibodies can neutralize the toxins of diphtheria and tetanus, and that
such antitoxins can even be administered passively to cure patients
already infected by these organisms. Here were two approaches that
seemed for a time to hold the promise of preventing or curing all of
the infectious diseases whose etiologic agents were being discovered
with great rapidity.

Ophthalmology was influenced by three components of the
developing research program of the young field of immunology, and
applied them in turn to the explanation of its own clinical disease
problems. The first of these was the "doctrine" of cytotoxic
antibodies. At the outset, the immune response had been viewed as
an evolutionary development for the protection of the individual
from harmful disease agents. Then came Jules Bordet, who showed in
1899[1] that antibodies could even be formed against erythrocytes,
which they destroyed (hemolysed) with the help of the nonspecific-
ally-acting serum factor complement. Pandora's box had been opened,
and investigators everywhere asked themselves why other tissues and

organs might not also stimulate an immune response that might account for the tissue destruction seen in so many diseases of unknown etiology and pathogenesis. Within a very short period, suspensions or extracts of almost every available tissue and organ were injected into animals to search for specific antibodies and for cytotoxicity, and theories were advanced to link the pathogenesis of one or another disease to this mechanism.

The second component of the immunological research program important to this discussion is the concept of autoimmunity. When Bordet reported on the significance of immune hemolysis, Paul Ehrlich and Julius Morgenroth wasted no time in testing whether an animal could form antibodies against its own erythrocytes. This they never observed, causing Ehrlich to advance the dictum of Horror Autotoxicus,[2] which held that even if autoantibodies could be demonstrated, internal regulatory mechanisms would operate to prevent self-destructive consequences. So great was Ehrlich's prestige that his concept was accepted as law. As a result, progress in autoimmune disease research was retarded for over 50 years,[3] and it was only the ophthalmologists who worked consistently on this problem during this period.

The third important component of the immunological research program that influenced ophthalmology was that of anaphylaxis and related disease mechanisms. In 1902, Paul Portier and Charles Richet reported that animals could be sensitized by a first exposure to antigen, such that a second challenge with the same antigen would lead to shock-like symptoms and even death.[4] Shortly thereafter, Maurice Arthus demonstrated that bland antigens injected repeatedly into the skin could cause local necrotizing lesions, a dermal antigen-antibody interaction thenceforth known as the Arthus phenomenon.[5] Finally, in 1906, Clemens von Pirquet and Bela Schick showed that the pathogenesis of human serum sickness was caused by an antibody response in the host to the injection of large quantities of foreign protein antigens.[6] Anaphylaxis became so popular that it penetrated into all branches of medicine, and not least into ophthalmological concepts of disease. This spread of interest was accelerated when it became apparent that those scourges of mankind, hayfever and asthma, were also related to anaphylactic mechanisms.

We shall now see how the field of ophthalmology was influenced by these three concepts. I shall discuss them in terms of their influence on the major trends of ocular immunopathology, but only carry the story up to the 1950s. After this, the explosion of interest and the progress made in each of these areas is too well known and too well documented in numerous texts' and symposium proceedings[8] to warrant repetition here.

SYMPATHETIC OPHTHALMIA

Ophthalmologists were not long in joining the new movement stimulated by the doctrine of cytotoxic antibodies. In 1907, Santucci drew attention to the possibility that sympathetic ophthalmia might be caused by the formation of cytotoxic antibodies following resorption of damaged ocular tissue in the first eye, which would then attack the hitherto normal contralateral eye.[9] Santucci presented experiments showing that injection of emulsified ocular tissue into rabbits and guinea pigs would cause endophthalmitis. No sooner had this thesis begun to attract attention than a counterclaim for priority appeared from the pen of S. Golowin in Russia,[10] who pointed out that he had advanced this idea in 1904,[11] in a Russian journal apparently unread in the West. Golowin claimed that the seat of attack in the sympathizing eye was the iris and ciliary body, and so named these antibodies "cyclotoxins."

It was then that the famous Elschnig of Prague entered the fray. Elschnig quickly became the leading advocate of an autoimmune pathogenesis of sympathetic ophthalmia.[12] He suggested that the resorption of antigen in the damaged eye led to a "hypersensitivity" that involved also the second eye. Thus, the mildest disturbance in the sensitized second eye might lead to inflammation and blindness. In the course of numerous animal experiments, Elschnig ultimately identified uveal pigment as the offending antigen. For many years, students of sympathetic ophthalmia continued to concentrate on uveal pigment, and Alan Woods[13] and Jonas Friedenwald[14] sought to show histopathologically and by the demonstration of positive skin tests employing uveal pigment as antigen that here was the true culprit. But a satisfactory animal model was not available, and progress was slow, until Collins published his landmark papers starting in 1949,[15] showing that uveal extracts injected in adjuvants would cause uveoretinitis in guinea pigs. These observations helped to ensure the modern revival of interest in autoimmune diseases and led to the exciting studies utilizing S-antigen, IRBP, and other components of the retinal outer segment to stimulate a disease in experimental animals that more and more resembles that seen in the human.

PHACOANAPHYLAXIS

A new chapter in the history of immunology was opened up by Paul Uhlenhuth when he reported[16] in 1903 that the antigens of the lens of the eye were organ-specific. This was the first intimation that unique antigens might exist within a single organ and, further, that they might be shared among widely divergent species. It was then shown by Kraus and coworkers,[17] and by Andrejew and Uhlenhuth[18] that these lens antigens could mediate both active and passive anaphylaxis in test animals. Uhlenhuth and Haendel then showed that a guinea pig could be rendered sensitive to its own lens protein and sent into anaphylactic shock with the proteins from any other lens.[19] These investigators drew no conclusions from their work that might be applied to clinical problems, although the ophthalmologist Paul Römer had earlier speculated that senile cataract formation might be mediated by autocytotoxic antibodies specific for the lens.[20] It was only when F.F. Krusius demonstrated that rupture of the lens capsule in a normal guinea pig would both sensitize the animal and serve also as the disease-producing challenge[21] that the true implications of this system for ocular disease became apparent.

In a comprehensive review of the subject in 1912, Römer and Gebb considered the broader implications of these findings in a most interesting way.[22] They asked whether autologous lens is really foreign in the guinea pig, or "whether the 'law of immunity research,' which Ehrlich has popularly termed horror autotoxicus, does not rather apply to the lens." Here, as early as 1912, was a foretaste of the later concept of the "sequestered antigen." If the body cannot respond to self, then all antigens able to stimulate an immune response must be foreign, i.e., normally sequestered somehow from contact with the host's immune system. But as true followers of Ehrlich, they finally came to the conclusion that lens is self, that it does stimulate an immune response, and that "We are rather convinced that the regulatory mechanism of the organism can and will refuse to serve under special conditions. And the investigation of these situations will further promote our understanding of pathological states." Interest in lens-induced immunogenic disease continued, and important contributions were made over the years. The clinical condition was named endophthalmitis phacoanaphylactica by Verhoeff and Lemoine in 1922,[23] and further investigation of antilens responses in patients with cataract was pursued by Burky and Woods.[24]

IMMUNOGENIC KERATITIS AND CORNEAL TRANSPLANTATION

It was Wessely[25] who first noticed that the injection of antigen intrastromally in the central cornea of a sensitized rabbit would produce an opaque ring of interstitial keratitis. This observation attracted much attention, especially of von Szily, who devoted an entire book[26] to the study of this phenomenon. It was finally Germuth, Maumenee, and coworkers,[27] employing modern technics such as immunofluorescent histochemical staining, who proved that the Wessely ring was in fact a true intracorneal Arthus reaction, i.e., an immune complex deposit with local fixation of complement and the release of pharmacologic agents that attracted polymorphonuclear leukocytes to the site.

Yet another approach to the problem of immunogenic interstitial keratitis stemmed from Robert Koch's tuberculin test, and from developments in the field of delayed hypersensitivity (cellular immunology) in which this test played so important a role. During the early period, when many new approaches to the diagnosis of tuberculosis were developed, Calmette proposed his "ophthalmo-reaction,"[28] in which tuberculin dropped on the eye of a sensitized individual would lead to a more-or-less severe conjunctivitis. While this test proved to be too dangerous, it did stimulate experiments using other ocular tissues, including the cornea. It was quickly found that intracorneal injection of tuberculin into sensitized guinea pigs would yield an interstitial keratitis, whereas injection of antigen into an anaphylactically sensitive animal would not lead to corneal inflammation. A different mechanism seemed to be involved, one that depended upon the normal avascularity of the cornea. Indeed, this difference was long used as one of the principal criteria to differentiate these two phenomena.

The history of attempts to transplant cornea to restore sight is a long one,[29] but it was only around the turn of this century that technical improvements in trephines and sutures permitted the ophthalmic surgeon to begin to realize success in this venture, employing what we now call allogeneic tissue. When, as frequently happened, a graft would fail, it was usually attributed to some unknown physiological factor. It remained for Peter Medawar to clarify the immunologic basis of allograft rejection in his elegant series of studies in the 1940s,[30] and these immediately caught the attention of transplant surgeons everywhere. It was Maumenee who was chiefly responsible for bringing these immune responses to the attention of ophthalmologists, and for bringing to the attention of the transplant immunologists the special characteristics of the cornea that allowed keratoplasty to succeed, while most other tissue and organ grafts failed.[31] Again, the important mechanism responsible for graft rejection was shown to be the cellular immune response mediated by effector lymphocytes, and the high success rate of allokeratoplasty was shown to reside in an immunological privilege of the cornea, due to its avascularity and lack of lymphatic drainage.[32]

IMMUNOGENIC UVEITIS

From the very outset, it had been demonstrated that the eye shared in the general hypersensitivity of the immunized or infected host, and that such sensitization could be induced by intraocular administration of antigen. But it remained for C. H. Sattler[33] to show that bland antigen introduced into the vitreous of the rabbit eye would cause a <u>local ocular hypersensitivity</u> also, an observation extended by the elegant studies of the Seegals.[34] Such a sensitized eye would respond with an acute anterior uveitis for many months thereafter to specific antigen, introduced intravenously or even by feeding. Here was a possible animal model of human recurrent nongranulomatous anterior uveitis that stimulated later workers to investigate its pathogenesis. Among the results of these studies was the finding that the eye could function as a highly efficient antibody producer. This emerged initially from studies on equine periodic ophthalmia, most notably by Witmer.[35]

With the finding that systemic hypersensitivity accompanies tuberculosis[36] and many other infectious diseases, many investigators wondered whether such immunologic components might not contribute to the pathogenesis of such granulomatous diseases of the eye as tuberculosis, syphilis, toxoplasmosis, and others. These considerations are well reviewed in the book of their foremost exponent, Alan Woods.[37]

ALLERGIC CONJUNCTIVITIS

We have already seen that the conjunctiva may become inflamed by instillation of tuberculin in the sensitized individual. With the finding that hayfever and asthma are also immunologic ("anaphylactic") reactions,[38] it became apparent that immunogenic conjunctivitis was a more general phenomenon, and clinicians became more interested in its pathogenesis and treatment. This stimulated research on the possible immunopathogenesis of such diseases as vernal catarrh". But perhaps the most interesting development along these lines was the suggestion that an immune reponse to the antigens of <u>Chlamydia trachomatis</u> might account for the primary lesions seen in trachoma[40] and in other follicular conjunctivitides.

REFERENCES

1. Bordet J (1899) Ann Inst Pasteur 12:688

2. Ehrlich P (1901) Verh 73 Ges Dtsch Naturforsch Aerzte

3. This hiatus is discussed by Silverstein AM (1989) A History of Immunology. Academic Press, New York, pp 160-189

4. Portier P, Richet C (1902) C R Soc Biol 54:170

5. Arthus M (1903) C R Soc Biol 55:817

6. von Pirquet C, Schick B (1906) Die Serumkrankheit. Deuticke, Vienna

7. See, e.g., Woods, AC (1933) Allergy and Immunity in Ophthalmology. Johns Hopkins Press, Baltimore; Theodore FH, Schlossman A, (1958) Ocular Allergy. Williams & Wilkins, Baltimore; Woods, AC (1956) Endogenous Uveitis. Williams & Wilkins, Baltimore; Böke W (1968) Immunpathologie des Auges. Karger, Basel; Rahi AHS, Garner A (1976) Immunopathology of the Eye. Blackwell, Oxford

8. Maumenee AE (1959) Uveitis. Survey Ophthalmol 4(part 2):212; Maumenee AE, Silverstein AM, eds. (1964) Immunopathology of Uveitis. Williams and Wilkins, Baltimore. See also the proceedings of the first four International Conferences on the Immunology and Immunopathology of the eye; and the National Eye Institute's three workshops on Immunology of the Eye. (1980-81) Information Retrieval, Washington

9. Santucci S (1906) Riv Ital Ottal Roma 2:213

10. Golowin S (1909) Klin Monatsbl Augenheilk 47:150

11. Golowin S (1904) Russky Vratch No. 22, May 29

12. Elschnig A (1910) von Graefes Arch Ophthalmol 75:459; 76:509; (1911) 78:549; 79:428

13. Woods AC (1917) Arch Ophthalmol 46:8; (1936) Am J Ophthalmol 19:9, 100

14. Friedenwald J (1934) Am J Ophthalmol 17:1008

15. Collins RC (1949) Am J Ophthalmol 32:1687; (1953) 36:150

16. Uhlenhuth P (1903) In: Festschrift zum 60 Geburtstag von Robert Koch. Fischer, Jena, pp 49-74

17. Kraus R, Doerr R, Sohma M (1908) Wien klin Wochenschr 21:1084

18. Andrejew P, Uhlenhuth P (1909) Arb Kaiserl Gesundheitsamte 30:450

19. Uhlenhuth P, Haendel (1910) Z Immunitätsforsch 4:761

20. Römer P, Gebb H (1905) von Graefes Arch Ophthalmol 60:175

21. Krusius FF (1910) Arch Augenheilk 67:6

22. Römer FF, Gebb H (1912) von Graefes Arch Ophthalmol 81:367, 387

23. Verhoeff FH, Lemoine AN (1922) Acta Int Cong Ophthalmol Washington 1:234

24. Burky EL, Woods AC (1931) Arch Ophthalmol 6:548; Burky EL (1934) Arch Ophthalmol 12:536

25. Wessely K (1911) Münch Med Wochenschr 58:1713

26. von Szily A (1914) Die Anaphylaxie in der Augenheilkunde. Ferdinand Enke, Stuttgart

27. Germuth FG, Maumenee AE, Senterfit LB, Pollack AD (1962) J. Exp. Med. 115:919-928

28. Calmette LCA (1907) C R Acad Sci 144:1324

29. See, e.g. Leigh AG (1966) Corneal Transplantation. Blackwell, London, pp 1-5

30. Medawar PB (1944) J Anat 78:176; (1945) J Anat 79:157

31. Maumenee AE (1955) Ann NY Acad Sci 59:453; see also Paufique L, Sourdille GF, Offret G (1948) Les Greffes de la Cornée (Kératoplasties). Masson, Paris

32. Billingham RE, Boswell T (1953) Proc Roy Soc London (Biol) 141:392

33. Sattler CH (1909) Arch Augenheilk 64:390

34. Seegal D, Seegal BH (1930) Proc Soc Exp Biol Med 27:390; (1931) J Exp Med 54:265

35. Goldmann H, Witmer RH (1954) Ophthalmologica Basel 127:323; Witmer RH (1953) Am J Ophthalmol 37:243; (1955) Arch Ophthalmol 53:811

36. Rich AR (1951) The Pathogenesis of Tuberculosis, 2nd ed. Charles C Thomas, Springfield, Illinois

37. Woods, AC (1961) Endogenous Inflammations of the Uveal Tract. Williams & Wilkins, Baltimore

38. Wolff-Eisner A (1906) Das Heufieber. Munich; Meltzer SJ (1910) J Am Med Assoc 55:1021

39. Oguchi M (1954) Acta Soc Opthalmol Japan 58:735

40. Dhermy P; Coscas G, Nataf R, Levaditi JC (1968) Int Rev Trachome pp 295-397

EDUCATIONAL LECTURES

© 1990 Elsevier Science Publishers (Biomedical Division)
Ocular Immunology Today. M. Usui, S. Ohno and K. Aoki, editors.

CLONAL ELIMINATION OF SELF-REACTIVE T-CELLS IN THE THYMUS OF IRRADIATION BONE MARROW CHIMERAS

KAZUNORI ONOÉ

Research Section of Pathology, Institute of Immunological Science, Hokkaido University, Sapporo, 060 (Japan)

INTRODUCTION

T cells do not react avidly with self antigens (1). However, to date various diseases including ocular ones (e.g. Behcet's disease, Vogt-Koyanagi-Harada disease) have been suggested to be caused at least to some degree by autoimmune mechanisms (2). Since T cells are thought to play a major role in discriminating between self and non-self antigens, mechanisms underlying the induction and maintenance of self-tolerance in T cell repertoire have been one of the most important subjects in basic immunology. Recently, it has been demonstrated that thymocytes bearing TCRs that react with self antigens are eliminated in the process of differentiation within the thymus (3-5).

In our previous studies (6,7), we have shown that T cells and thymocytes obtained from allogeneic bone marrow (BM) chimeras were specifically unresponsive against both donor and recipient antigens when evaluated by ability to initiate GVHR. No suppressor mechanisms could be shown to exist that might explain the tolerant state of the T cells. We, thus, considered that clonal elimination was also a most probable explanation for the mechanisms involved in specific tolerance induction in the chimera system.

In the present study, we analyzed differentiation process of thymocytes and tolerant state of T cells obtained from allogeneic BM chimera mice. We show herein the characteristics of cell components which contribute to clonal elimination of T cells positive for V beta 6 of the T cell antigen receptor (TCR) whose expression is strongly associated with T cell recognition of both I-E and Mls-1^a antigens (8).

MATERIALS AND METHODS

Chimera. Irradiation BM chimeras were prepared by a method described elsewhere (6,9). For convenience chimeras prepared by injecting B10 (H-2^b, Mls-1^b) BM cells into irradiated (1,000R) AKR (H-2^k, Mls-1^a) mice will be referred to as [B10 → AKR]. Other chimeras established with different combinations will be expressed according to this nomenclature.

Surface marker analysis. FACS analysis was carried out basically according to Fukushi et al. (9) and Iwabuchi et al. (10). In some experiments, three color analysis was carried out as previously described (11).

Proliferative responses. Thymocytes were co-cultured with APC and various reagents, i.e. 2C11 (anti-CD3 mAb), Con A or PMA + murine rIL-2 as described elsewhere (12).

RESULTS

Sequential changes of surface phenotypes of thymocytes from chimeras. At first we analyzed sequentially surface phenotypes of donor-derived thymocytes from [B10 → AKR] chimeras. Prior to analysis of expression of CD4 and/or CD8 antigens, thymocytes were treated with anti-Thy 1.1 + C to completely eliminate the recipient, AKR, cells.

At day 9 after reconstitution most of cells in the thymocyte population were shown to be CD4$^-$8$^-$ (Fig.1). More than 90% of these thymocytes were IL-2R$^+$ (data not shown). At day 14, however, 86% of thymocytes were CD4$^+$8$^+$ and the proportion of CD4$^-$8$^-$ cells was reduced to 9%. At day 28, the proportion of CD4$^+$8$^-$ or CD4$^-$8$^+$ single positive (SP) cells markedly increased.

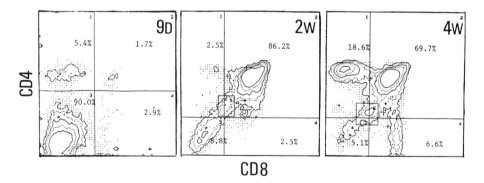

Fig.1 FACS analysis of CD4 and/or CD8 expressions on donor-derived thymocytes from [B10 → AKR] chimeras. The percentages of subpopulations in each fraction are indicated.

None of cells showed recipient, Thy 1.1, phenotype. Further, by day 21 a significant number of thymocytes became to express CD3 and TCR (data not shown and (12)). Thus, these findings indicate that mature thymocytes appear after 2 wk following reconstitution. <u>Sequential changes in the responsiveness of thymocytes to various stimuli</u>. We then analyzed the responses to anti-CD3 (2C11), PMA + rIL-2 or Con A plus 3,000R-irradiated APC from AKR mice in thymocytes obtained from [B10 → AKR] chimeras at various periods after reconstitution. As shown in Fig.2, the thymocytes showed only negligible proliferative responses to 2C11, PMA + IL-2 or Con A at 2 wk. Thereafter, responses to Con A gradually increased and reaching a plateau at day 28. This finding is compatible with our previous report (13). The responses to PMA + rIL-2 or 2C11, on the other hand, were detectable around 4 wk after reconstitution and reached a plateau at day 35. Thus, the latter responsiveness appeared to lag behind that to Con A.

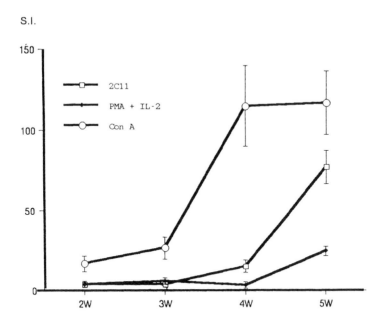

Fig. 2. Sequential analysis of proliferative responses in thymocytes from [B10→AKR] chimeras to 2C11, PMA + rIL-2 or Con A.

Clonal elimination of V beta 6[+] mature thymocytes in chimeras where I-E[−] or I-E[+] and Mls-1[b] mice were donors and AKR (I-E[+], Mls-1[a]) were recipients. We then analyzed expressions of V beta 6 and V beta 8 TCR on CD4[+]8[−] or CD4[−]8[+] single positive (SP) thymocytes from various kinds of chimeras. The V beta 6 TCR specific for I-E and Mls-1[a] antigens are not expressed on mature T cells in recipient, AKR, strain because of clonal elimination, while donor mice lacking Mls-1[a] antigens have a substantial proportion of V beta 6 bright positive T cells (Table I)(14). The expression of V beta 8 TCR serves as a positive control for determination of the stage of thymocyte differentiation.

As shown in Table I, when the proportion of V beta 6[+] SP thymocytes were compared between [E[−]→ AKR] and [E[+]→ AKR] in which I-E[−] or I-E[+] mice were donors, respectively, almost complete elimination of V beta 6[+] cells was seen only in thymuses from latter [E[+]→ AKR] chimeras 5 wk after reconstitution. By contrast, significant numbers of V beta 6[+] cells were detected in SP thymocyte populations from [E[−] → AKR] chimeras, although the proportions varied chimera by chimera. The variation appeared to be dependent on H-2 haplotype of donor strain of mice (9). Significant differences were not seen in proportions of V beta 8[+] cells among various chimeras.

Table I
FREQUENCY OF V BETA 8[+] OR 6[+] CELLS IN SP THYMOCYTES FROM NORMAL MICE OR CHIMERAS

Mice	Donor I-E	Donor Mls	V beta 8/CD3(%)	V beta 6/CD3(%)
B10	−	b	24.8 ± 0.3	8.2 ± 0.2
B10.AQR	+	b	24.6 ± 0.6	9.5 ± 0.1
SWR	−	b	−*	6.5 ± 0.3
AKR	+	a	23.7 ± 0.2	0.6 ± 0.1
[B10 → AKR]	−	b	19.7 ± 0.3	4.3 ± 0.5
[SWR → AKR]	−	b	−*	9.5 ± 0.6
[B10.AQR → AKR]	+	b	21.8 ± 0.4	0.9 ± 0.2
[B10.BR → AKR]	+	b	21.6 ± 0.3	0.6 ± 0.2

* SWR mice lack TCR of V beta 8 family.

Clonal elimination of V beta 6+ mature thymocytes in chimeras where I-E and Mls-1a antigens were expressed separately on either donor or recipient cells. Prior experiments suggest that donor-derived I-E+ cells are crucial for elimination of V beta 6+ cells from donor derived SP thymocytes. To analyze the characteristics of Mls-1a positive cells, we then prepared [B10.BR(BR)→DBA/1] and [DBA → B10.BR(BR)] chimeras in which DBA/1 (I-E⁻) mice were used as a source of cells positive for Mls-1a antigens.

As shown in Table II, significant numbers of V beta 6+ cells were detected in both B10.BR and DBA/1 mice. However, 5 wk after reconstitution the V beta 6+ cells were almost completely eliminated in [BR → DBA/1] chimeras. By contrast, in [DBA/1 → BR] chimeras the proportion of V beta 6+ cells fell within the same range as that of normal donor mice. These findings demonstrate again that BM-derived I-E+ cells are crucial for clonal elimination of V beta 6+ T cells and indicate that for deletion of V beta 6+ cells, Mls-1a antigens need not exist on the same cells as those on which I-E molecules are expressed. It seems that in [BR → DBA/1] chimeras Mls-1a antigens from DBA/1 cells were transferred to I-E+ cells of donor, B10.BR, BM origin as previously proposed by Speiser et al. (15).

Table II

FREQUENCY OF V BETA 6+ CELLS IN SP THYMOCYTES FROM CHIMERAS IN WHICH I-E AND MLS ANTIGENS ARE EXPRESSED ON DIFFERENT CELLS

Mice	Donor		Recipient		V beta 6/TCR(%)
	I-E	Mls-1	I-E	Mls-1	
B10.BR(BR)	+	b			8.0 ± 0.3
DBA/1	−	a			4.2 ± 0.4
[BR→DBA/1]	+	b	−	a	0.9 ± 0.3
[DBA/1→BR]	−	a	+	b	4.5 ± 0.2
[BR→[BR→DBA/1]]	+	b	−	a	3.6 ± 0.7
[AQR→AKR]	+	b	+	a	0.8 ± 0.4
[BR→[AQR→AKR]]	+	b	+	a	9.4 ± 1.2

Also presented in this table are data which show that in [BR→ [BR → DBA/1]] double chimeras which had been prepared by reconstituting lethally (1,000R) irradiated [BR→DBA/1] chimeras 14 wk after the first BM transplantation with T-cell depleted BM cells from B10.BR mice, complete elimination of V beta 6[+] cells did not occur. This finding suggests that cells expressing Mls-1[a] antigens did not exist in sufficient number in the recipient, [BR→ DBA/1], chimeras when the second reconstitution was performed. Similar result was obtained with [BR→[AQR→AKR]] double BM chimeras (Tabale II). Thus, the result with these double chimeras, [BR→ [BR→DBA/1]] or [BR→[AQR→AKR]], indicates that DBA/1 or AKR cells bearing Mls-1[a] antigens are relatively radio-sensitive. Such cells appear to belong to hematopoietic and/or lymphopoietic lineages.

DISCUSSION

In the present communication we have investigated cell components involved in clonal elimination of V beta 6[+] cells in SP mature thymocytes from allogeneic BM chimeras. V beta 6 of TCR correlates with reactivity to I-E and Mls-1[a] antigens (8). We demonstrated that the I-E[+] cells from BM origin are crucial for elimination of V beta 6[+] cells among SP thymocytes. Since substantial numbers of BM-derived I-E[+] cells, macrophages and/or dendritic cells, were detectable only in the thymic medulla 2 wk after reconstitution and beyond (9,16), the elimination appeared to occur at the medulla after this stage, when small proportion of CD4[+]8[-] or CD4[-]8[+] SP thymocytes began to appear in the thymus. A direct evidence for this postulate was obtained from immunohistochemical analyses (9). A significant number of V beta 6[+] cells were found in the thymic medulla of [BR→DBA/1] chimeras 2 wk after reconstitution, while none of V beta 6[+] cells could be seen at 3 wk. At these stages, however, the thymocytes did not show significant proliferative responses to a stimulus by anti-CD3 mAb plus APC, although a substantial proportion of the thymocytes expressed CD3 and TCR molecules (12).

Concerning which of Mls-1[a] positive cells are involved in clonal elimination, it is clear that cells bearing Mls-1[a] antigens need not to express simultaneously I-E antigens. In our prior study (9), we showed that Mls-1[a] positive cells might be of either donor or recipient lineages in the presence of I-E[+] cells derived from donor BM. The Mls-1[a] positive cells, however, were shown to be radio-sensitive by the experiment of double BM chimeras (e.g. [BR→ [BR→ DBA/1]]). Such cells bearing Mls-1[a] antigens and contributing to the elimination of V beta 6^+ thymocytes were demonstrated to be the cells which had existed in $[BR \rightarrow DBA/1]$ chimeras for a sufficient period but were the cells which decreased immediately in number after the second total body irradiation followed by BM transplantation. Thus, these cells appear to belong to hematopoietic and/or lymphopoitic lineages.

The present findings, thus, suggest that both $I-E^+$ cells and $Mls-1^a$ positive cells in the thymus which are responsible for elimination of V beta 6^+ T cells are the cells derived from BM.

ACKNOWLEDGEMENTS

This work was supported in part by Grant-in-Aid for Scientific Research from Ministry of Education, Science and Culture, The Special Grant-in -Aid for Promotion of Education and Science in Hokkaido University Provided by the Ministry of Education, Science and Culture, Japan. I thank Ms M. Konishi for preparation of the manuscript.

REFERENCES

1.Marrack P, Kappler J (1987) Science 238:1073

2.Nussenblatt RB, Grey I, Ballintine EJ, Wacker WB (1980) Am J Ophthalmol 89:173

3.Marrack P, Lo D, Brinster R, Palmiter R, Burkly L, Flavell RH, Kappler J (1988) Cell 53:627

4.MacDonald HR, Pedrazzini T, Schneider R, Louis JA, Zinkernagel RM, Hengartner H (1988) J Exp Med 167:2005

5.Kisielow P, Blüthmann H, Staerz UD, Steinmetz M, von Boehmer H (1988) Nature 333:742

6.Onoé K, Fernandes G, Good RA (1980) J Exp Med 151:115

7.Onoé K, Iwabuchi K, Iwabuchi C, Arase H, Hatakeyama S, Wambua PP, Fukushi N, Negishi I, Good RA, Ogasawara K (1989) Immunobiol 179:172

8.Payne J, Huber BT, Cannon NA, Schneider R, Schilham MW, Acha-Orbea H, MacDonald HR, Hengartner H (1988) Proc Natl Acad Sci USA 85:7695

9.Fukushi N, Wang B, Arase H, Ogasawara K, Good RA, Onoé K (in press) Eur J Immunol

10.Iwabuchi K, Negishi I, Arase H, Iwabuchi C, Ogasawara K, Good RA, Onoé K (1989) Proc Natl Acad Sci USA 86:5089

11.Arase H, Fukushi N, Hatakeyama S, Ogasawara K, Iwabuchi K,

Iwabuchi C, Negishi I, Good RA, Onoė K (in press) Immunobiol

12.Ogasawara K, Fukushi N, Arase H, Iwabuchi C, Hatakeyama S, Iwabuchi K, Good RA, Onoė K (in press) Immunobiol

13.Onoė K, Fernandes G, Shen FW, Good RA (1982) Cell Immunol 68:207

14.Hengartner H, Odermatt B, Schneider R, Schreyer M, Wälle G, MacDonald HR, Zinkernagel RM (1988) Nature 336:388

15.Speiser DE, Schneider R, Hengartner H, MacDonald HR, Zinkernagel RM (1989) J Exp Med 170:595

16.Hatakeyama S, Ogasawara K, Fukushi N, Iwabuchi C, Iwabuchi K, Wang B, Kajiwara M, Good RA, Onoė K (in press) Acta Pathol Jpn

© 1990 Elsevier Science Publishers (Biomedical Division)
Ocular Immunology Today. M. Usui, S. Ohno and K. Aoki, editors.

THE ROLE OF LYMPHOCYTE FUNCTIONING ANTIGEN (LFA) IN IMMUNE RESPONSE

KO OKUMURA AND HIDEO YAGITA

Department of Immunology, Juntendo University School of Medicine, 2-1-1 Hongo Bunkyo-ku, Tokyo 113, Japan

1. INTRODUCTION

Cell involved in immune-reactions display a variety of surface molecules that are responsible for specific effector or recognition functions. Besides the molecules of primary importance in the recognition of antigen, such as the T cell receptor complex, several accessory molecules have been demonstrated to play an important role in regulating immune responses. The recently accumulating knowledge about the structure and function of those molecules, which has been obtained from molecular and cellular biological studies, provided several new approaches to understand the immunological disturbances accompanied to various kinds of diseases. Since those molecules called lymphocyte functioning antigen(LFA) have been known to play crucial role in lymphoctye differentiation as well as final effector phase of immunereactions, such as target lysis or target killing, the understandings of the regulation of LFA expression and signal transduction mechanisms through LFA provide extremely useful tools for the future immunotherapy of the disease. By introducing our trial to study the significance or LFA in various immune-reactions, the involvement of LFA in disease manifestation was discussed.

2. THE ROLE OF MURINE LFA(CD2,LFA-1,VLA)

To characterize the biological functions of LFA, we are mostly focussing the animal experimental model by utilizing cDNA of LFA or monoclonal antibodies against mouse or rat LFA which have been prepared by us or our collaborators (1-3).

In order to investigate the functional role of CD2 molecule in a TCR/CD3-independent system, we introduced the full length murine CD2 cDNA (CD2FL) prepared from pMCD2-2 into a murine LGL clone, SPB2.4, lacking CD2 and TCR/CD3. We examined the cytotoxicity of SPB2.4 and its CD2 transfectant (SPB2.4-CD2FL) against various target cell lines, and found that the cytotoxicity against a target, P815, was reproducibly augmented by the introduction of CD2. This augmentation was perfectly abrogated by an anti-murine CD2 mAb which blocks murine CD2-mediated cellular adhesion. The augmented cytotoxicity of the CD2 transfectant against P815 and its blocking by the anti-CD2 mAb were accompanied with an increase in conjugated formation and its abrogation by the anti-CD2 mAb. Cell surface expression of murine LFA-3 in P815 could not be directly tested by the lack of a mAb reagent for this molecule, however, expression of the putative murine LFA-3 mRNA has been demonstrated by cross-hybridization with the human LFA-3 cDNA probe. This suggests that the cellular interaction between SPB2.4-CD2FL and P815 is mediated by the intercellular binding between CD2 and LFA-3. Recently, it has been demonstrated that CD2-as well as TCR/CD3-mediated activation resulted in the enhancement of LFA-1-mediated cell adhesion, which constitutes another predominant cellular interaction pathway than CD2. However, the conjugate formation as well as the cytotoxicity of SPB2.4-CD2FL against P815 was not inhibited by anti-LFA-1 mAbs at all. Therefore, the cellular interaction between SPB2.4-CD2FL and P815, which led to the augmented cytotoxicity, appeared to be solely mediated by the introduced CD2 molecule. Addition to anti-CD2, we recently established monoclonal antibody which could inhibit this CD2/LFA-1-independent cellular interactions. One of these mAbs, mAb 1.4.4, inhibited the CD2/LFA-1-independent LAK cell cytotoxicity and target cell binding at the effector site. The antigen recognized by mAb 1.4.4 was not expressed on thymocytes and spleen cells but appears to be a very late activation (VLA) antigen as its expression could be induced after prolonged (7-14 days) stimulations with mitogens, alloantigens or IL-2 in vitro. The 1.4.4 antigen was a heterodimer composed of non-covalently linked 130 and 90 kDa subunits, and the 130 kDa subunit was cleaved into 110 and 25 kDa fragments under a reducing condition. These VLA integrin-like characters of the 1.4.4 antigen prompted us to test the possibility that it was an extracellular matrix (ECM) receptor. 1.4.4 mAb efficiently inhibited the LAK cell binding to fibronectin (FN), fibrinogen, and vitronectin, indicating that the 1.4.4 antigen is a murine lymphocyte integrin. Although integrin superfamily proteins have been extensively characterized in humans, VLA-like expression pattern, molecular nature, and ECM ligand specificity of the 1.4.4 antigen did not fit with any member of the human intergrins so far.

3. EFFECT OF ANTI-ICAM-1 ON IN VIVO IMMUNE REACTIONS.

As above mentioned, various kinds of LFA molecules have been revealed to be involved in lymphocyte-target, and/or lymphocyte-macrophage interactions by in vitro experimental systems. To understand more directly the role of these molecules in immuno-pathological reactions in vivo, we administrated the monoclonal antibodies to the experimental animals which cause well known immuno pathological reactions namely, adjuvant arthritis and the rejection reaction against transplanted heart. Since rat systems are rather convenient than mouse for the studies of above immune reaction, we chosen monoclonal antibody against rat ICAM-1 which has been known as a ligand molecule ʕf LFA-1 of T or NK cell, for the in vivo experiments.

Five mg/kg of anti-rat ICAM-1 was injected at the start of experiment when 0.25mg of Freund's complete adjuvant was injected to the one hind footpad. Then, by two day interval, the same amount of mAb was succeedingly administered. The control rat which received the same amount mAb having activities for DNP showed typical inflamatory swelling after ten days in the opposite hind foot as well as the foot received FCA at two weeks after the start experiment. Swelling reached peak at 13 days and persisted more than 30 days. Whereas, the rat received anti-ICAM-1 did not develop any inflamatory reaction in opposite hind foot throughout the experiment and the slight inflamatory reaction was observed only hind foot received FCA. These results clearly showed the involvement of LFA-1 and ICAM-1 interactions in allergic inflamation caused by lymphocytes, although it is not clear whether the inhibition is due to the effect of mAb on inductive phase or effecter phase.

To investigate the significance of such LFA in in vivo immune reactions furthermore, the effect of anti-ICAM-1 was also determined by their inhibitory activities on the allo-heart graft rejection in the combination of Fisher and Lewis rat strains. The mAb (1mg/kg) was administered daily after the cardiograft surgery. The control group showed prominent rejection phenomenon at 9-12 days after the operation and the grafted hearts of all control recipients have lost their functions until 13 days of the experiment. On the contrary, the group received anti-ICAM-1 has not shown the rejection reaction until more than 25 days. During the course of antibody administration, donor heart has maintained their function. Pathological examination revealed that, despite of mononuclear cell infiltration to the heart muscle, there are few necrotic area in heart muscles which were treated by mAb. Thus, the significance of LFA in allergic reaction in vivo is becoming clearer and it was suggested that the way to regulate LFA and ligands interactions has some clue to find out the clinical tools to control immunological reactions.

4. FINAL EFFECTER MOLECULE "PERFORIN" IN IMMUNE REACTION.

We have been also focussing on the final effector molecules of lymphocyte in various kinds of immune reactions. Including cytokines, several molecules has been known as a candidate of final effect molecules of lymphocyte. Perforin (pore-forming protein, PFP or cytolysin) is one of the candidates for effector molecules responsible for cell-mediated cytolysis. Perforin binds to a cell membrane in the presence of Ca^{2+}, and polymerizes to construct lethal doughnut-like channels. Perforin have previously been found to be associated with the cytoplasmic granules of CTL and NK cells. By the studies using mouse, human and rat perforin cDNA, it has been confirmed that the expression of perforin gene is highly restricted to the cytolytic cells (4). Recent studies on cytotoxic lymphocytes in vivo showed that mouse perforin was detected in the peritoneal exudate lymphocytes (PEL) CTL elicited by allogenic tumor cells, the tissue infiltrating lymphocytes of the mice infected with lymphocytic choriomeningitis virus (LCMV), and those of nonobese diabetic (NOD) mice. In these studies, perforin was predominantly in blastic CD8 T cells and asialo GM_1^+ NK cells. These results further stress that perforin is an important cytolytic mediator of the cytotoxic cells. By utilizing newly established mAb reactive with mouse and human perforin (5), histochemical examination revealed that perforin containing CD8+ cells are the major populations in the allograft rejection reaction of the kidney. Although still we did not succeeded to establish mAb which is able to neutralize the perforin activities, the mAb which we established is useful tool to understand the final effector mechanisms of allergic reactions including various kinds of immunological eye disease.

5.REFERENCES

(1) Yagita, H., Nakamura, T., Karasuyama, H., Okumura,K.. (1989) Proc. Natl. Acad.Sci.USA.86;645-649

(2) Nakamura, T., Takahashi, K., Fukazawa, T., Koyanagi, M., Yokoyama, A., Kato, H.,Yagita, H., Okumura, K. (1990) J.Immunol. in press

(3) Tamatani, T. Miyasaka, M. (1990) Int. Immunol. 2:165-171

(4) Shinkai, Y., Takio K. Okumura, K. (1988) Nature 334:525-527

(5) Kawasaki, A . , Shinkai, Y., Kuwana, Y., Furuya, A., Iigo, Y., Hanai, N.,Ito,S.,Yagita, H., Okumura, K. Int. Immunol. in press

ALLERGY

© 1990 Elsevier Science Publishers (Biomedical Division)
Ocular Immunology Today. M. Usui, S. Ohno and K. Aoki, editors.

TEAR SPECIFIC IgE IN THE DIAGNOSIS OF ALLERGIC HAY FEVER TYPE CONJUNCTIVITIS

A.G. SECCHI, A. LEONARDI, E. DANIOTTI, G. CARNIEL and I.A. FREGONA.

Institute of Ophthalmology, University of Padova, School of Medicine. Padova, Italy.

INTRODUCTION

Allergic hay fever type conjunctivitis and, to a lesser extent, vernal keratoconjunctivitis (VKC) may develop without any correlation with a systemic hypersensitivity, being the only manifestation of an allergic condition.

The finding of high levels of specific IgE in tears from allergic patients suggests the hypothesis of a local production of specific antibodies (1). The possibility of a conjunctival hypersensitivity to specific antigens not involved in a systemic sensitization should, therefore, be taken into con sideration by the evaluation of both systemic (skin test, serum specific IgE -sFAST-) and local (conjunctival provocation test -CPT-, tear specific IgE -tFAST-) allergometric tests.

MATERIALS AND METHODS

A group of 81 patients with both history and clinical picture suggestive of allergic hay fever type conjunctivitis, and a group of 15 patients affected by VKC were tested for skin test reactivity. Levels of specific serum and tear IgE were also analyzed in both group of patients using a fluorescence enzyme immunoassay (3M Diagnostic System, Santa Clara, CA, distributed by Eurospital Pharma, Trieste, Italy). In the group of hay fever patients, 32 CPTs were performed during the inactive phase of the inflammation. The choice of allergens was made according to the results of skin/sFAST/tFAST tests, or to the clinical history. Three dilutions of each allergen (10,100,1000 AU/ml) were made from the basic solution (Lofarma, Milano, Italy) at the time of testing. Criteria for a positive CPT were:development of itching and/or burning and/or tearing, with or without conjunctival hyperaemia and/or oedema. Additional CPTs in the same patients using different antigens were performed at weekly intervals

Correlations between skin test and tFAST,sFAST and tFAST (in both group of patients), and between tFAST and CPT (in the hay fever group only) were analysed using the agreement coefficient (Cohen's K). Values below 0,4 were considered to represent poor agreement.

A total of 163 tear specific IgE determinations were performed. In the hay fever group, the correlation between the results of skin test and tFAST showed an agreement in 62% of the cases, either positive (42%) or negative (20%) (table 1). The remaining 38% were discordant: 28% of the patients were skin test negative, but tFAST positive to the same antigen; 10%, skin test positive, were negative at tFAST. The Cohen's coefficent showed a poor agreement between these two tests with a K=0,22.

TABLE 1

SKIN TEST vs tFAST IN HAY FEVER

	tFAST +	tFAST -	
skin +	42% (40)	10% (10)	K = 0,22
skin -	28% (27)	20% (19)	

In the same patients, the correlation between sFAST and tFAST showed an agreement in 65% of the cases (table 2). Of the discordant 35%, 30% were positive only to tFAST and 5% only to sFAST. The Cohen's coefficent showed again a poor correlation between the two tests with a K = 0,33.

TABLE 2

sFAST vs tFAST IN HAY FEVER

	tFAST +	tFAST -	
sFAST +	39% (43)	5% (6)	
sFAST -	30% (33)	28% (26)	K = 0,33

In the group of VKC patients skin and tFAST were discordant in 52% of the cases which were all skin test negative and tFAST positive (table 3). In the same group, the correlation between sFAST and tFAST showed an agreement in 59% of the cases, 32% positive and 27% negative. In 36% of the cases, a negative sFAST concurred with a positive tFAST; in 5% of the cases sFAST was positive and tFAST negative (table 4). The Cohen's coefficent in the VKC group showed again a poor agreement.

TABLE 3

SKIN TEST vs tFAST IN VKC

	tFAST +	tFAST -	
skin +	20% (5)	0% (0)	K = 0,17
skin -	52% (13)	28% (7)	

TABLE 4

sFAST vs tFAST IN VKC

	tFAST +	tFAST -	
sFAST +	32% (7)	5% (1)	K = 0,25
sFAST -	36% (8)	27% (6)	

The correlation between CPT and tFAST showed an agreement in 87,5% of the cases (table 5). 9,5% of cases, which were tFAST positive, resulted negative to the CPT, and 3% of the cases, which were tFAST negative, responded positively to the CPT. The Cohen's coefficent showed a good agreement between the two tests.

TABLE 5

CPT vs tFAST IN HAY FEVER

	tFAST +	tFAST -	
CPT +	78% (25)	3% (1)	K = 0,53
CPT -	9,5% (3)	9,5% (3)	

DISCUSSION

A suggestive personal and family history, associated with relevant clinical symptoms and signs, allow a first approach to the diagnosis of allergic conjuctivitis. A panel of allergometric tests has, however, to be performed in order to confirm the diagnosis, and establish a specific
lergens (2-3).

A high percentage of hay fever type conjunctivitis may develop without any history or clinical evidence of allergic rhinitis, and it is known that the conjunctiva may be the only affected organ in subjects with systemic sensitization or, conversely, it may represent the only sensitized tissue. Specific IgE antibodies have been detected in tears of patients with vernal conjunctivitis, associated with little or no IgE in the serum (1-4). In the present study we have shown that a selective finding of IgE in tears may occur also in patients with a hay fever conjunctivitis, supporting the theory of a local production of specific antibodies (5-6).

The correlation between skin test/serum specific specific IgE, which reveal a systemic sensitization,and tear specific IgE showed a poor agreement in both hay fever and VKC groups. Systemic allergometric tests,should, therefore, not be considered per se entirely reliable in the diagnosis of allergic conjunctivitis,because they may not reveal those situations (30% in our series) characterized by a preferential, or unique, conjunctival reactivity. The good agreement between CPT and FAST confirm the possibility of an exclusively local sensitization. A CPT and tFAST negative with skin test and sFAST positive does not exclude the allergic pathogenesis of he conjunctival disorder; it may only indicate, in fact, that the allergens involved in the conjunctival sensitization may be different from those responsible for the systemic sensitization. It may also be very important to know which allergen is involved in a local sensitization when one takes into consideration the therapeutic possibility of a local desensitization.

The detection of specific IgE in tears, and the conjunctival provocation test, should be considered important complements in the diagnostic protocols of suspected allergic conjunctivitis.

REFERENCES

1. Ballow M, Mendelson L (1980) Specific immunoglobulin E antibodies in tear secretion of patients with vernal conjunctivitis. I Allergy Clin Immunol 66:112-118

2. Secchi AG, Fregona IA, De Carli M (1990) Allergic conjunctivitis. In Falagiani (ed) pollinosis,CRC Press Inc Publ (in press)

3. Secchi AG, Fregona IA, De Carli M (1990) The role of the conjunctival provocation test in the management of allergic conjunctivitis. In Falagiani (ed) Pollinosis. CRC Press Inc Publ (in press)

4. Sompolinsky D, Samara Z, Zavaro A, Barishak Y (1984) Allergen-specific immunoglobulin E antibodies in tears and serum of vernal conjunctivitis patients. Int Arch Allergy Appl Immunol, 75:317-321

5. Leonardi A, Daniotti E, Carniel G et al (1989) I test allergometrici sistemici e lacrimali nella diagnosi di congiuntivite allergica. Proocedings 69th Congress SOI, Roma

6. Liotet S, Warnet VN, Arrata M (1986) Lacrimal immunoglobulin E and allergic conjunctivitis. Ophthalmologica 186:31-34

© 1990 Elsevier Science Publishers (Biomedical Division)
Ocular Immunology Today. M. Usui, S. Ohno and K. Aoki, editors.

MANAGEMENT OF SEVERE ATOPIC KERATOCONJUNCTIVITIS

C. STEPHEN FOSTER, MARGARITA C. CALONGE
Immunology Service, Department of Ophthalmology, Massachusetts Eye and Ear Infirmary, Harvard Medical School, Boston, Massachusetts 02114 (USA)

INTRODUCTION

Atopy is a common condition, affecting 10 to 20% of the population (1, 2). Atopic phenomena are entirely or partially responsible for several disorders of the ocular surface, including hay fever conjunctivitis (HFC) or allergic conjunctivitis, giant papillary conjunctivitis, vernal keratoconjunctivitis (VKC), and *atopic keratoconjunctivitis (AKC)*. Only in the last two conditions the cornea is actively involved (2). AKC includes multifactor ocular surface disorders in a context of atopic dermatitis. In addition to the characteristic skin changes, patients may also have asthma, hay fever, urticaria, migraine headaches, and rhinitis (1, 3). The reported incidence of ocular involvement in atopic dermatitis is between 25% (1, 4) and 42% (5). AKC is always bilateral and symptoms include itching, burning, tearing, and an abundant mucoid discharge. The disease may include lid eczema, chronic blepharitis, cicatrizing conjunctivitis and compromized vision from corneal scarring and neovascularization (5, 6). Successful care of the atopic patient is complex and frequently highly fragmented with a failure in longitudinal care by one physician.

MATERIAL AND METHODS

We have cared for *45 patients* with AKC in the Immunology Service of the Massachusetts Eye and Ear Infirmary between 1980 and 1989. The criteria for making the diagnosis of AKC were a history of blepharoconjunctivitis and/or keratoconjunctivitis in a patient with atopic dermatitis (with or without asthma and/or hay fever), and no identifiable cause for the ocular inflammation other than atopy.

RESULTS

Patient age ranged from 9 to 76 years old, with a mean of 46.2 years. Nineteen were male and 26 were female. Forty four patients were caucasian and one was black. The patients were followed for a mean of 40.2 months (range 3 to 171 months). All patients had atopic eczema, fifteen had asthma (past or current), 29 had hay fever, and one had urticaria. In addition to AKC, another atopic ocular manifestation was found in 31 patients. Eleven patients had VKC, and 29 HFC.

Allergies were reported by 32 patients: to air-borne allergens by 24 patients, to drugs by 18, to food by 12, to wool by three patients, to glued paper by one, and to cosmetics by one. Seasonal exacerbations of ocular inflammation were reported and/or observed in 33.3%.

A positive family history of atopy was elicited in 29 of our patients, 23 of whom had HFC in addition to AKC. The most frequent family finding was hay fever (43.5%), and atopic dermatitis (43.5%), asthma (26.1%), food hypersensitivity (8.7%), and urticaria (4.4%).

Associated ocular pathology

Cataracts were present in 17 patients (30 eyes): these were judged to be age related in four patients (seven eyes), steroid-induced in 8 patients (13 eyes), and atopic and steroid-related in 5 patients (ten eyes). Bilateral open angle glaucoma was discovered in two patients; three other cases (five eyes) of steroid-related glaucoma were detected, and two more were detected after cataract surgery. Ten patients experienced herpetic ocular disease; two patients with extraocular.

Herpes simplex virus manifestations experienced not only keratitis but also uveitis. Rosacea-related blepharoconjunctivitis was present in eight patients and was an important factor in the ocular pathology in one case. Retinal detachment had ocurred several years after intracapsular cataract extraction in five patients, but had had no apparent antecedent in a sixth patient.

Clinical findings

Best corrected *visual acuity* at the time of first visit with us was 20/40 or better in 40 eyes (44.4%), between 20/50 and 20/100 in 23 eyes (25.6%), and 20/200 or worse in 27 eyes (30.0%). Reasons for visual acuity 20/50 or worse at our first examination were attributable to AKC in 30 eyes (33.3%). Visual acuity at the last follow-up improved by two Snellen lines or better in 14 eyes (15.6%), remained the same in 50 eyes (55.6%), and decreased by two or more Snellen lines in 26 eyes (28.9%).

Conjunctival pathology attributable to AKC is shown in Table 1. One of the conjunctival manifestations in many of our patients was particularly remarkable: subepithelial fibrosis was seen in 26 patients, thirteen of whom had frank fornix foreshortening and/or symblepharon formation. Because of this, some of the patients
were referred to us as possible candidates for immunosuppressive chemotherapy for ocular cicatricial pemphigoid.

TABLE 1
CONJUNCTIVAL MANIFESTATIONS IN PATIENTS WITH AKC

	No. of patients (%)
Subepithelial fibrosis	26 (57.8)
Mucus excess	20 (44.4)
Papillae	20 (44.4)
Fornix foreshortening	13 (28.9)
Symblepharon	12 (26.7)
Giant papillae	11 (24.4)

Corneal complications (Table 2) were the most devastating problem in this group of patients. Thirty four of the 45 (75.6%) patients developed severe keratopathy. Neovascularization was present in 17. Lipid deposition was present in two patients, one of whom developed peripheral ulcerative keratitis. The other developed gelatinous hypertrophy in the limbal area. Keratoconus was present in three patients (four eyes). *Persistent epithelial defects (PED)* were common, occurring in 21 eyes of 17 patients. PED following surgery (penetrating keratoplasty) were encountered eight times. The mean duration of PED was 38.6 days (range from 7 to 360 days). Visual acuities prior to the start of the PED were 20/40 or better in eight eyes (38.1%), between 20/50 and 20/100 in seven eyes (33.3%), and 20/200 or worse in 6 eyes (28.6%). Visual acuities after the last episode were 20/40 or better in 3 eyes (14.3%), between 20/50 and 20/100 in 5 eyes (23.8%), and 20/200 or worse in 13 eyes (61.9%). Therefore, vision decreased by two or more Snellen lines in 13 eyes (61.9%), improved in two eyes (9.5%), and remained unchanged in the remainding 6 eyes (28.6%). The variable treatments employed were designed to eliminate or minimize atopic inflammation and conspiratorial factors such as sicca, exposure, trichiasis and infection, and to encourage surface re-epithelization. Infectious corneal ulcerations in the course of a PED developed in four patients, with perforation in two of them. Cyanoacrylate tissue adhesive and bandage soft contact lens, with eventual penetrating keratoplasty was employed in these cases. One patient was managed by lamellar grafting, followed by penetrating keratoplasty for visual rehabilitation.

TABLE 2
CORNEAL ABNORMALITIES IN AKC PATIENTS

	No. of patients (%)
Superficial punctate keratitis	24 (53.3)
Scarring	24 (53.3)
Neovascularization	17 (37.8)
Persistent epithelial defects	17 (37.8)
Sectorial thinning	6 (13.3)
Keratoconus	3 (6.7)
Vernal shield ulcer	2 (4.4)
Filamentary keratitis	2 (4.4)

Multisystem therapy is required for long term success with these patients. A strict environmental control form the basis of the therapy. We suggest maximization of systemic antihistamine therapy in order to maintain quiescence of skin and eye inflammation. Hydroxazine, Terfenadine or Astemizole have been efective in our hands. Topical medication was limited to 4% cromolyn sodium four times a day. We advocate short-term 1% methylprednisolone for inflammatory flare-ups and for peri-operative therapy. In summary, this study demonstrates the chronicity, complexity of treatment and potentially blinding consequences of AKC.

REFERENCES
1. Braude LS, Chandler JW (1984) Atopic corneal disease. Int Ophthalmol Clin 24:145
2. Buckley RJ (1988) In: Cavanagh HD (eds) The Cornea: Transactions of the World Congress of the Cornea III. New York, Raven Press, Ltd, pp 435
3. Carr RD, Berke M, Becker SW (1964) Incidence of atopy in the general population. Arch Dermatol 89:27
4. Jay JL (1981) Clinical features and diagnosis of adult atopic keratoconjunctivitis and the effect of treatment with sodium cromoglycate. Br J Ophthalmol 65:335
5. Garrity JA, Liesegang TJ (1984) Ocular complications of atopic dermatitis. Can J Ophthalmol 19:21
6. Hogan MJ (1953) Atopic keratoconjunctivitis. Am J Ophthalmol 36:937

© 1990 Elsevier Science Publishers (Biomedical Division)
Ocular Immunology Today. M. Usui, S. Ohno and K. Aoki, editors.

TOPICAL CYCLOSPORINE-A IN THE TREATMENT OF VERNAL AND OTHER IMMUNOLOGYCALLY
MEDIATED KERATOCONJUNCTIVITIS

A.G. SECCHI, M.S. TOGNON and A. LEONARDI

Institute of Ophthalmology, University of Padova, School of Medicine
Padova, Italy.

INTRODUCTION

Topical Cyclosporine-A (Cy-A) has already been found useful in a short-term
open treatment of vernal keratoconjunctivitis (VKC), as reported by Ben Ezra
et al (1); Holland et al., more recently, have shown that it may also be active
in the treatment of ligneous conjunctivitis, an inflammatory condition whose
pathogenesis seems to be related to immunopathological, possibly type IV, disorders (2). The present report deals with the effect of topical Cy-A in the long
term open treatment of a group of patients affected by vernal KC, and in a mixed population of patients suffering for different immunopathologically mediated corneo-conjunctival inflammations.

MATERIALS AND METHODS

The first group of patients was made of 11 patients, 7-27 years of age, affected by the tarsal conjunctival and/or the limbal type of vernal KC; all of them
were at least partially sensitive only to high dosages of topical and/or systemic steroids. The second group of patients was made of two cases of catarrhal
KC, two cases of giant papillary conjunctivitis (GPC) in contact lens wearers,
two cases of pemphigoid, and two cases of atopic KC. They were between 11 and 60
years old and some of the inflammatory conditions (catarrhal and GPC) were partially sensitive to high dosages of topical steroids, the others being insensi-
tive to any kind of therapy.

Cy-A for topical use was prepared under sterile conditions from Sandimmun
(Sandoz;Basel,Switzerland) for intravenous use, at a 2% concentration in castor
oil. The drug was given four times/day, one drop in the lower fornix, for four
to eleven months in the first group of patients, and for three to more than
twelve months in the second.

Signs and symptoms of the diseases were graded according to an arbitrary score
(Table 1), and recorded at time 0, day 15th, day 30th, then monthly through the
whole lenght of the treatment.

TABLE 1
 SCORING SYSTEM FOR SYMPTOMS AND SIGNS

Symptoms: 1.itching 2.photophobia 3.tearing 4.dryness
          5.foreign body sensation 6.mucous discharge

  0=absent 1=mild 2=moderate 3=severe 4=very severe
          (with a total of 24 available points/eye)

Signs: 1. conjunctival hyperemia (bulbar)
          2. conjunctival hyperemia (superior tarsal)
          3. conjunctival hyperemia (inferior tarsal)
          4. conjunctival chemosis   5. secretion/exudate
          6. corneal/limbal infiltrates
          7. follicoles   8. papillae   9. giant papillae

  0=absent   1=present   (with a total of 9 available points/eye)

In four patients (two VKC, one GPC, one atopic) the systemic levels of cyclo-sporinemia have been measured at day 30th; the test has been performed by RIA with monoclonal antibodies.

RESULTS

Table 2 shows the results of the trial in the vernal KC patients as far as symptoms and signs are concerned. Both improved significantly within the first 15 days of trial, and even more thereafter.

In the course of the treatment, three patients (27%) needed occasionally additional therapy with topical steroids (1-2% dexamethason, or milder drugs, 2-4 times/days, 3-8 days).

Three patients (27%) are still in treatment. Five patients (45%) underwent a relapse of the disease within 2-4 months from the end of the trial; two of them are again, successfully, in treatment with topical Cy-A; three are now well controlled with 4% disodiumchromoglycate, which previously was almost completely ineffective. Three patients (27%) showed no relapse after 4-5 months from the end of the trial.

Table 3 shows the results of our trial in the miscellaneous KC patients population. Topical Cy-A proved to be effective also in these cases, inducing a significant improvement in boths symptoms and signs of the diseases within the 15th day of treatment.

Topical Cy-A was most effective on the limbal/corneal infiltrates characteristic of catarrhal KC, as it was in the limbal cases of vernal KC and, at a rather lessere extent, in the cases of atopic KC.

TABLE 2
  TOPICAL TREATMENT OF VERNAL KERATOCONJUNCTIVITIS
  WITH CYCLOSPORINE-A

A. BEHAVIOUR OF SYMPTOMS

	Age		A Sympt. Time 0	B Sympt. day 15	C Sympt. end treatm.	months of treatment
1.	12 y	OD+OS	12/48	6/48	0/48	7
2.	11 y	OD+OS	40/48	20/48	0/48	4
3.	17 y	OD+OS	24/48	16/48	0/48	6
4.	7 y	OD+OS	24/48	0/48	0/48	4
5.	10 y	OD+OS	30/48	10/48	0/48	7
6.	11 y	OD+OS	32/48	4/48	0/48	7
7.	27 y	OD+OS	36/48	18/48	2/48	11
8.	26 y	OD+OS	23/48	10/48	14/48	4
9.	12 y	OD+OS	21/48	5/48	0/48	7
10.	7 y	OD+OS	14/48	8/48	2/48	6
11	7 y	OD+OS	34/48	8/48	6/48	5

mean +/-S E   26.36±2.68   9.36±1.87   2.18±1.31

Stat. evaluation: A versus B $p < 0.01$
                  A versus C $p < 0.01$
                  b versus C $p < 0.01$

B. BEHAVIOUR OF SIGNS

	Age		D signs Time 0	E signs day 15	F signs end treatm.	months of treatment
1.	12 y	OD+OS	9/18	4/18	3/18	7
2.	11 y	OD+OS	12/18	11/18	4/18	4
3.	17 y	OD+OS	16/18	14/18	2/18	6
4.	7 y	OD+OS	10/18	4/18	4/18	4
5.	10 y	OD+OS	14/18	6/18	4/18	7
6.	11 y	OD+OS	16/18	6/18	4/18	7
7.	27 y	OD+OS	12/18	6/18	6/18	11
8.	26 y	OD+OS	16/18	12/18	4/18	4
9.	12 y	OD+OS	16/18	6/18	2/18	7
10.	7 y	OD+OS	10/18	7/18	4/18	6
11	7 y	OD+OS	18/18	12/18	10/18	5

mean +/-S E   13.54±0.93   8.00±1.07   4.00±0.66

Stat. evaluation: D versus E $p < 0.01$
                  D versus F $p < 0.01$
                  E versus F $p < 0.01$

TABLE 3
TOPICAL TREATMENT OF MISCELLANEOUS KERATOCONJUNCTIVITIS
WITH CYCLOSPORINE-A

A. BEHAVIOUR OF SYMPTOMS

	Age	A Sympt. Time 0	B Sympt. day 15	C Sympt. end treatm.	months of treatment
CATARRHAL:	1. 17y OD+OS	13/48	0/48	0/18	3
	2. 11y OD+OS	21/48	9/48	3/18	5
GPC:	3. 27y OD+OS	12/48	4/48	4/18	3
	4. 21y OD+OS	21/48	6/48	6/18	3
PEMPHIGOID:	5. 56y OD+OS	33/48	17/48	2/18	>12
	6. 60y OD+OS	21/48	8/48	4/18	>12
AKC:	7. 42y OD+OS	27/48	13/48	9/18	12
	8. 42y OD+OS	22/48	18/48	10/18	3

mean +/-S E   21.25±2.41 9.37±2.22 4.75±1.21

Stat. evaluation: A versus B $p < 0.01$
                  A versus C $p < 0.01$
                  B versus C   n.s.

B. BEHAVIOUR OF SIGNS

	Age	D signs Time 0	E signs day 15	F signs end treatm.	months of treatment
CATARRHAL:	1. 17y OD+OS	14/18	6/18	4/18	3
	2. 11y OD+OS	14/18	2/18	2/18	5
GPC:	3. 27y OD+OS	6/18	1/18	1/18	3
	4. 21y OD+OS	8/18	3/18	3/18	3
PEMPHIGOID:	5. 56y OD+OS	16/18	14/18	12/18	>12
	6. 60y OD+OS	7/18	4/18	4/18	>12
AKC:	7. 42y OD+OS	11/18	5/18	3/18	12
	8. 42y OD+OS	16/18	14/18	12/18	3

mean +/-S E   11.5±1.45 6.1±1.81 5.1±1.54

Stat. evaluation: D versus E $p < 0.01$
                  D versus F $p < 0.01$
                  E versus F   n.s.

GPC in contact lens wearers responded very well to the treatment, which had to be stopped because of the smeary oily nature of the drops, uncomfortable for the patients vision.

The two cases of pemphigoid showed a satisfactory results as far as symptoms and background signs of inflammation were concerned; the conjunctival sinechiae, in fact, were probably too consolidated to undergo significant morphological changes upon medical treatment.

All of the second group patients, with the exception of the two GPC, are still in treatment.

Side effects: sixteen out of the nineteen patients (84%) reported some burning upon instillation of the drug, milder after the first few days of treatment. Two patients (10%) showed punctate corneal epithelial defects, healed after suspension of the treatment for a few days. IOP was never affected.

The level of cyclosporineamia measured in four patients after 30 days of treatment, was always below the minimum detectable by RIA with monoclonal antibodies; topical treatment, therefore, is not followed by any systemic accumulation of the drug.

DISCUSSION

Experimental studies have demonstrated that the topical administration of Cy-A allows significant levels of the drug in the corneal epithelium and stroma, in the sclera, and in the conjunctiva (3,4,5). The use of topical Cy-A in immunologically mediated corneo-conjunctival diseases, where cell-mediated immunopathologies seem to play a major pathogenic role, is therefore rational.

Our long-term open trial indicates that Cy-A is effective in controlling the symptoms/signs of both tarsal conjunctival and limbal types of vernal KC, and of other immunologically mediated KC. Symptoms were seen to respond more readily; limbal and recent corneal infiltrates were, among the signs, most sensitive to the treatment; other signs like papillary hyperplasia or giant papillae showed, within the terms of our trial, less relevant changes.

Topical Cy-A does not seem to cure vernal KC, since almost 50% of our patients relapsed within few months from the suspension of the treatment. It has demonstrated, however, 1. an excellent antinflammatory activity; 2. the possibility of long term and/or repeated cycles of therapy without important side effects; 3. a substantial capability of behaving as a substitute, or at least as an excellent sparing factor, for steroids.

Topical Cy-A, in conclusion, may represent an important therapeutical tool in the treatment of a variety of frequent and severe immunopathologies of the outer eye, so far sensitive only -and not always- to strong steroids.

REFERENCES

1. Ben Ezra D, Pe'er J, Brodsky M and Cohen E (1986) Cyclosporine eyedrops for the treatment of severe vernal keratoconjunctivitis. Am J Ophthal 101: 278-282

2. Holland EJ, Chan CC, Kuwabara T, Palestine AG, Rowsey JJ and Nussenblatt RB (1989) Immunohistologic findings and results of treatment with Cyclosporine in ligeous conjunctivitis. Am J Ophthal 107:160-166

3. Mosteller MW, Gebhardt BM, Hamilton AM and Kaufmann HE (1985) Penetration of topical Cyclosporine into the rabbit cornea, aqueous humor, and serum. Arch Ophthal 103:101-102

4. Wiederholt M, Kossendrup D, Schulz W and Hoffman F (1986) Pharmacokinetic of topical Cyclosporine A in the rabbit eye. Invest Ophthal Vis Sci 27:519-524

5. Bell TAG and Hunniset AG (1986) Cyclosporine A: tissue levels following topical and systemic administration to rabbits. Br J Ophthal 70:852-855

© 1990 Elsevier Science Publishers (Biomedical Division)
Ocular Immunology Today. M. Usui, S. Ohno and K. Aoki, editors.

CONJUNCTIVAL MAST CELL SUBTYPES IN VERNAL KERATOCONJUNCTIVITIS

K.F. TABBARA,[*] A.A. IRANI,[+] S.I. BUTRUS,[°] and L.B. SCHWARTZ[+]
*Dept. of Ophthalmology, King Saud University, Riyadh, Saudi Arabia
+Medical College of Virginia, Richmond, Virginia, U.S.A.
°Georgetown University, Washington, D.C., U.S.A.

Vernal keratoconjunctivitis (VKC) is a severe form of ocular allergy which may cause visual impairment or blindness. The disease, which affects mainly children and young adults, has a worldwide distribution but is more common in hot countries. The symptom of VKC include redness, tearing, foreign body sensation, photophobia, itching, burning, irritation and a thick stringy mucoid discharge. Symptoms may be evident all year round, but the intensity increases during the warm and hot seasons.

VKC causes major discomfort and distress to sufferers. Furthermore, because children with VKC may be absent from school for days or even weeks, it can also interfere with their education.

VKC is frequently associated with other atopic diseases, such as asthma, allergic rhinitis and atopic dermatitis, and with a family history of atopy. Patients with this disease show elevated IgE levels (including allergen specific IgE) in serum and tears, elevated histamine levels in tears, mast cells in the conjunctival epithelium and substantia propria, and peptido-leukotrienes and other potent inflammatory mediators.

Furthermore, VKC has been associated with hyper IgE syndrome.[1] These findings confirm the atopic nature of VKC which has classically been referred to as an immediate Type I IgE-mediated hypersensitivity disorder of the ocular surface.[1] However, there is now evidence indicating that the pathogenesis of VKC involves more than one immune reaction.[2,3]

Mast cells appear to play an important role in the initiation and propagation of the inflammatory reaction in patients with VKC.[2,4,5] The products of the mast cells and other cells cause the signs and symptoms of VKC. Mast cells possess receptors on their cell membranes for the Fc portion of the IgE molecule and the presence of specific antigens causes mast cell stimulation. Phospholipase A_2 causes hydrolysis of membrane phospholipids (eg. phosphatidylcholine and alkylacyl glycerophosphatidylcholine) with subsequent liberation of arachidonic acid and platelet activation factor (PAF). Arachidonic acid is then metabolized via two pathways; the cyclo-oxygenase pathway resulting in the production of prostaglandins (such as PGD_2) and the 5-lipoxygenase pathway leading to the generation of hydroxy-eicosatetranenoic acid and peptidoleukotrienes (for example LTC_4 LTD_4 and

LTE_4). These membrane lipid products are potent inflammatory mediators. In addition to the membrane lipid-derived mediators, mast cells contain granules that store inflammatory mediators, such as histamine, proteases, proteoglycans and peptides. On stimulation, the mast cell undergoes degranulation resulting in the release of these active mediators with subsequent initiation of inflammatory reactions.

Two subtypes of mast cells have been recognized in humans.[4,6] These have been described according to their neutral protease composition, T lymphocyte dependency and ultrastructural characteristics. Table 1 shows the differences between the two subtypes of mast cells: MC^T contains tryptase but no chymase and MC^{TC} contains both tryptase and chymase.

TABLE 1

DIFFERENCES BETWEEN MAST CELL SUBTYPES

| | Mast Cell TC | |
	(MC^T)	(MC^{TC})
T lymphocyte dependency	Yes	No
Degranulation by 48/80	No	Yes
Protease	Tryptase	Tryptase and chymase
Staining	Alcian blue	Alcian blue and saffranin
Location	Mucosa of alveoli and small intestine	Skin and submucosa of small intestine

The distribution of the two subtypes has been studied in the conjunctival tissue of patients with VKC giant papillary conjunctivitis (GPC) and normal subjects.[7] Seven patients with VKC, six with GPC and 19 normal controls were included in the study. Conjunctival tissue specimens were fixed in Carnoy's fixative (60% absolute ethanol, 30% chloroform, 10% glacial acetic acid) for 24 hours, embedded in paraffin, and cut into 4 um thick sections. Double sequential immunohistochemical staining for the detection of MC^T and MC^{TC} was performed using mouse monoclonal antichymase antibody and mouse and monoclonal antitryptase antibody. Mast cells of each subtype were counted by a diagnosis-masked investigator and the concentration of cells per mm^3 of tissue was determined.

There were no mast cells in the conjunctival epithelium of normal subjects. In contrast, there was a marked increase in the number of mast

45

cells in the conjunctival epithelium of VKC patients with a mean of 7994 ($\pm$ 2120) mast cells/mm^3. In patients with VKC, MC^T and MC^{TC} were detected in both the epithelium and substantia propria. In patients with VKC, ninety six percent of the mast cells in the conjunctival epithelium were TC mast cells and 4% were T mast cells. On the other hand, 82% of the mast cells in the substantia propria were TC mast cells and 18% were T mast cells. In patients with giant papillary conjunctivitis (GPC), all mast cells observed were MC^{TC} and no MC^T were seen in either the epithelium or substantia propria. In all subjects (VKC, GPC and controls)MC^{TC} were detected in the substantia propria of the conjunctiva. These results show that MC^{TC} are the predominant cell type in the conjunctiva. A significant increase in the number of MC^T is seen in the conjunctival epithelium and substantia propria of VKC patients but not in GPC patients or normal subjects.

The distribution of mast cell subtypes may contribute to the distinct clinical pictures of the various allergic ocular diseases. It is possible that the subtypes react differently to therapeutic compounds and this will have important consequences on the treatment of such diseases.

REFERENCES

1. Butrus SI, Leung DYM, Gellis S, et al. Vernal conjunctivitis in the hyperimmunoglubulinemia E syndrome. Ophthalmol 1984; 91:1213-1216.

2. Buckley RJ. Vernal keratoconjunctivitis. Int Ophthalmol Clinics 1988; 28(4):303-308.

3. Allansmith MR, Ross RN. Mast cells and the eye. In Kay AB (Ed) Allergy and inflammation. San Diego. Academic Press, London 1987; 20:307-322.

4. Irani AA, Schecter NM, Craig SS, et al. Two types of human mast cells that have distinct neutral protease compositions. Proc Natl Acad Sci USA 1986; 83:4464-68.

5. Schwartz LB, Irani AA, Roller K, et al. Quantitation of histamine, tryptase and chymase in dispersed human T and TC mast cells. J Immunol 1987; 138:2611-15.

6. Irani AA, Craig SS, De Blois G, et al. Deficiency of the tryptase positive chymase negative mast cell type in gastrointestinal mucosa of patients with defective T lymphocyte function. J Immunol 1987; 138:4381-86.

7. Irani AA, Butrus SI, Tabbara KF, Schwartz LB. Human conjunctival mast cells: distribution of MC^T and MC^{TC} cells in vernal conjunctivitis and giant papillary conjunctivitis. In press.

© 1990 Elsevier Science Publishers (Biomedical Division)
Ocular Immunology Today. M. Usui, S. Ohno and K. Aoki, editors.

CONJUNCTIVAL PROVOCATION TEST IN ALLERGIC DISORDERS

MICHIYO SAKASHITA*,YAYOI NAKAGAWA,REI TADA AND TAKENOSUKE YUASA
Osaka Prefectural Habikino Hospital,Habikino City,Osaka 583 (Japan)*
Dept. of Ophthalmology,Osaka University Medical School,Osaka(Japan)

For diagnosis of causative antigens in cases with allergic disorders of the conjunctiva,skin tests and serum RAST are used. These results not always show true antigens of the diseases. Provocation tests with specific antigens are useful to decide true antigens of conjunctivitis (1,2); preparation of antigen extracts are not easy and results obtained in several clinics cannot be compared with each other,because antigens used in each clinics are different.

We preferred commercial antigens available in Japan for scratch tests,and after dialyzing and diluting the antigens,conjunctival provocation tests were performed. Provocation tests may have possibilities to be a method to clarify mechanisms of conjunctival allergy and to evaluate effects of antiallergic agents clinically used. Provocation tests were performed before and after treatment and the results were discussed.

MATERIALS AND METHODS

Commercial antigen extracts for scratch tests (Torii Phamaceutical Co.,Tokyo) were dialyzed in phosphate buffered saline (PBS,0.005M,pH7.4) and diluted to 10 to 10^5 folds with PBS in final concentration. These antigens were preserved in plastic tubes containing 100ul at -20 C until clinical use. Used antigens were house dust mite,orchard grass,Japanese cedar,candida and alternaria.

Conjunctival provocation tests were performed in cases with allergic disorders of the conjunctiva,including allergic conjunctivitis (AC),vernal keratoconjunctivitis (VKC),and giant papillary conjunctivitis (GPC). After 5 to 10 minutes of instillation with 10 ul of antigen solution,itching and/or hyperemia were elicited in cases with positive reactions. In patients without these responces,antigens of higher concentration were challenged. The lowest concentration of antigens with which a case showed positive signs was determined as the threshold concentration of antigens in the provocation tests.

Cases with allergic conjunctivitis were treated with eye drops of 2% disodium cromoglycate or 0.1% of fluorometholone for two weeks. Before and after the treatment,provocation tests were done and the threshold concentration of provoking antigens was measured.

48

RESULTS

TABLE 1. THRESHOLD CONCENTRATION OF ANTIGENS IN PROVOCATION TEST

Antigen dilution	$X10^1$	$X10^2$	$X10^3$	$X10^4$	$X10^5$	Total
House dust mite	11	28	22	7	0	68
Orchard grass	1	7	15	4	0	27
Japanese cedar	5	10	6	1	0	22
Moulds	n.d.	1	4	4	0	9

TABLE 2. PROVOCATION AND SERUM RAST OF HOUSE DUST MITE
Number of case:AC-VKC-GPC

Provocation test	Antigen dilution	RAST score 0(-)	1(+-)	2(+)	3(++)	4(+++)
Negative		9-1-4	0-1-0	2-0-1	0-1-0	0-0-0
Positive	$X10^1$	4-0-0	0-0-0	0-0-0	1-2-0	1-2-0
	$X10^2$	5-1-0	1-0-0	3-1-0	3-3-0	7-1-0
	$X10^3$	5-1-0	1-1-0	2-0-0	4-0-1	5-1-0
	$X10^4$	1-0-0	0-0-0	2-0-0	2-0-0	2-0-0

TABLE 3. PROVOCATION AND RAST OF JAPANESE CEDAR AND ORCHARD GRASS
Number of cases:Japanese cedar-orchard grass

Provocation test	Antigen dilution	RAST score 0(-)	1(+-)	2(+)	3(++)	4(+++)
Negative		3-5	0-0	1-0	2-0	0-0
Positive	$X10^1$	1-1	0-0	0-0	4-0	0-0
	$X10^2$	1-1	0-0	4-1	2-2	1-1
	$X10^3$	1-0	0-0	2-2	3-6	0-3
	$X10^4$	0-0	0-0	0-1	1-1	0-1

The maximal frequency in the threshold concentration of provocation was seen in dilution of 10^2 folds in house dust mite and Japanese cedar pollens, 10^3 in orchard grass pollens and 10^{3-4} in moulds, respectively (Table 1).

In cases sensitive to house dust mite, relationship between the provocation tests and serum RAST is shown in Table 2. Seventeen cases were positive in the provocation tests and negative in serum RAST; on the contrary, there were only 4 cases with negative provocation and positive RAST. The same relationship in cases suspected pollen allergies is shown in Table 3. These tests were performed in a

TABLE 4. ASSOCIATION BETWEEN PROVOCATION TEST AND SERUM RAST

Provocation	+	+	-		+	+	-	
Serum RAST	+	-	+	Coincidence				
Skin test					+	-	+	Coincidence
House dust mite	43	19	4	65%	44	10	8	71%
Orchard grass	19	2	0	90	14	8	1	61
Japanese cedar	17	3	3	74	16	1	5	73
Moulds	5	3	0	63	7	2	6	47

TABLE 5. EFFECTS OF TREATMENTS AND THRESHOLD OF PROVOCATION TEST

Provocation threshold	Symptoms after treatment		
	Improved	Unchanged	Worsened
Elevated	11	5	0
Unchanged	8	6	0
Lowered	3	2	0

year with abundant pollens of orchard grass and scanty ones of Japanese cedar. In several patients suspected pollinosis of Japanese cedar, dissociation of the results in these tests were found; these dissociation were observed only in two cases sensitive to orchard grass pollens.

In cases sensitive to orchard grass pollens and moulds, the results of serum RAST were more closely related to the provocation tests than those of skin tests; rates of coincidence between the provocation tests and serum RAST were equal to those between provocation and skin tests in house dust mite and Japanese cedar (Table 4). Skin tests of mould antigens were seemed not to be reliable in allergic disorders of the conjunctiva.

Effects of treatments and deviation of the threshold of the provocation tests were shown in Table 5. In 17 out of 35 cases, these two factors were concomitant; in 15 cases, one of the factors was unchanged, although the other changed. In three cases, in spite of improvement in clinical symptoms, the threshold of the provocation lowered.

DISCUSSION

Commercial antigens for scratch tests can easily obtained in Japan and prepared for the provocation tests by dialyzing in PBS in our method. The technique of the tests is simple and every ophthalmologist can utilize this tests in his clinical

50

procedure;the results obtained in different clinics can be discussed on the basis
of a standardized antigens and methods (3).

There were some cases in which skin tests or serum RAST were negative and
antigens of conjunctivitis were found only with the conjunctival provocation
tests. On the contrary,in several cases,ocular provocation tests with RAST-
positive antigens failed to elicit conjunctival inflammation. In latter cases,
these antigens seemed to produce IgE antibodies in the conjunctival tissues,if
sufficient amount of antigens stimulated the local immune system of the cases.
These phenomena of dissociation between two tests have been noticed (4), and
provocation tests are useful in cases in which conjunctival antigens were found
only with those methods.

In a season of pollinosis,in which abundant pollens were scattered, the results
of conjunctival provocation tests and serum RAST closely related each other;
a dissociation between the results of two tests was revealed in a season with
small amount of pollens produced. In cases with lowered hypersensitivity due to
decrease of antigens invading in the conjunctival sac,effects of treatments,or
reducing of sensitivity of the conjunctival tissues,the threshold of provocation
usually elevated and vice versa.

Influences of treatments to the provocation tests were not constant;in some
cases effectively treated,conjunctival itching occurred without an increase of
challenging antigens. As to effects of treatments,transition of subjective
symptoms and fluctuation of the threshold in the provocation were not identical
phenomena in the immediate type of allergy;these dissociations of the results
may not be unreasonable.

REFERENCES
1. Stenis-Aarniara BSM,Malmberg CHO,Holopainen EEA (1978) Clin Allergy 8:403-409
2. Akiyama K,Yui Y,Shida T (1981) Clin Allergy 11: 343-351
3. Sakashita M,Takagi T,Nakagawa,Tada R,Hagihara M,Inoue A,Yuasa T (1988)
   Acta Soc Ophthalmol Jpn 92: 806-810
4. Malmberg CHO,Holopainen EEA,Steinus-Aaniala BSM (1978) Clin Allergy 8:397-402

© 1990 Elsevier Science Publishers (Biomedical Division)
Ocular Immunology Today. M. Usui, S. Ohno and K. Aoki, editors.

CHEMICAL WEAPONS MAY TRIGGER VERNAL CONJUNCTIVITIS IN SUSCEPTIBLE SUBJECTS:
THREE CASE REPORTS

MOHAMMAD P. DAFTARIAN; M. A. ZAREH; H. A. SHAHRIARI; A. FARHODI; M. RASTIN.
Zahedan Medical Sciences University, P.O. Box 98135-396, Zahedan (Iran)

INTRODUCTION

The Alkylating agents such as mustard gas, interfere with DNA duplication and
are most effective in rapidly dividing cells. Tissues vary in their ability to
repair DNA after alkylation, which accounts for their differing sensitivities to
this group of agents. Depending on the time and dose of exposure, antibody production and delayed type hypersensitivity may become reduced or enhanced (1, 2, 3,
6, 7, 9).

On the other hand, mustard gas (most widely used chemical weapon) is categorised
as a "hapten" based on its physical and chemical properties: And may be able to
bind to carriers and become an Immunogen (6, 9, 12). It is reported that some
Iranian casualties (during Gulf War) have developed Urticaria after second
exposure to mustard gas (7, 8, 9, 10, 11, 12).

MATERIAL AND METHODS

Among 68 casualties which we studied and were exposed to chemical weapons
during the Gulf War (1986-87), six casualties were atopic patients. Atopic
patient was defined as a patient with high specific IgE antibody in the serum by
EIA as well as a positive skin test, elevated total IgE and clinical history of
allergy (2, 3, 4). These casualties were admitted to Loghman-Hakim Hospital
(Tehran), except one* who admitted to the Ophthalmic Center, Zahedan Medical
Sciences University. Out of the six patients three had shown conjunctivitis.
They were 23, 24 and 28 years old (all males)

In this study the total IgE was estimated by Enzyme Immuno Assay (5). The
titers of allergen specific IgE was estimated by the method of ELISA (Enzym
Linked Immuno Sorbant Assay). Skin prick test for common enviromental allergens
allergens was also performed (4, 5). The Serum Samples were collected and stored
at - 20 C and the skin tests were performed on the same day. The clinical history
of allergy was taken into consideration. The skin prick test was performed on the
volar surface of the forearm, the reactions were compared to a saline and histamine control. The area of more than 3 mm in diameter comparing to that of negative control was considered positive. The Allergen specific IgE was scored as
one to four depending on the amount of absorbance, compared to that of reference
disks which were incubated with the known positive sera.

* This patient was exposed to the gases used at the Haj Ceremony (1986).

All nasal and conjunctival secretions and epithelial scraping specimens were collected and stained with Wright-Giemsa stain.

The tests were carried out for eighteen patients as control who were exposed to chemical weapons but none of them were atopic.

CASE 1: A 24 years old, Iranian patient who was exposed to sulphur mustard gas for about 20 minutes. His father is suffering from allergic asthma, his sister has shown urticaria and he himself has had a mild seasonal Rhinitis.

CASE 2: A 23 years old, Iranian patient who was exposed twice to sulphur mustard gas about five minutes for each. His son is suffering from atopic eczema (his wife is not atopic), his brother has shown rhinitis and he himself is suffering from seasonal allergic asthma.

CASE 3: A 28 years old Iranian patient who was exposed to the gases used at the Haj Ceremony in 1986, for 10 minutes. His mother has been suffering from mild allergic asthma and his father has shown Urticaria.

RESULTS

The results of this study are summerized in table I, II and III.

Severe itching , photophobia, blurring, limbal hypertropy, lacrimation along with a white ropy secretion, and conjunctival excraping containing high numbers of eosinophils were common signs shown by the above patients after exposure to chemical weapons.

TABLE I

TOTAL* IgE OF PATIENTS** & THE RESULT OF EXAMINATION OF PARASITES

Patients	Total IgE	Parasite
A.M.	490 IU/ml	Negative X(3)
K.E.	400 IU/ml	Negative X(3)***
H.A.N.	540 IU/ml	Negative X(3)

* Total IgE of controls were less than 200 IU/ml.

** After exposure.

*** For three times and three days.

TABLE II

POSITIVE ALLERGEN SPECIFIC IgE & SKIN PRICK TEST[*]

Patients	Elisa R.S.IgE[**]	Class	Skin prick test	Wheal and flare
A.M.	Phleum pratense	III	Cat fur	5---7
	Cat fur	II	S.V.G	5---7
	S.V.G[***]	III	Phleum pratense	5---9
K.E.	Lolium SPP.	III	B_5	7---15
	Phleum pratense	III	B_3	5---9
	Salix SPP	III	Cat fur	4---6
	Artemisia SPP	II	d (mite)	5---5
	Cat fur	II		
H.A.N.	Corylus SPP	IV	B_2	3---7
	Artemisia V.	IV	B_3	5---5
	Plane	III	B_5	5---20
			House dust	5---17

* Allergen Specific IgE was performed from pharmacia and Allergens from Pharmacia and Bencard.

** A.S.IgE: Allergen Specific IgE.

*** S.V.G. Sweet Vernal Grass.

TABLE III

((Atopic diseases: After exposure and previous Allergic reactions in pateints))

Patients	Previous	After exposure
A.M.	Rhinitis (Moderate and seasonal)	Vernal conjunctivitis
K.E.	Allergic Asthma (seasonal)	Vernal conjunctivitis
H.A.N	Allergic Asthma (mild)	Vernal conjunctivitis and Rhinitis

According to these observations it has been supposed that chemical weapons (especially mustard gas) may trigger some related mechanisms in atopic patients due to their genetical and physiopathological charactristics.

54

REFERENCES

1. Helen Chapel et al.(1984) Essentials of clinical Immunology. P.372.

2. Stites P.D. (1987) Basic and clinical Immunology P.350.

3. P.J. Lachman (1982) Clinical Aspect of Immunology PP 531-2.

4. Nelson (1984) What is atopy post gradute medicine 76-1.

5. M. Ali (1980) Correlation of the dianostic skin test with the Immuno penoxidose ... Annals of Allergy Vol. 45 P 63.

6. R. Farid etail (1988) Respiratory complications of sulfur mustard poisoning ... Abstracts of The First International Medical Congress on Chemical Warfare Agents in Iran* Article No.23.

7. S. Enshayeh (1988) Skin manifestation of Mustard Gases. Abstracts of the First International Medical Congress on Chemical Warfare Agents in Iran.* Article No.37.

8. M. Mehzad (1988) Pathological study of skin lesions in chemical casualties. Abstracts of the First International Medical Congress on Chemical Warfare Agents in Iran* Article No.78.

9. M. M. Lari (1988) Nitrogen Mustard. Abstracts of the Warfare Agents in Iran* Article No.48.

10. M. Balali (1988) Report of Late toxic effects of sulfur mustard poisoning. Abstracts of chemical Warfare Agents in Iran* Article No.65

11. U.K. Helm (1988) Cutaneous Lesions Produced by Mustard Gas. Abstracts of chemical Warfare Agents in Iran* Article No.90.

12. Rezaei Poor R. (1988). Immunogenicity of Mustard Gas. Abstracts of First International Medical Congress on Chemical Warfare Agents in Iran.* Article No. 28.

* In abstracts of the First International Medical Congress on Chemical Warfare Agents in Iran, 1988; Mashad University of Medical Sciences.

CYTOKINES

© 1990 Elsevier Science Publishers (Biomedical Division)
Ocular Immunology Today. M. Usui, S. Ohno and K. Aoki, editors.

GAMMA INTERFERON PRODUCTION BY PERIPHERAL BLOOD LYMPHOCYTES FROM PATIENTS WITH HLA B27 ANTERIOR UVEITIS

DENIS WAKEFIELD, ELIZABETH TOMPSETT, PETER M[C]CLUSKEY, DAVID ABI-HANNA, NICHOLAS HAWKINS AND JOHN McSHANE.

Laboratory of Ocular Immunology, School of Pathology, University of NSW. PO Box 1, Kensington, NSW, 2033. Australia.

INTRODUCTION

Anterior uveitis (AU) is a common inflammatory eye disease [1]. It is usually idiopathic with approximately half of the patients possessing the HLA B27 antigen [2]. We, and others, have previously shown that a proportion of patients with AU have evidence of preceding infection due to *chlamydia, yersinia* and other gram negative bacteria [3,4,5]. Similarly, we have shown that anterior uveal cells, with the exception of vascular endothelium, do not normally express class 1 HLA antigens [6], although these cells may be induced to express such antigens under the influence of gamma interferon (IFN-γ) and other cytokines. Furthermore, the level of expression of class 1 antigens on diseased uveal tissue correlates with the level of IFN-γ in the aqueous humor of patients with AU [7].

In order to further investigate the possible relationship between the immune response to gram negative bacteria and IFN-γ we analysed the amount of interferon produced by peripheral blood lymphocytes from patients with anterior uveitis in response to a variety of gram negative bacteria (*Salmonella, Shigella, Klebsiella* and *E. coli*).

METHODS

Peripheral blood was collected from 13 patients with acute AU, (six were HLA B27) and 13 age and sex matched controls (7 were HLA B27). Peripheral blood mononuclear (PBMN) cells were separated by Ficoll Hypaque differential centrifugation. These cells (2×10^6 cells/ml) were then incubated with heat killed micro-organisms (*Klebsiella pneumoniae, Shigella flexneri, Salmonella typhimurium* and *E. coli*) at a concentration of 5×10^8 bacteria per ml for 7 days and the supernatants collected and assayed for IFN-γ concentration. Interferon levels were measured using a radioimmunoassay (Centocor, USA). The lymphocyte transformation response to these microbial antigens was also assessed as previously described[3].

RESULTS

The results of these investigations indicate that HLA B27 positive individuals, whether they have anterior uveitis or not, produced significantly more INF-γ in response to *klebsiella, shigella* and *E. coli* antigens, than HLA B27 negative individuals. (p<0.05 for each antigen). There was no difference between controls except that HLA B27 subjects produced significantly more IFN-γ than non HLA B27 individuals in response to *salmonella*.

TABLE 1

LYMPHOCYTE PRODUCTION OF INTERFERON-γ IN PATIENTS WITH UVEITIS

Production of IFN-γ in U/ml from peripheral blood lymphocytes from patients with uveitis and control groups. Data is shown for both HLA B27 +ve and HLA B27 -ve subgroups. The standard deviation of each result is shown in brackets.

Patients	Microbial Antigen				
	Klebsiella	Shigella	Salmonella	E.coli	Nil
Uveitis					
B27 +ve	49 (13)	47 (12)	42 (10)	38 (9)	2 (2)
B27 -ve	15 (3)	23 (12)	38 (7)	22 (6)	3 (2)
Total	28 (9)	28 (9)	36 (9)	22 (8)	3 (1)
Control					
B27 +ve	32 (8)	34 (7)	53 (7)	29 (5)	4 (2)
B27 -ve	23 (7)	19 (5)	29 (7)	15 (5)	1 (1)
Total	29 (8)	27 (6)	35 (7)	21 (5)	3 (2)

DISCUSSION

The peripheral blood lymphocytes of HLA B27 positive individuals produce more IFN-γ in response to a number of gram negative bacteria than do individuals who do not possess this HLA antigen. This increased production of IFN-γ was observed irrespective of the disease status of the patients and was seen in response to bacteria previously implicated in the pathogenesis of anterior uveitis (*klebsiella* and *shigella*) and also in response to *E coli*, a ubiquitous gram negative bacteria not implicated in triggering acute attacks of AU.

IFN-γ may play an important role in the production of uveal inflammation. As a site for persistent immunologically mediated inflammation the uvea is characterised by the presence of a large number of lymphocytes and macrophages. In other inflammatory diseases such as rheumatoid arthritis, these cells have been shown to produce a large number of secreted products, prominent amongst which are the cytokines. In the case of rheumatoid synovium the cytokines produced by macrophages (IL-1, IL-6, IL-8, GM-CSF, TNF-α, M-CSF, PDGF, IGF, EGF, TGF-β) appear to predominate over those secreted by T cells (IFN-γ, IL-2, IL-6, GM-CSF, TNF-α, TGF-β) [8]. Whether this is the pattern that occurs in all forms of synovitis, or in AU, remains to be determined.

There is increasing evidence based on in vitro, and a limited amount of in vivo data, that cytokines play a pivotal role in the pathogenesis of uveitis. In a recent study we showed that the level of IFN-γ in the aqueous humor of a group of patients with AU correlated with the degree of expression of HLA antigens on iris cells [7]. The induction of HLA antigens on uveal cells may be due to a number of cytokines and it remains to be shown which ones play a dominant role in vivo in patients with AU. We have examined the effects of a number of different cytokines, and combinations of cytokines, for their effect on HLA antigen expression on uveal cells. These experiments have revealed that IFN-γ is the most potent inducer of Class I and Class II HLA antigen expression and that combinations of cytokines were additive in there effect on Class I expression [9]. Combinations of IFN-γ with TNF produced an enhancement of Class I HLA antigen which was more than the additive effect of the two cytokines alone. Moreover, we have shown that iris cells in biopsies from patients with AU, but not from patients with senile cataract, express abundant Class I HLA antigens. These observations, and those of others, suggest that uveal autoimmunity may only be possible following HLA antigen induction on specific target tissues , and that IFN-γ, along with other cytokines, may be involved. Similarly, Hooks et al [10] have demonstrated the presence of IFN-γ and IL-2 in the eyes of patients with posterior uveitis associated with infiltration by T cells and local induction of class II HLA antigens. Further evidence for a role for IFN-γ in the pathogenesis of AU has been provided by our demonstration of increased serum neopterin levels in patients with acute AU [11] and Kotake's [12] results showing increased interferon and oligo-2',5'-adenylate synthetase activity in peripheral blood lymphocytes of patients with uveitis complicating Behcet's syndrome, Vogt Koyonagi Harada syndrome and sarcoidosis.

REFERENCES

1. Wakefield D, Dunlop I, McCluskey P, Penny R. Uveitis: aetiology and disease associations in an Australian population. Aust. NZ J Ophthalmol 1986, 14; 181-187.

2. Wakefield D, Abi-Hanna D. HLA antigens and there significance in the pathogenesis of anterior uveitis. Curr Eye Res. 1986, 5; 465-471.

3. Wakefield D and Penny R. The role of chlamydia in HLA B27 anterior uveitis. In: Immunology and Immunopathology of the Eye. Masson Pub. USA 1985.

4. Wakefield D, Stahlberg T, Freston J, Buckley R. Anterior Uveitis and Yersinia Infection. Arch. Ophthalmol 1989 (in press)

5. Sarri KM, Laitinen O, Leirisalo and Sarri R. 1980. Ocular inflammation associated with yersinia infection. Am J Ophthalmol. 89, 84-95.

6. Abi-Hanna D, Wakefield D. HLA antigens in Ocular Tissue. Transplant. 1988, 45(3); 610-613.

7. Abi-Hanna D, McClusky P and Wakefield D. HLA antigens in the iris and aqueous humor interferon levels in anterior uveitis. Invest Ophthalmol Vis Science. 1989 30: 5 990-994

8. Lipsky P E, Davies LS, Cush JJ and Oppenheim Marks N. The role of cytokines in the pathogenesis of rheumatoid arthritis. Springer Semin Immunopath 1989, 11: 123-162.

9. Abi-Hanna D and Wakefield D. Expression of HLA antigens on the human uvea. Br. J.Rheum. 1988; 27 (supp II) 68-71.

10. Hooks JJ, Chan CC and Dietrich D. Identification of lymphokines, IFN-γ and IL-2 in inflammatory eye disease. Invest Ophthalmol Vis Sci. 1988, 29 (9) 1444-51.

11. Abi-Hanna D and Wakefield D. Increased serum neopterin levels in patients with acute anterior uveitis. Cur Eye Res, 1988, 7(5); 497-502.

12. Kotake S. Investigation of interferon and oligo-2',5'-adenylate systems of endogenous uveitis. Hokkaido Igaku Zasshi. 1988, 63 (3), 398-406.

© 1990 Elsevier Science Publishers (Biomedical Division)
Ocular Immunology Today. M. Usui, S. Ohno and K. Aoki, editors.

OCULAR INFLAMMATION STIMULATED BY INTRAVITREAL INJECTION OF
INTERLEUKIN-8.

MICHAEL R. FERRICK[§], MONTY H. OPPENHEIM, STEPHAN R. THURAU*, CARL P.
HERBORT, CLAUS O. C. ZACHARIAE[†], CHI-CHAO CHAN, AND KOUJI MATSUSHIMA[†].
Laboratory of Immunology, National Eye Institute, [†]Laboratory of Immunoregulation, National
Cancer Institute, and [§]Howard Hughes Medical Institute. *S.R.T. receives a scholarship from the
German Research Council (DFG). Address correspondence to Michael R. Ferrick, National Eye
Institute, 9000 Rockville Pike, Building 10, Room 10N206, Bethesda, MD 20892 U.S.A.

INTRODUCTION

Accumulation of leukocytes in a tissue is thought to be the result of the release of specific
chemotactic mediators in the area of inflammation. One of these factors, Interleukin-8 (IL-8),
selectively activates polymorphonuclear neutrophils and T-lymphocytes[1]. IL-8 has been referred to
as monocyte-derived neutrophil chemotactic factor (MDNCF), neutrophil-activating peptide-1
(NAP-1), and neutrophil-activating factor (NAF)[2]. Among its various properties are IL-8's ability to
cause the chemotaxis of neutrophils, neutrophil shape change, exocytosis of neutrophilic granules,
surface expression of adhesion molecules, respiratory burst, and a rise in cytosolic $[Ca^{2+}]$ within the
neutrophil[3]. Peripheral blood monocytes, alveolar macrophages, endothelial cells, fibroblasts,
epithelial cells, and hepatoma cells all are capable of elaborating IL-8[3,4]. LPS is a stimulus for the
first three types of cells, and $TNF\alpha$ and IL-1 are each independent stimuli for all six cell types[3]. IL-8
has in vivo inflammatory activity in the skin[5]. In order to further elucidate the mechanisms of ocular
inflammation[6,7], purified, human recombinant IL-8 was injected intravitreally into rats. IL-8 does
cause an inflammation characterized by the influx of neutrophils into the iris, ciliary body, cornea,
posterior chamber, and anterior chamber of the injected eye.

MATERIALS AND METHODS

Animals / Procedures

Male F344 Fischer rats were purchased from Charles River Laboratories (Raleigh, North
Carolina) and used at age 7-9 weeks. Animals were anesthetized with a combination of ketamine (10
mg) and xylazine (8 mg) given intramuscularly and proparacaine given topically to the eye.
Paracentesis of the anterior chamber was performed, and a volume of 10 μL was injected using a
30-gauge needle inserted through the pars plana into the central vitreous[8]. Each animal was injected
with sterile balanced salt solution in its right eye and IL-8 in its left eye. The volume was measured
with a Hamilton 50 μL syringe. After the injection gentamicin ophthalmic ointment was applied.

Cytokine

Purified human recombinant IL-8 was diluted in sterile balanced salt solution (Endosol from Entravision) and injected intravitreally in total doses of 1 pg, 100 pg, 10 ng, and 1 μg[9].

Cell counts, Histology, and Protein Concentration

Animals were euthenized with CO_2 at different intervals after injection, and 6 μL of aqueous humour was aspirated. Leukocytes in 2 μL were stained with Wright's stain and were counted. 4 μL were used for protein concentration determination by Bradford-Lowry Method. Eyes from animals not used for aspiration were enucleated and fixed in 4% gluteraldehyde and 10% formalin. Sections through the vertical plane were stained with conventional hematoxylin and eosin.

RESULTS

The intravitreal injection of 10 ng of IL-8 produced a significant influx of neutrophils into the anterior chamber of the rat eye at 20 hours after injection. The eyes injected with IL-8 have more leukocytes than the control eye in 10 out of 11 animals (Figure 1). Histology confirms that these cells are almost exclusively polymorphonuclear neutrophils. In IL-8 injected eyes these cells can be found in the iris, ciliary body, cornea, posterior chamber, and anterior chamber. Severity of ocular inflammation, assessed by histological examination, in IL-8 and control eyes correlates with cell count data (data not shown).

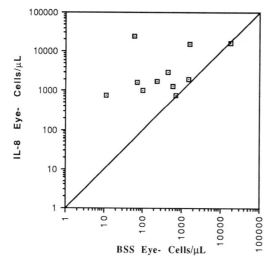

Figure 1. Each point represents number of leukocytes in aqueous humour from 1 animal. 10 μL of BSS OD and 10 ng of IL-8 in 10 μL OS. Cell counts for each eye on respective axes. Statistics: $p < .05$ by Wilcox Signed Rank.

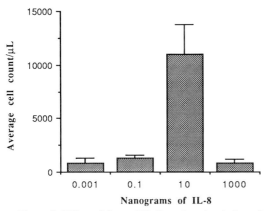

Figure 2. Effect of dose of IL-8 on the stimulation of ocular inflammation.
Leukocytes in 1 μL of anterior chamber aqueous were counted.
SEM indicated by bars.

The presence of protein in the aqueous humour is indicative of plasma leakage from blood vessels in an inflammatory condition. Protein concentration was not significantly higher in the IL-8 injected eyes compared to the control eyes (data not shown). The most effective dose of IL-8 appears to be approximately 10 nanograms, and 1 μg causes an inflammation similar to the lowest dose tested, 1 pg (Figure 2). The peak activity of intravitreal IL-8 is between 10 and 24 hours after the injection, and IL-8 induced neutrophil infiltration is subsiding at 48 hours (Figure 3).

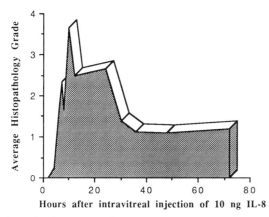

Figure 3. Time course of IL-8 activity. Eyes were graded on a scale from 0 to 4 determined by the number of neutrophils in ocular tissues.

DISCUSSION

The present study indicates that intravitreal IL-8 does induce significant neutrophil infiltration in the iris, ciliary body, cornea, posterior chamber, and anterior chamber between 10 and 24 hours after the injection. The time course of intraocular IL-8 is much longer than has been reported for this cytokine injected into the dermis[5]. In the dermis IL-8 causes the influx of neutrophils by 30 minutes, and the neutrophils are leaving by 3 hours. In the eye it is not until about 48 hours that IL-8 induced inflammation is subsiding. Morphological differences between the vitreous and the dermis are what most likely account for the disparate time courses. The dermis is a much more vascular tissue with better circulation than the vitreous gel. Intravitreal IL-8 follows a classical bell shaped dose response curve with the peak dose lying at approximately 10 ng. Since exogenous IL-8 does have activity in the eye, it may be involved in ocular inflammatory conditions. Cytokines such as IL-1 and TNFα stimulate a more general inflammatory reaction by causing the activation of a variety of cells which then, among their other functions, release a cascade of other cytokines[2,6,7]. One of the cytokines that is produced is IL-8, and it is the IL-8 which has the more direct action of activating the neutrophils and, as has been recently described, T-lymphocytes[1,2]. It is the various cytokines with more specific functions, such as IL-8, which mediate some of the effects of IL-1 and TNFα. In order to further understand the role of IL-8 in ocular inflammation, it will be necessary to study the production of endogenous IL-8 in the eye.

REFERENCES

1. Larsen CG, Anderson AO, Appella E, Oppenheim JJ, Matsushima K (1989) Science 243:1464-1466

2. Matsushima K, Oppenheim JJ (1989) Cytokine 1:2-13

3. Baggiolini M, Walz A, Kunkel SL (1989) Journal of Clinical Investigation 84:1045-1049

4. Larsen CG, Anderson AO, Oppenheim JJ, Matsushima K (1989) Immunology 68:31-36

5. Rampart M, Van Damme J, Zonnekeyn L, Herman AG (1989) American Journal of Pathology 135:21-25

6. Rosenbaum JT, Samples JR, Hefeneider SH, Howes EL (1987) Archives of Ophthalmology 105:1117-1120

7. Rosenbaum JT, Howes EL, Rubin RM, Samples JR (1988) American Journal of Pathology 133:47-53

8. Forrester JV, Worgul BV, Merriam GR Jr. (1980) Albrecht von Graefes Archiv für Klinische und Experimentelle Ophthalmologie 213:221-233

9. Furuta R, Yamagishi J, Kotani H, Sakamoto F, Fukui T, Matsui Y, Sohmura Y, Yamada M, Yoshimura T, Larsen CG, Oppenheim JJ, Matsushima K (1989) Journal of Biochemistry 106:436-441

© 1990 Elsevier Science Publishers (Biomedical Division)
Ocular Immunology Today. M. Usui, S. Ohno and K. Aoki, editors.

IN VIVO TREATMENT OF EXPERIMENTAL UVEORETINITIS WITH MONOCLONAL ANTIBODY TO GAMMA-INTERFERON

L. R. ATALLA, S. YOSER, N. A. RAO

Doheny Eye Institute, Los Angeles, California (USA)

INTRODUCTION

Interferons have been found to possess both inhibitory and enhancing immunomodulating properties. Interferons activate cells of the macrophage-monocyte series. They also modulate certain cell surface characteristics likely to be of immuno-logical significance. In particular, gamma interferon (IFN-y) appears to be the most active in enhancing H-2 antigen expression, increasing the number of Ia bearing thymocytes and inducing HLA-A,B and C. Pursuing the hypothesis that IFN-y plays a crucial role in the pathogenesis of autoimmune processes, blocking the effect of IFN-y might down regulate such a process.

Theoretically MAbs to IFN-y should be able to selectively inhibit the functions of gamma interferon that contribute to autoimmune disease. Accordingly, we studied the effect of different doses of MAbs against IFN-y on the development of experimental autoimmune uveitis (EAU).

MATERIALS AND METHODS

Female Lewis rats were immunized with HSA 320 synthetic peptide of human retinal S-antigen of the following sequence: DTNLASSTIIKEGIDRTVLG. Each animal received foot-pad injection of 50 μg of the antigen in CFA. The animals were divided into 4 groups that were treated differently. Animals in the first group were injected with the R4-6A2 MAb rat anti-mouse gamma interferon, in a dose of 1.4 mg/injection. The second group received the same antibody in a lower dose of 0.5 mg/injection. The last 2 groups were control-treated wih IgG 1.4 mg/injection and Dulbecco's Modified Eagle's Medium (DMEM) respectively. Treatment were done I.P. on day 1 as regards the antigen injection and continued every day for 6 days. All groups were sacrificed on day 15 after the peptide administration and eyes were submitted for histological studies. In groups 1 and 3 spleens were used for lympocyte transformation assay and sera for ELISA.

Anti-gamma interferon antibody preparation: R4-6A2 cell line that produces antibody reactive to gamma interferon was obtained from American Type Culture Collection (Rockville, MD). Dulbecco's Modified Eagle's medium with 4.5 g IL glucose and non-essential amino acids, 90%; Fetal bovine serum, 10% was used for cell cultures. Cells were split repeatedly till enough volume was reached. Supernatants were appropriately prepared and stored at -70° C. Antibody specifity was tested as described earlier.[1]

Lymphocyte proliferation assay: Spleen cells 2 x 10^5/well were incubated with S-antigen and Con A in different dilutions for 4 days. Cells were pulsed with 1.0 μci ^{3}H-thymidine per well for 6 hours. The cultures were harvested, counted and stimulation indecies were calculated.

Anti-gamma interferon antibody titers: Anti-y interferon antibody titers were determined by ELISA. Briefly plates were coated with the antigen (50 ng/well) then washed and appropriate serum dilutions were added and incubated at 37° C with CO_2 5%. After incubation, plates were washed and incubated again with perioxidase-conjugated anti-rat IgG. Color was developed by the substrate o-phenylendiamine and 3% H_2O_2 and the color intensity was measured by absorbance at 490 nm.

RESULTS

Histopathologically the following results were obtained:

-In Group 1 (treated with anti-interferon gamma 1.4 mg/ injection), one of nineteen rats developed uveoretinitis; this animal had only mild disease.

-In Group 2 (treated with anti-interferon gamma 0.5 mg/injection, four of eight rats demonstrated severe uveoretinitis; one other rat had mild disease.

-In Groups 3 and 4 (controls), all twenty animals showed severe uveitis and retinitis.

Lymphocyte stimulation indices were markedly diminished in Group 1 animals versus the control group ($p < 0.05$).

Anti-S-antibody titers were markedly diminished in Group 1 animals versus the control group ($p < 0.0001$).

DISCUSSION

IFN-y has been established as the prototype lymphokine to induce enhancement of synthesis and surface expression of MHC class II antigens in a wide variety of cell types, both in vitro and in vivo.[2] Moreover, in vivo administration of mAbs specific for an IA and IE region of MHC class II proved successful in abrogation of several autoimmune diseases.[3] Blocking of IFN-y might inhibit the propagation of autoimmune process. The results of this study showed dramatic inhibition of EAU using a relatively high dose of the mAbs (1.4 mg/injection). On the other hand, treatment with Dulbecco medium or irrelevant antibody (IgG) did not prevent the development of the disease. Monoclonal anti-IFN gamma may down regulate class II MHC antigen expression that could be initiated by IFN gamma. This down regulatory effect alone and/or accompanied by enhanced T-suppressor subpopulation activity may be responsible for immune regulation In considering potential theraputic applications of IFN-y[4], this lymphokine should not be considered exempt from possible untoward consequences. The present study with other observations [5-6], suggest that IFN-y may be contra-indicated in patients with certain autoimmune diseases. Conversely, we have shown that in vivo therapy with monoclonal anti-IFN-y can significantly alter the course of EAU in rats.

CONCLUSION

-Antibodies to gamma-interferon can suppress the development of
 experimental autoimmune uveitis (EAU).
-The suppression of EAU by antibodies to gamma-interferon is dose
 dependent, a high dose (1.4 mg/injection) was significantly more
 effective than a low dose (0.5 mg/injection).
-Gamma-interferon plays a significant role in the development of
 EAU.
-New strategies will likely aim at blocking the contribution of
 cytokines in the development and regulation of autoimmune
 disorders, including uveitis.

REFERENCES

1. McMaster WR and Williams AR. Identification of Ia glycoproteins in rat thymus and purification from rat spleen.
Eur J Immunol (1979) 9:426.

2. Wong, GHW, Clark-Lewis I, McKinn-Besdikin TL, Harris AW and
Schrader JW. Interferon gamma indices enhanced expression of
Ia and H-2 antigens on B lymphoid, macrophages and myeloid
cell lines. J Immunol (1983) 131:788.

3. Steinman L, Rosenbaum JT, Sriram S and McDevitt HO: In vivo
effects of antibodies to immune response gene products:
Prevention of experimental allergic encephalitis. Proc Natl
Acad Sci USA (1981) 78:7111.

4. Nathan CF, Kaplana G, Lewis WR, Nustrat A, Witmer MD, Sherwin
SA, Job CK, Horowitz CR, Steinman RM, and Cohn ZA. Local and
systemic effects of intradermal recombinant interferon-y in
patients with Lepromatous leprosy. N Engl J Med (1986) 315:6.

5. Pantitch HS, Haley AS, Hirsch RL and Johnson KP. A trail
gamma interferon in multiple sclerosis: clinical results.
Neurology (1986) 36:285 (suppl. 1).

6. Jacob CO, van der Meide PH and McDevitt HO. In vivo treatment
of (NZB x NZW) F1 lupus-like nephritis with monoclonal
antibody to y-interferon. J Exp Med (1987) 16:798-803.

© 1990 Elsevier Science Publishers (Biomedical Division)
Ocular Immunology Today. M. Usui, S. Ohno and K. Aoki, editors.

INTERLEUKIN-1β IN MONOCYTE CULTURE SUPERNATANTS AND CEREBROSPINAL FLUID OF
PATIENTS WITH VOGT-KOYANAGI-HARADA DISEASE

KOTARO ETO[1,2],YASUHIDE SANEYOSHI[1],REIKO OGUSHI[1],HIROSHI SHOUJI[3],
HISAHARU YOSHIOKA[1],MITCHEL MITSUO YOKOYAMA[2]

Department of [1]Ophthalmology,[2]Immunology,[3]Internal medicine,Kurume University
School of Medicine,Kurume,(Japan)

INTRODUCTION

Interleukin-1(IL-1) is a macrophage-derived protein which is known to activate
lymphocytes and mediates a wide range of biological activities. Recently,
biochemical purification and molecular cloning of cDNA of murine and human IL-1
have shown that there are at least two distinct forms of IL-1. IL-1α presents
in cell membrane of macrophage and IL-1β is serect as soluble form from the cells.

Vogt-Koyanagi-Harada(VKH) disease is a bilateral panuveitis with exudative
retinal detachment, associated with polyosis, and meningial sign. In VKH,
lymphocyte transformation test showed positive uptake of ^{3}H-tymidine, cytotoxic
T lymphocytes have the capability of specifically affecting the melanoma cells,
and interferon(IFN) and interleukin-2(IL-2) levels in serum are found to be
elevated. These results indicate that the T lymphocytes are thougt to be activated by factor which may presents in serum of patients with VKH. In this paper,
the levels of IL-1β in sera, supernatants of monocyte cultures and CSF of
patients with VKH were measured by sandwich immunoassay.

MATERIAL AND METHOD

  Patients. Twenty-three VKH(13 active and 10 inactive cases) and these patients
included 11 males and 12 females with age between 19 and 48 years are admitted
to the Ophthalmology Clinic of Kurume University Hospital. Thirteen active cases
were fresh VKH within two weeks prior to the present analysis and 10 contlols (5
 males and 5 female) were also examined. Cerebrospinal fluids(CSF) of patients
of VKH and CSF of controls were obtained from Department of Anesthesiology of
Kurume University Hospital

  Supernatants of cultured monocyte. Monocnuclear cells were isolated from
heparinized blood of patients and healthy controls by density gradients centrifugation on Ficoll-Hypaque solution and the cells were washed three times in phosphate buffered saline (PBS). Mononuclear cells were cultured in RPMI 1640 medium
(Gibuco) with 10% human AB serum at 37°C with 5% CO_2 for 1 hour. The cells were
placed on plastic Petri dishes and non-adherent cells were sucked off, and
monocytes were suspended (2×10^5 cells/ml) in RPMI 1640 with 10% human AB serum
supplemented. The monocytes were incubated at 37°C for 24 hours in presence or

absence of 10μg/ml lipopolysaccharide (LPS). The culture supernatants were harvested and then stored at -80°C prior to use.

Sandwich enzyme immunoassay for IL-1β. IL-1β in sera, supernatants of cultured monocytes and CSF was measured by commercial test kit(Otsuka Pharmaceutical Co.,Ltd.,Japan). One microgram per ml of mouse anti-human IL-1β monoclonal antibody was incubated on a 96 wells microplate for over night. After washing three times in PBS, added 1% bovine serum albumin (250μl) used as blocking regent and incubated for 4 hours, and washed three times again. Two hundred microlitters of recombinant hIL-1β or test samples were added to plate and then incubated over night. After washing three times in PBS, 1% rabbit anti-IL-1β serum (100μl) added to the plate, incubated 2 hours and washed three times. Anti-rabbit IL-1β IgG Fab'-peroxidase conjugate (100μl) added and then incubated 2 hours and washed three times. Peroxidase activity was assayed using a substrate buffer with o-phenylene diamine and the enzymatic reaction was stopped by adding 1N H_2SO_4. Fluorecence intensity was measured by auto-reader (Sanko Junyaku Co.,Ltd.), using 492 nm for emission.

RESULTS

The levels of IL-1β in sera were not found to be significantly difference between active cases in VKH however, three cases (two actives andone inactive) showed higher levels than that of other samples (Fig.1).

IL- 1β levels in the monocyte culture supernatants without LPS stimulation were elevated in the patients group as compared to the healthy controls(p 0.05)

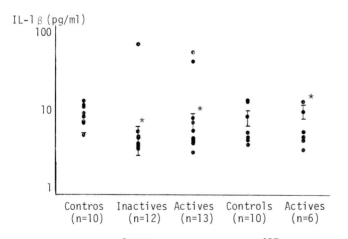

IL-1 β (pg/ml)

| Contros | Inactives | Actives | Controls | Actives |
| (n=10) | (n=12) | (n=13) | (n=10) | (n=6) |

Serum   CSF

Fig. 1 The levels of IL-1βin serum and cereblospinal fluids
    * p>0.05

(Fig.2). Furethermore, IL-1β levels in the supernatants of cultured monocytes which stimulated with LPS were also elevated in the patients when the results were compared with the controls (p<0.05). Particularly, in the supernatants of of active VKH cases after the monocytes stimulated with LPS a significant elevation (p<0.01) of IL-1β was noticed (Fig.3). IL-1β in CSF of VKH patients was not elevated as compared to the controls.

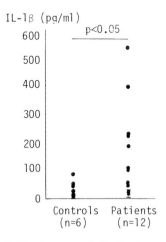

Fig.2 The levels of IL-1β in monocyte culture supernatants without LPS

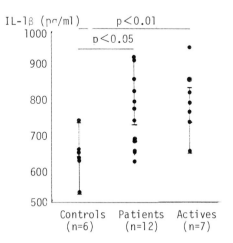

Fig.3 The levels of IL-1β in monocyte culture supernatants with stimulated LPS

DISCUSSION

IL-1β, one of the biologically active lymphokines with a characteristcs of lymphocyte activation found in serum, CSF and supernatants of cultured monocytes was assayes by ELISA in patients with VKH disease and controls. The IL-1β levels in the supernatants of cultured monocytes of the patients with VKH after culturing with or without LPS were found to be significantly elevated when the results were compared with the controls. These data indicated that the monocytes of the patients could be stimulated in vivo by facter(s) which is not identified yet. The elevated IL-1β derived from the activated monocytes may react with cells, namely T lymphocytes possessing the receptor to the cell surface membrane. Due to the results of IL-1β and its receptor binding a variety of lymphokines including IL-2, IFN etc could be released from the activated T lymphocyte which could initiate cytotoxic T cells. The immuno net network is possibly activated based on the exposure of melanocyte autoantigen stimulates immune cells, particulary $CD4^+2H4^+$ lymphocytes. The stimulated $CD4^+2H4^+$ cells may be activated and released IL-2 and γ-IFN which could initiate the induction of cytotxic T cells which could effect to to melanocytes to be altered Therefor the elevation of Il-1β may considered to be a disease entity of VKH.

ACKNOWLEDGEMENTS

 We greatfully acknowledge Prof.T Muteki, Department of Anesthesiology, Kurume University Hospital who provided CSF of the control group of this study.

REFERENCE

1. Lomedioco PT, Gulber U, Hellman CP (1984) Nature 312: pp458-462

2. Mizel sb, Mizel D (1981) J Immunology 126: pp834-837

3. Maezawa N,Yano A, Taniguchi M (1982) OphthalmolgiKa L85; pp179-186

4. Ohno S (1984) Elsevier Science Publishers B.V.,Amsterdum,pp401-405

%. Iwata M, Kitano S (1989) Acta Soc Ophthal 83: pp1025-1031

INDUCING ENDOPHTHALMITIS BY INTERLEUKIN 1

TOSHIO KATAYAMA and HISAKO FUJIWARA
Department of Ophthalmology, Kawasaki Hospital, Kawasaki Medical School
2 - 1 - 80 Nakasange, Okayama 700 (Japan)

INTRODUCTION

Interleukin 1 (IL - 1) was initially described as products of monocytes and macrophages. IL - 1 stimulates thymocyte proliferation, interleukin 2 production, and function of platelet activating factor (PAF)[1,2].

We studied IL - 1 induced inflammation in rabbit eyes. Anti - inflammatory effects of prostaglandin (PG) synthesis inhibitor, corticosteroid and PAF antagonist were examined in IL - 1 induced endophthalmitis.

METERIALS AND METHODS

The animals used were white rabbits weighing about 1.5 kg. We used recombinant IL - 1 beta (R & D) for IL - 1 and the PAF receptor antagonist (CV - 3988, Takeda) for the PAF antagonist. As the PG synthesis inhibitor, we used 0.5 % indomethacin eye drops (Indomerol®, Senju), for steroid eye drops, we used 0.1 % betamethasone (Rinderon A®, Shionogi). To determine the protein level in the anterior aqueous humor, we used the Bio - Rad Protein Assay method and to determine the PGE_2 level in the anterior aqueous humor, we used the PGE_2 [^{125}I] RIA KIT (NEN).

1) Inducing Endophthalmitis by IL - 1

We dissolved 10, 100, 500, and 1000 U of IL - 1 into 25 μl of lactated Ringer's solution and then injected it into the vitreous. 25 μl of lactated Ringer's solution without IL - 1 was injected into the other eye as the control. We had been observing the eye reaction for six hours, then the aqueous humor was harvested and both the protein levels and PGE_2 levels were measured.

2) Effects of the PAF Antagonist

Before IL - 1 injection PAF antagonist was given at a dose of 10mg/kg intravenously and the same amount of this drug was given every two hours arter IL - 1 injection. Six hours after IL - 1 injection, we measured the protein levels and the PGE_2 levels in the aqueous humor.

3) Effects of the PG Synthesis Inhibitor

Indomethacin or steroid was given topically every sixty minutes starting three hours before IL - 1 injection and this administration was continued after IL - 1 injection. Six hours after IL - 1 injection, the protein levels and the PGE₂ levels in the aqueous humor were measured.

RESULTS
  1) Induction of IL – 1 Endophthalmitis
(1) Changes in the Anterior Eye Based on a Dosage of IL – 1
  No changes were observed in the anterior eye in the control and the 10U group. Dose – dependent changes including hyperemia of the iris, edema of the iris, and turbidity of the anterior chamber were observed in the 100U dosage or above groups. Fibrin exudation was observed in half of the animals at a dose of 1000U.
(2) Protein Level in the Anterior Aqueous Humor
  The protein level in the controls was 0.19 ± 0.01 mg/ml (mean ± S.D.) and at doses of 500U or above a marked increase (P < 0.01) in the protein level was observed.
(3) PGE₂ Level in the Anterior Aqueous Humor
  The PGE₂ level in the controls was 5.75 ± 2.33 pg/ml and in the 500U or above groups a marked increase (P < 0.01) in PGE₂ level was observed.

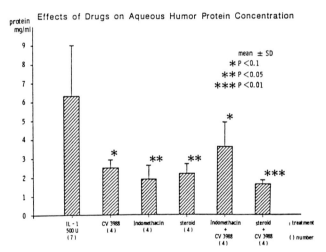

Fig. 1.
    Aqueous humor protein levels were slightly decreased after intravenous injection of CV 3988 (P<0.1).
    Combined administration of steroid and CV 3988 further reduced in aqueous humor protein level (P<0.01).

2) Effects of the PAF Antagonist, PG Synthesis Inhibitor, and Steroid
(1) Protein Level in the Anterior Aqueous Humor (Fig. 1)

The PAF antagonist decreased the protein level to 2.50 ± 0.35 mg/ml ($P < 0.1$), indomethacin eye drops to 1.96 ± 0.73 mg/ml ($P < 0.05$) and steroid eye drops to 2.23 ± 0.45 mg/ml ($P < 0.05$).

Combined administration of the PAF antagonist and indomethacin decreased the protein level to 3.63 ± 1.30 mg/ml ($P < 0.1$); combined administration of the PAF antagonist and steroid eye drops decreased the protein level to 1.76 ± 0.06 mg/ml ($P < 0.01$).

(2) PGE₂ Level in the Anterior Aqueous Humor (Fig. 2)

The PAF antagonist had no effect on the PGE_2 level (49.9 ± 36.2 pg/ml). Indomethacin eye drops decreased the PGE_2 level to 1.67 ± 1.50 pg/ml ($P < 0.01$), and steroid eye drops decreased this level to 18.2 ± 15.1 pg/ml ($P < 0.05$).

Combined administration of the PAF antagonist and indomethacin eye drops decreased the PGE_2 level to 1.20 ± 0.96 pg/ml ($P < 0.01$); combined administration of the PAF antagonist and steroid eye drops decreased it to 9.53 ± 4.61 pg/ml ($P < 0.05$).

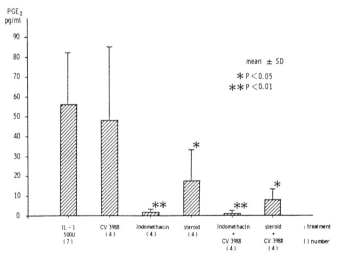

Effects of Drugs on Aqueous Humor PGE₂ Concentration

Fig. 2.
Aqueous humor PGE₂ levels were not decreased after intravenous injection of CV 3988.
Combined administration of indomethacin and CV 3988 further reduced in aqueous PGE₂ level ($P < 0.01$)

CONCLUSION

We were able to induce endophthalmitis by intravitreous injection of IL − 1 similar to previous reports[3,4,5]. This inflammation was characterized by an inflammation centering on the anterior portion of the eye.

The protein and PGE_2 levels showed significant increases ($P < 0.01$) at doses of 500U or above of IL − 1.

The PAF antagonist acted to decrease the protein level in the anterior aqueous humor but it did not decrease the PGE_2 level. The PG synthesis inhibitor decreased both the protein level and the PGE_2 level. Combined administration of the PAF antagonist and the PG synthesis inhibitor further reduced both the protein level and the PGE_2 level.

These facts suggest the possibility that PAF and PG act as mediators of endophthalmitis due to IL − 1.

Acknowledgments

This study was supported by a Grant for Scientific Research (No. 62570804, 1989) from the Ministry of Education, Japan.

REFERENCES

1. Mantovani A, Dejana E (1987) Modulation of endothelial function by interleukin 1. Biochem Pharmacol 36 : 301 − 305

2. Oppenheim JJ, Kovacs EJ, Matsushima K, Durum SK (1986) There is more than one interleukin 1. Immunol Today 7 : 45 − 56

3. Bhattacherjee P, Henderson B (1987) Inflammatory responses to intraocularly injected interleukin 1. Curr Eye Res 6 : 929 − 934

4. Rosenbaum JT, Samples JR, Hefeneider SH, Howes EL (1987) Ocular inflammatory effects of intravitreal interleukin 1. Arch Ophthalmol 105 : 1117 − 1120

5. Rubin RM, Rosenbaum JT (1988) A platelet activating factor antagonist inhibits interleukin 1 − induced inflammation. Biochem Biophys Res Commun 154 : 429 − 436

© 1990 Elsevier Science Publishers (Biomedical Division)
Ocular Immunology Today. M. Usui, S. Ohno and K. Aoki, editors.

SOLUBLE INTERLEUKIN-2 RECEPTOR LEVELS IN PATIENTS WITH UVEITIS

JAMES T. ROSENBAUM, M.D.[1] ; MORRIS E. TILDEN, M.D.[2]; and ANTONY BAKKE, M.D.[3]

Departments of Ophthalmology, Medicine, and Cell Biology[1]; Department of Ophthalmology[2]; and Department of Clinical Pathology[3], Oregon Health Sciences University, 3181 S.W. Sam Jackson Park Road, Portland, Oregon 97201

INTRODUCTION

Inflammation in the eye, similar to inflammation elsewhere in the body, is the result of an immune response regulated by an intricate balance of homeo-statically controlled signals passing between different subsets of effector cells. Much of this regulation is accomplished by secreted peptides known as interleukins.

One of the first interleukins to be identified was Interleukin-2 (IL-2), or T-cell growth factor (1). IL-2 is a cytokine whose primary function is to induce the proliferation and activation of T-cells (2), B-cells (3,4), and natural killer (NK) cells (5,6). It is also induces the expression of IL-1 in monocytes and histiocytes (7), and co-induces (with IL-1) expression of interferon-gamma in T-cells (8,9).

IL-2 binds to a discreet receptor (10). The increased detection of a soluble IL-2 receptor (sIL-2R) in serum may represent a characteristic marker for T-cell activation. Elevated levels of sIL-2R have been reported in such disparate diseases as tuberculosis (11), atopic eczema (12), Hodgkin's and non-Hodgkin's lymphoma (13,14), solid tumors (15), rheumatoid arthritis (16, 17), systemic lupus erythematosus (18), HIV infection (19), chronic renal failure (20), and type 1 diabetes (21). In diseases such as rheumatoid arthritis, systemic lupus, and primary Sjogren's syndrome, the degree of ele-vation appears to correlate with disease activity (17,18,22). Many forms of uveitis appear to be immunologically mediated in both experimental models and clinical disease states (23). Since elevated levels of sIL-2R are frequently found in patients with "autoimmune" diseases, we have assessed the clinical utility of the measurement of sIL-2R levels in patients with active uveitis.

METHODS

Patients were attending the Uveitis Clinic, Department of Ophthalmology, Oregon Health Sciences University. All patients were seen by one of us (JTR). Normal controls were 21 consecutive Red Cross blood donors. Soluble IL-2R levels were determined by a sandwich ELISA assay (T Cell Sciences, Cambridge, MA) employing two monoclonal antibodies directed against two different epitopes of the 55kD Tac protein, one of the two components of the IL-2 receptor. Results are reported as mean units/ml $\pm$ the standard error.

Statistical comparisons were performed by Student's T-test.

RESULTS

Detectable levels of sIL-2R were significantly elevated in patients with
uveitis (mean=707 + 40, n=101) relative to healthy controls (mean=568 + 57,
n=21, p< 0.025). The average age of patients was 41 + 16 years including 41
males and 60 females, while the average age of controls was 46 + 14 including
13 males and 8 females. In the patients with uveitis, overall mean levels of
sIL-2R were similar in males and females (668 + 63 vs 734 + 49, p> 0.1)

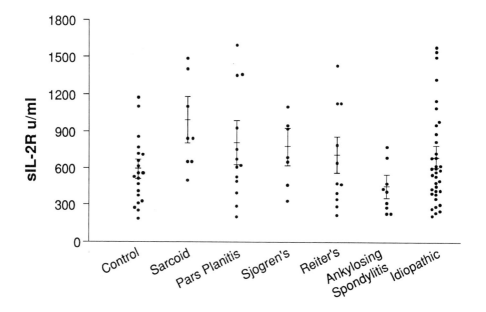

Fig. 1. sIL-2R levels in patients with uveitis

Levels of sIL-2R in patients with uveitis were further analyzed on the basis
of distinct disease subsets (Figure 1). Patients with sarcoidosis had the
highest, consistent level (mean=933 + 129, n=8, p< 0.01 relative to control).
Elevated levels also tended to be present in patients with pars planitis
(mean=753 + 121, n=13, p< 0.1) as well as in patients with suspected Sjogren's
syndrome (24) (dry eyes and bilateral, chronic uveitis) (mean=728 + 104, n=7,
p< 0.1). Most of these latter patients had not undergone minor salivary gland
biopsy. Of the three patients with a more definite diagnosis on the basis of
minor salivary gland biopsy the mean level was 813 + 144 (p=0.055 relative to
control). Elevated levels were not consistently found among patients with
Reiter's syndrome (mean=666 + 103, n=11) or patients with ankylosing

spondylitis (mean=427 ± 64, n=9). Although the number of patients studied was small, elevated levels were not found in two patients with toxoplasmosis, two patients with Fuch's heterochromic cyclitis, or two patients with Birdshot choroidopathy. In contrast, marked elevations (greater than three standard deviations above the mean of healthy controls) were seen in one patient with syphilis in the setting of HIV infection, one patient with suspected interstitial nephritis, and two patients with iritis typical of juvenile rheumatoid arthritis and minimal joint disease. In addition one of two patients with acute multifocal placoid pigmentary epitheliopathy had a marked elevation. In all, 18% of the 101 patients studied had levels greater than two standard deviations above the mean value. Patients who could not be placed into a distinct clinical diagnostic group were termed idiopathic.

Patients with bilateral involvement had significantly elevated sIL-R levels (mean=814 ± 65, n=46) when compared to those with only unilateral involvement (mean=617 ± 45, n=55, p< 0.01). The location of ocular inflammation did not appear to influence sIL-2R levels, however. Patients with anterior (mean=684 ± 59, n=45), posterior (mean=687 ± 87, n=14), combined anterior and posterior (mean=752 ± 80, n=29), or chorioretinal (mean=755 ± 133, n=11) involvement were not significantly different (p> 0.1). Likewise, sIL-2R levels in those with acute onset of uveitis (mean=658 ± 55, n=53) were not significantly different from those with insidious onset (mean=773 ± 56, n=47, p> 0.1). There also appears to be no correlation between sIL-2R levels and age, duration of disease, or visual acuity (r< 0.1 in all cases).

DISCUSSION

This study indicates a statistically increased level of sIL-2R in patients with uveitis. However, the vast majority of patients fell within a normal range. Therefore, the data should not be interpreted as indicating a diagnostic utility for this test. Previous studies have shown systemic immunologic abnormalities in many patients with uveitis. For example, approximately 25% of patients with uveitis have elevated antinuclear antibody levels (25,26). In one study on peripheral blood lymphocytes from patients with uveitis, increased expression of IL-2R was found in 16 of 24 patients (27). IL-2 has also been detected in the uvea in an immunohistologic study of uveitis (2).

Soluble IL-2R levels were most consistently elevated among patients with sarcoid, a disease with known systemic immunologic abnormalities. Levels were not elevated among patients with Reiter's syndrome or ankylosing spondylitis, in contrast to levels reported in other immunologically mediated joint diseases such as rheumatoid arthritis and systemic lupus (16,18). The increased levels in patients with bilateral disease may reflect the `systemic' nature of a bilateral ophthalmologic process. However, the unilateral group includes all the patients with ankylosing spondylitis and Reiter's syndrome who have a systemic process without elevated sIL-2R levels.

Our study confirms the ability to detect systemic immunologic abnormalities among a subset of patients with uveitis.

ACKNOWLEDGEMENTS

Supported in part by grant number EY06484 from the National Eye Institute.

REFERENCES

1. Gillis S, Ferm MM, Ou W, Smith KA (1978) J Immunol 120:2027-2032

2. Hooks JJ, Chan CC, Detrick B (1988) Investigative Ophthalmology and Visual Science 29:1444-1451

3. Waldmann TA, Goldman CK, Robb RJ, et al (1984) J Exp Med 160:1450-1466

4. Zubler RH, Lowenthal JW, Erard F, Hashimoto N, Devos R, MacDonald R (1984) J Exp Med 160:1170-1183

5. Anegon I, Cuturi MC, Trinchieri G, Perussia B (1988) J Exp Med 167:452-472

6. Aribia M-HB, Leroy E, Lantz O, et al (1987) J Immunol 139:443-451

7. Numerof RP, Aronson FR, Mier JW (1988) J Immunol 141:4250-4257

8. Reem GH, Cook DM (1984) Science 225:429-430

9. Wilson AB, Harris JM, Coombs RRA (1988) Cellular Immunology 113:130-142

10. Robb RJ, Munck A, Smith KA (1981) J Exp Med 154:1455-1474

11. Brown AE, Reiker KT, Webster HK (1989) Am Rev Respir Dis 139:1036-1038

12. Colver GB, Symons JA, Duff GW (1989) Br Med J 298:1426-1428

13. Chilosi M, Semenzato G, Vinante F, et al (1989) Am J Clin Path 92:186-191

14. Lissoni P, Barni S, Rovelli F, Crispino S, Tancini G (1988) Int J Biol Markers 3:273-274

15. Rovelli F, Lissoni P, Crispino S, Barni S (1988) Tumori 74:633-637

16. Keystone EC, Snow KM, Bombardier C, Chang C-H, Nelson DL, Rubin LA (1988) Arth Rheum 31:844-849

17. Symons JA, Wood NC, Di Giovine FS, Duff GW (1988) J Immunol 141:2612-2618

18. Manoussakis MN, Papadopoulos GK, Drosos AA, Moutsopoulos HM (1989) Clin Immunol Immunopath 50:321-332

19. Lang JM, Cocumaros G, Levy S, Falkenrodt A (1988) Immunol Lett 19:99-102

20. Takamatsu T, Yasuda N, Ohno T, Kanoh T (1988) Tohoku J Exp Med 155:343-347

21. Giordano C, Galluzo A, Marco A, Panto F (1988) Diabetes Res 8:135-138

22. Semenzato G, Bambara LM, Biasi D, Frigo A (1988) J Clin Immunol 8:447-452

23. Nussenblatt RB Palestine AG (1989) Uveitis: Fundamentals and Clinical Practice Yearbook Medical Publishers, Chicago, pp 1-447

24. Rosenbaum JT, Bennett RM (1987) Am J Ophthalmol 104:346-352

25. Epstein WV, Tan M, Easterbrook M (1971) New Engl J Med 285:1502-1506

26. Glass D et al (1980) J Clin Invest 66:426-429

27. Deschenes J, Char DH, Kaleta S (1988) Br J Ophthalmol 72:83-87

© 1990 Elsevier Science Publishers (Biomedical Division)
Ocular Immunology Today. M. Usui, S. Ohno and K. Aoki, editors.

IMMUNE PRIVILEGE AND ITS REGULATION BY IMMUNOSUPPRESSIVE GROWTH FACTORS IN AQUEOUS HUMOR

SCOTT W. COUSINS AND J. WAYNE STREILEIN

Departments of Ophthalmology, Bascom Palmer Eye Institute and of Microbiology and Immunology, University of Miami School of Medicine, Miami Florida (USA) 33136

INTRODUCTION

Over the past 15 years, this and other laboratories have described the characteristics of immune privilege of the anterior chamber. Most of the experimental evidence documents the deviant immune response that occurs after immunization of animals via the anterior chamber, a phenomenon termed Anterior Chamber Associated Immune Deviation (ACAID).[1] However, recently we have observed that immune privilege is also extended to include the expression of immunity within the anterior chamber. That is, certain immune effector functions are inhibited within the normal anterior chamber as compared to conventional, extraocular sites. These observations have led us to postulate that the normal anterior chamber is a generalized immunosuppressive microenvironment, the composition of which is multifactorial, including the presence of unique cells and molecules. This report will briefly summarize our current concepts regarding the role of immunosuppressive growth factors in the maintenance of immune privilege.

IMMUNE PRIVILEGE OF THE AC IS EXTENDED TO THE EXPRESSION OF IMMUNITY

We sought to determine whether certain aspects of immune privilege might not also operate upon the expression of immune responses within the AC. We reasoned the AC should be relatively resistant to immunologic stimuli that cause immune-mediated inflammation within conventional sites. Using a mouse model, we have demonstrated that the AC is resistant to the inflammation produced by the local adoptive transfer of immune effectors in two different models of immune mediated inflammation.[2] Adoptive transfer of primed lymphocytes plus antigen-pulsed antigen presenting cells into the subconjunctival space resulted in the production of a moderate conjunctival inflammatory response. However, the transfer of a similar inoculum into the AC failed to produce a clinically significant inflammatory response. Similar results were detected after the local adoptive transfer of alloantigen-responsive effectors (local graft versus host reaction). In fact, the mouse AC failed to sustain antigen-specific immune-mediated inflammation even after direct intraocular challenge with antigen in a previously immunized animal, although the same mice expressed normal immune-mediated inflammation within the skin and subconjunctival sites, and remained susceptible to the direct action of inflammatory mediators within the AC. Thus, the AC demonstrates a qualitative resistance to certain immune-mediated effector functions.

AQUEOUS HUMOR CONTAINS FACTORS WHICH INHIBIT LYMPHOCYTE FUNCTION IN VITRO AND IN VIVO

In an attempt to further explain the mechanism of this inhibition, we postulated that the AC is a generalized immunosuppressive microenvironment. We suspected that soluble immunosuppressive growth factors within the aqueous humor were an important component of this microenvironment. For decades, investigators have attempted to prove that normal aqueous humor contains growth inhibitory factors, but their characterization has remained elusive. Recently, our laboratory has demonstrated that normal aqueous humor was a potent inhibitor of certain in vitro assays for lymphocyte function, including antigen-induced, mitogen-induced and cytokine-induced cellular proliferation. Indeed, dose response curves performed in various assays demonstrated that the maximal inhibition occurred at 25-50% concentrations of aqueous humor, but inhibition was still identifiable in some assay with concentrations as low as 1-5%. Even at the highest concentrations, aqueous humor failed to alter the function of "mature" cytotoxic T cells was unaffected.[3] These observations suggested that aqueous humor contains factors capable of regulating some, but not all, lymphocyte functions in vitro.

Recently, we have demonstrated that the antiproliferative activity of aqueous humor functions in vivo as well. Using the same local adoptive transfer models described previously, we sought to determine if the diminished clinical inflammatory response was associated with diminished proliferation of the effector lymphocytes in vivo. We developed a method to measure proliferation of cells recovered from injected eyes using a technique called DNA analysis by flow cytometry. Cellular infiltrates from enucleated mouse eyes were simultaneously stained for DNA content (with a fluorescent dye,

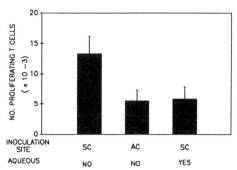

Figure 1. T cell proliferation 48 hours after adoptive transfer of Mycobacteria-primed lymphocytes into the subconjunctiva (SC) or anterior chamber (AC), with or without aqueous humor pretreatment.

propidium iodide) and T cell surface markers (with a fluorescein-labelled anti-Thy 1.2 antibody). Using a flow cytometer, we were able to identify T lymphocyte proliferation within the various inflamed sites (Fig. 1). A high number of proliferating T cells was observed in the subconjunctival site after local adoptive transfer of Mycobacteria-primed lymph node cells. In contrast, when similar cells were transferred into the mouse anterior chamber, only a few proliferating T cells were detected. Importantly, pretreatment of the adoptive transfer inoculum with 25% aqueous humor, prior to transfer into the subconjunctival space, abolished the clinical inflammatory response and markedly decreased the number of proliferating T cells. A similar observation was noted for the adoptive transfer of local graft versus host reactions. Thus, we conclude that normal aqueous humor can inhibit T cell proliferation and function in vivo.

IDENTIFICATION OF THE IMMUNOSUPPRESSIVE FACTOR(S) IN AQUEOUS HUMOR

These observations led us to attempt to identify the immunosuppressive factor(s) within normal aqueous humor. Partial purification of the inhibitors in aqueous humor by HPLC revealed that at least one important molecule was present within the 20 to 30 kD molecular weight fractions, although preliminary data suggest others are also present. Recently, a widely distributed polypeptide cytokine called transforming growth factor-β (TGF-β) has been characterized and has been reported to display immunosuppressive properties not unlike aqueous humor. We sought to determine if TGF-β might be one of the immunoregulatory molecules in aqueous humor. Indeed, aqueous humor from man, rabbits, mice, pigs and cows contained large amounts of both active and latent TGF-β (Table 1) as measured by bioassay or immunoblotting. In addition, TGF-β eluted in the same fractions containing the 20-30 kD inhibitor. Subsequent bioassay revealed that TGF-β was the relevant inhibitor in those fractions. We have shown that the aqueous humor concentrations of TGF-β are adequate to explain much of the immunosuppressive properties in aqueous humor (Fig. 2). Also, neutralizing antibodies to TGF-β2 were effective in reversing 50-70% of the activity of normal aqueous humor (depending upon the assay tested), but the neutralization was even more impressive if latent TGF-β had previously been activated prior to assay. Therefore, we have concluded

TABLE 1: Quantitative determination of TGF-β concentration in pooled aqueous humor from various species

Source of Aqueous Humor	Amount of TGF-β		Relative Amt‡	
	Mature*	Total†	%β1	%β2
Human	450	1170	20	80
Rabbit	470	1400	6	94
Bovine	< 20	1130	ND	ND
Porcine	< 20	490	ND	ND
Mouse	ND	1120	ND	ND

*Mature refers to TGF-β bioactivity (pg/ml) in unmanipulated aqueous humor as measured in the CCL 64 mink epithelial cell bioassay. ND indicates assay not done.
†Total refers to TGF-β bioactivity (pg/ml) after transient acidification of aqueous, activating any latent TGF-β.
‡Refers to relative amount of two forms TGF-β1 versus TGF-β2, as determined by specific neutralizing antisera.

that TGF-β in aqueous humor is one of the important immunoregulatory factors, although others remain to be characterized.

CELLULAR SOURCE OF THE IMMUNOSUPPRESSIVE FACTORS IN AQUEOUS HUMOR

The presence of immunosuppressive factors in aqueous humor suggests local synthesis by cells within the AC. In fact, serum contains mostly TGF-β1; the predominance of TGF-β2 in aqueous humor supports the notion of intraocular production of this factor. We have reported that cell lines produced from explants of normal iris and ciliary body display extremely interesting properties. Among these properties include the capacity to directly inhibit lymphocyte activation in various in vitro assays.[4] Additionally, these cells secrete potent immunosuppressive factors into the culture medium which mimic the properties of aqueous humor (Fig. 2). Although TGF-β is one of the factors, other potent molecules are also contributing to the inhibition. These types of experiments indicate that many of the endogenous ocular cells, such as the ciliary epithelium, corneal endothelium or resident cells within the iris stroma, might have the capacity to regulate ocular immune privilege by their secretion of immunoregulatory molecules.

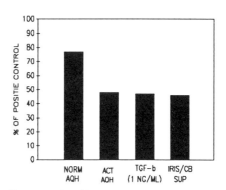

Figure 2. Inhibition of IL-2 production by a T cell hybridoma after incubation with 25% normal aqueous humor, 25% acid-activated aqueous humor, TGF-β or supernatants from cultures conditioned by iris/ciliary body cells.

LOSS OF IMMUNE PRIVILEGE AND OCULAR INFLAMMATION

If the anterior chamber is immunosuppressive, how does immune-mediated inflammation occur during uveitis? We reasoned that the local presence of certain immunoregulatory cytokines might be capable of antagonizing the immunosuppressive environment, thus enabling the expression of normal immunity. Interferon gamma (IFN-γ) is a cytokine that possess numerous regulatory functions, including the capacity to upregulate class II MHC molecules, recruit new antigen presenting cells into the eye and reverse some of the effects of TGF-β. In high doses, IFN-γ is an inflammatory mediator. However, when low doses (i.e., 100 units per eye) are injected into the AC, no clinical or histologic evidence for inflammation is detected. Yet, important physiologic changes were induced. Within 72 hours after injection, the density of class II positive APC had nearly doubled within the iris, suggesting both local upregulation as well as recruitment from the blood. When we performed an experiment to assess the expression of delayed hypersensitivity in a IFN-γ treated eye, the AC was found to express vigorous antigen specific inflammation, either to direct antigen challenge or to the local adoptive transfer of effector cells. Immune privilege had been abolished by the IFN-γ pretreatment.

CONCLUSIONS AND SPECULATION

Our interpretation of this series of experiments is that immune privilege in the anterior chamber is actively-produced (by factors and cells), highly-regulated and capable of being abolished (by immunopotentiating cytokines). Normally, the anterior chamber is protected from the expression of immune-mediated inflammation. However, events may conspire against the AC to alter this environment and make it susceptible to the same effector responses that other sites routinely experience. The efficiency with which the endogenous ocular cells can re-establish the privileged environment might serve to regulate exacerbations and remissions of intraocular inflammation.

A number of intriguing questions are raised by these experiments. How is immune privilege regulated and abolished in vivo? What is the role of T cell cytokines in this regulatory process? Do genetic differences exist in the local ocular regulation of cytokine production? In addition, the high number of proliferating T cells within sites of immune-mediated inflammation are greater than would be predicted on the basis of the number of antigen-specific cells adoptively transferred. What is the antigen-specificity of these proliferating cells? Are they contributing to the inflammatory process? These questions are the basis for our current experiments.

REFERENCES

1. Streilein JW (1987) FASEB J 1: 199
2. Cousins SW, Streilein JW (1989) Inv Ophthalmol Vis Sci (supp) 30:440
3. Kaiser CJ, Ksander BR, Streilein JW (1989) Reg Immunol 2: 42
4. Williamson JSP, Bradley D, Streilein JW (1989) Immunology 67:96

© 1990 Elsevier Science Publishers (Biomedical Division)
Ocular Immunology Today. M. Usui, S. Ohno and K. Aoki, editors.

THE ROLE OF TUMOR NECROSIS FACTOR IN ENDOTOXIN INDUCED UVEITIS

YOSHIHITO TANOUCHI, SATOSHI MIKI, TOMOKO OTANI, KEIKO YAMAGUCHI
AND YASUO MIMURA
Department of Ophthalmology, Tokushima University School of
Medicine, Tokushima 770 (Japan)

INTRODUCTION

It is well known that systemic injection of endotoxin induces
uveitis in rats and rabbits[1,2]. Systemic administration of endotoxin also produce transient granulocytopenia followed by a
marked granulocytosis and disseminated intravascular coagulation[3].
However, little is known concerning what role leukocytes play in
the onset of uveitis after endotoxin administration. On the other
hand, tumor necrosis factor (TNF) is a cytokine that acts to
monocytes, leukocytes and vascular endothelium[4]. We studied the
systemic and ocular changes present in endotoxin induced
uveitis (EIU) of rats and rabbits.

MATERIALS AND METHODS

Treatment of animals

Experiment 1. Salmonella typhimurium endotoxin(100μg/rat) was inoculated into the footpad of female Lewis rats(b.w.ca170g, 8 weeks
old). The eyes were examined with a slit lamp biomicroscope,
and peripheral blood and aqueous humor samples were obtained at
0.5, 1.5, 3, 6, 12, 24 and 48 hours after endotoxin injection.

Experiment 2. Salmonella typhimurium endotoxin (200μg/kg) was
injected intravenously two times with 24 hours intervening in black
rabbits. The aqueous flare was examined and peripheral blood was
obtained regularly.

Number of leukocytes and protein concentration

The number of leukocytes in the peripheral blood and aqueous
humor were counted by Burker Turk counting chamber. Protein concentration of aqueous humor was assayed by monitoring the absorbance of Coomassie Brilliant Blue G-250 binding protein at 595 nm.

Aqueous flare

Aqueous flare was examined by using a laser-flare cell meter
(Kowa FC-1000). Flare was shown as photon count.

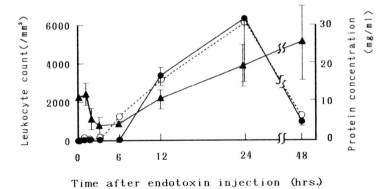

Time after endotoxin injection (hrs.)

Fig. 1 Time course of the leukocyte count in the peripheral
blood(▲) and in the aqueous humor(●), and protein concentration
in the aqueous humor(○) following endotoxin administration.

Table 1 The time course of serum TNF
levels following endotoxin administration

Time after endotoxin administration (hours)	Serum TNF (IU/ml)
0	N.D.
0.5	198±117
1.5	3499±612
3	0.25±0.09
6	N.D.

Table 2 Time course of the aqueous flare and leukocyte count in the
peripheral blood following endotoxin administration

Time after endotoxin administration	Photon count (/msec)		Leukocyte count (/mm³)	
	1st.	2nd.	1st.	2nd.
0	15± 9	204±226	3725±1121	6845±2664
0.5	18± 20	845±417	2506± 908	2838± 685
1.5	193±136	1110±497	963± 266	2513±1107
3	224±170	1230±520	1320± 587	2780±1317
6	292±115	1030±508	2819±1631	4719±2528
12	289±126	1127±596	6500±4142	5250±1893
24	204±226	779±579	6845±2664	6838±3443

TNF activity

Actinomycin D(1μg/ml)-treated mouse fibroblast L-929 cells(6x10^6 cells/ml) were incubated with serially diluted serum for 18 hours at 37°C and lysis was determined by staining unlysed cells with crystal violet. TNF activity was measured by monitoring the absorbance at 600 nm.

Histopathology

Rats were sacrificed 3 and 24 hours after endotoxin injection. Eye, lung, liver and skin were removed, fixed in 10% neutral buffered formalin, embedded in paraffin and stained with hematoxylin and eosin.

Rabbits were sacrificed 3 hours after the first and the second injection of endotoxin. Eye, lung, liver and kidney were removed, fixed, embedded and stained with phosphotungstic acid hematoxylin.

RESULTS

Experiment 1.

Endotoxin administration induced iris hyperemia at 3 hours and inflammation peaked at 24 hours. The number of leukocytes in peripheral blood decreased to one third that of the controls during 3 to 6 hours following endotoxin administration, but increased thereafter with the number of leukocytes and protein concentration in the aqueous humor (Fig. 1). Serum TNF peaked at 1.5 hours and then rapidly decreased (Table 1). More leukocytes could be found in endotoxin treated rats than in the controls in the small vessels of the iris, lung, liver and skin. Some of them were attached to the vascular endothelium.

Experiment 2.

The aqueous flare increased at 1.5 hours, attaining maximum intensity at 6 hours. The number of leukocytes in the peripheral blood decreased at 1.5 hours with subsequent leukocytosis within 12 hours following the first administration of endotoxin. After the second injection of endotoxin, the aqueous flare peaked in three hours and was 5 times as high as the first peak (Table 2). Serum TNF activity peaked at 1 hour following the first endotoxin administration and showed the same behavior after the second endotoxin injection (Table 3). Fibrin formation in the small vessels of systemic organs within 3 hours following the second administration of endotoxin could be detected histopathologically.

Table 3 The time course of serum TNF levels following
endotoxin administration

Time after endotoxin administration	TNF activity (IU/ml)	
	1st.	2nd.
0	N.D.	N.D.
0.5	225±169	16±9
1	979±257	120±55
1.5	766±212	178±94
2	442±258	79±54
3	28±19	13±5
6	N.D.	N.D.

DISCUSSION

Endotoxin stimulates the formation of macrophages which in turn
produce TNF[5]. In Experiment 1, the number of leukocytes in
peripheral blood decreased during three to six hours after endotoxin administration and more leukocytes were observed than in
controls in the small vessels of systemic organ. Serum TNF reached
a peak at 1.5 hours following endotoxin administration. In Experiment 2, the number of leukocytes in the peripheral blood decreased
at almost the same time as the peak of serum TNF activity was
observed. TNF may have enhanced the adherence of neutrophils,
monocytes and lymphocytes to the vascular endothelium which was
damaged by chemical mediators such as prostaglandins, platelet activating factor, histamine and serotonin released from leukocytes.
These factors may have disrupted the blood aqueous barrier in the
early period, inducing EIU as a result.

REFERENCES

1. Bhattacherjee P, Phylactos A (1977) Eur J Pharmacol 44:75-80
2. Rosenbaum JT, McDevitt HO, Guss RB, et al (1980) Nature 286:
   611-613
3. Morrison DC, Ulevitch RJ (1978) Am J Pathol 93:527-617
4. Gemsa D (1987) Immunobiology 175:1-143
5. Beutler B, Greenwald D, Hulmes JD, et al (1985) Nature 316:
   552-554

© 1990 Elsevier Science Publishers (Biomedical Division)
Ocular Immunology Today. M. Usui, S. Ohno and K. Aoki, editors.

REGULATION OF LYMPHOCYTE PROLIFERATION
BY RESIDENT OCULAR CELLS

PHILIP L. HOOPER, THOMAS A. FERGUSON, HENRY J. KAPLAN

Department of Ophthalmology and Visual Science, Washington University, St. Louis, Missouri 63110

Co-culture of single cell suspensions prepared from murine uveal tissue with lymphocytes results in marked inhibition of cellular proliferation as measured by ^{3}H incorporation. This inhibition is not H-2 restricted and is mediated by a soluble factor. Pretreatment of uveal cells with cycloheximide or paraformaldehyde blocked the inhibition, but pre-incubation with mitomycin did not. This suggests that protein synthesis and membrane turnover by uveal cells is required to produce this factor, although the ocular cells themselves do not need to proliferate.

Introduction of antigen into the anterior chamber of the eye results in inhibition of the systemic DTH response to that antigen, while antibody production and cytotoxicity are augmented. This phenomenon has been described by a number of authors using a variety of antigens including allogeneic tissue grafts, viruses, tumor cells, and haptens.

The underlying mechanism of the inhibited DTH has been extensively studied and involves the following steps after antigen introduction into the eye[1]:

1) Secretion of a soluble factor from the eye into the serum.

2) Production of antigen specific T cells within the spleen as a result of the presence of this factor.

3) Induction of antigen specific inhibition of DTH by either these T cells or by a soluble factor released by the cells.

Little is known about the distinctive milieu of the eye which results in the initiation of the cascade leading to altered immunoreactivity. We have performed a series of experiments which demonstrate that resident ocular cells within the iris,ciliary body and choroid are capable of influencing lymphocyte proliferation in vitro.

MATERIALS AND METHODS
Preparation of Ocular Tissue

Immediately following death, donor animals were perfused with 30cc of cold HBSS through a cardiac puncture. Eyes were enucleated, placed in cold HBSS, and dissected into two sections at the limbus. The iris, choroid/ciliary body, and retina were separated from remaining ocular tissue and single cell suspensions prepared by enzymatic digestion. For digestion, we utilized a mixture of collagenase type II (1mg/ml), trypsin inhibitor (4mg/ml), and DNAase (0.1mg/ml) in HBSS. Following digestion the cell suspensions were washed twice in HBSS and viable cells counted.

Lymphocyte Proliferation Assays

1) Mixed Lymphocyte Cultures (MLC) were performed with Balb/c splenocytes as responders and C57BL/6 splenocytes as stimulators. Stimulator lymphocytes were pretreated with mitomycin c or were irradiated with 3000 rad prior to use. Cells were seeded at the concentrations shown in complete RPMI with 10% FCS and were incubated for 96 hours. Culture wells were pulsed with 1 microCurie of ^{3}H thymidine for the final 12 hours of the incubation period.

2) Antigen specific proliferation assays utilized primed lymphocytes prepared from lymph nodes of Balb/c mice which had previously been immunized with 100 micrograms of HEL in CFA. Conditions of incubation were identical to that used for the MLC.

3) Clone proliferation assays utilized the murine conalbumin/ H-2^k specific Th2 clone D10.G4.1 which had been rested for 7 days prior to use. Feeder lymphocytes were C3H splenocytes. Wells were incubated for 72 hours and received 1 microCurie of ^{3}H thymidine for the final 12 hours of incubation.

RESULTS

The effect of ocular uveal tissue on lymphocyte proliferation was compared to the effect of a non-uveal tissue (retina). Subsequently, the mechanism by which inhibition was produced was explored.

Effects of ocular cell suspensions on antigen specific lymphocyte proliferation

Single cell suspensions prepared from retina, iris and choroid of the H-2 disparate mice Balb/c (H-2^d) and C3H (H-2^k) were seeded at a concentration of 1×10^5 cells/well into wells of a 96 well tissue culture plate containing 2×10^5 primed Balb/c lymphocytes and 50 micrograms of antigen in a total volume of 200 microliters. Our results (Figure 1) showed that uveal cells from both strains inhibited the proliferation of the primed lymphocytes and that inhibition was independent of the H-2 haplotype of the ocular cell donor (p $\leq$0.05). The tissue specific nature of the inhibition was demonstrated by the fact that an equal number of retinal cells failed to produce inhibition.

Figure 1

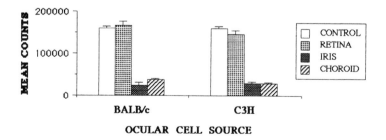

Cellular mechanisms underlying inhibition

In order to assess whether uveal cells need to proliferate to inhibit lymphocyte proliferation, mitomycin c (mito) was used to pre-treat the ocular cell suspension. The results (Figure 2) did not demonstrate any significant difference in the inhibition following mitomycin c treatment. The importance of protein synthesis and membrane turnover in the production of inhibition was demonstrated by experiments utilizing cycloheximide (cyclo), and paraformaldehyde (para) pre-treatment. (Figures 3,4).

Figure 2

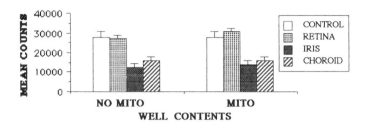

Figure 3

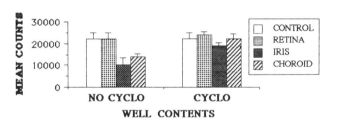

Figure 4

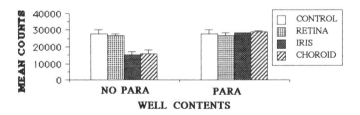

Demonstration of a Soluble Factor

The presence of a soluble inhibitory factor was demonstrated 2 ways. In the first experiment,(data not shown), 100 microliters of supernatant from a 200 microliter well containing ocular cells, responder, and stimulator lymphocytes was transferred at 48 hours to a well containing responder and stimulator lymphocytes only. Significant inhibition of proliferation was observed only in wells receiving the supernatant of wells containing uveal cells. The second experiment (Figure 6) utilized a 0.45 micron membrane which separated ocular cells and lymphocytes. This experiment demonstrated that inhibition could be transferred across a semipermiable membrane.

Figure 6

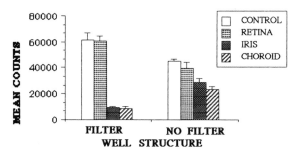

DISCUSSION

The data presented in this paper demonstrate that cells resident within the iris, ciliary body and choroid are capable of producing soluble factors which suppress lymphocyte proliferation in vitro. Proliferation of the ocular cells is not required to produce this factor, which appears to be a protein. Although the stimulus to the ocular cells which results in the production of the factor is unclear, our data suggest that it is independent of antigen processing by the ocular cells and the MHC. Further studies will identify if this factor is similar to inhibitors described in aqueous and vitreous, and whether it plays a role in the events leading to suppression of systemic immune responses in vivo.

REFERENCES

1.Ferguson TA, Kaplan HJ (1987) J. Immunol. 139:346

ANIMAL MODELS

© 1990 Elsevier Science Publishers (Biomedical Division)
Ocular Immunology Today. M. Usui, S. Ohno and K. Aoki, editors.

ANDROGEN TREATMENT OF AUTOIMMUNE DISEASE IN LACRIMAL GLANDS OF MRL/Mp-lpr/lpr AND NZB/NZW F1 MICE

HIROKO ARIGA, ANA CRISTINA L.M. VENDRAMINI, ELCIO H. SATO, CYNTHIA SOO, JOAN A. EDWARDS AND DAVID A. SULLIVAN

Department of Ophthalmology, Harvard Medical School and Immunology Unit, Eye Research Institute, 20 Staniford Street, Boston, MA, USA 02114

INTRODUCTION

Autoimmune diseases often manifest a sexual dichotomy, with estrogens exacerbating immunopathology in females and androgens suppressing autoimmune severity in males (1). In fact, androgen treatment has been utilized to significantly curtail autoimmune sequelae in animal models of systemic lupus erythematosus, thyroiditis, polyarthritis and myasthenia gravis, as well as the human disorder, idiopathic thrombocytopenic purpura (1). Quite possibly, androgen administration may also serve as an effective therapy for Sjögren's syndrome. This syndrome is an autoimmune disorder found almost entirely in females and is associated with alterations in T cell distribution (2), pronounced lymphocytic infiltration into the lacrimal gland, disruption of acinar and ductal epithelium and keratoconjunctivitis sicca (3). Given that androgens improve T cell function (4), regulate lacrimal gland immunity and modulate lacrimal structure and function (5), these hormones may have therapeutic potential.

The purpose of the current study was to determine, by using mouse models of Sjögren's syndrome, whether androgen treatment might suppress autoimmune expression in the lacrimal gland. Experiments also evaluated the impact of testosterone on the populations of total, helper and suppressor/cytotoxic T cells, B cells and Ia positive lymphoyctes in lacrimal tissue infiltrates.

MATERIALS AND METHODS (6-8)

Age-matched female MRL/Mp-lpr/lpr (MRL/lpr; 4-5 months old) and NZB/NZW F1 (F1; 6 months old) mice (n= 6-11/treatment group) were administered subcutaneous implants of placebo (cholesterol, methyl cellulose, lactose)- or testosterone (10 mg or 25 mg)-containing pellets after the onset of disease. These pellets were designed for gradual release of physiological (10 mg) or supraphysiological (25 mg) amounts of testosterone over a 3 week period; pellets were reimplanted every 17 days to maintain hormone levels. Lacrimal glands, and for comparison, submandibular glands, were obtained from sacrificed mice before androgen therapy (pretreatment controls) and following 34 (MRL/lpr) or 51 (F1) days of continuous testosterone exposure. For morphological analysis, tissues were fixed in 10% buffered formalin, dehydrated, embedded in

Historesin, cut into 3 μm sections (4 sections/gland) and stained with hematoxylin and eosin. Sections were evaluated with a Zeiss image analysis system to precisely determine the percentage of lymphocyte infiltration (% = [area of lymphocyte infiltration/area of entire section] x 100), as well as to quantitate acinar area and density. For immunoperoxidase examination, lacrimal glands of MRL/lpr mice were frozen in liquid nitrogen, transferred to OCT compound and cut into 6 μm sections at -20°C. Sections were fixed in acetone, blocked with rabbit serum, avidin and biotin solutions and exposed to rat IgG monoclonal antibodies to Thy 1.2 (total T cells), L3T4 (helper T cells), Lyt 2 (suppressor/cytotoxic T cells), IgM heavy chain (B cells) or Ia antigen. After appropriate incubation periods and washes, sections were successively treated with biotinylated rabbit IgG, which had been pretreated with mouse liver powder, an avidin/biotin complex and developed with hydrogen peroxide and 3-amino-9-ethylcarbazole. Sections were then placed in paraformaldehyde, stained with Gill's hematoxylin, dipped in a lithium carbonate solution and preserved in Biomeda's Crystal Mount. Quantitation of the percentage of cells positive for specific surface markers was performed by microscopic analysis ($\pm$ 5%). Data was statistically analyzed by using Student's t test.

RESULTS (6-8)

Lacrimal glands of F1 and MRL/lpr mice exhibited marked differences in autoimmune expression before the initiation of testosterone treatment. Glands from MRL/lpr animals (pretreatment) harboured extensive regions of lymphocyte infiltration, whereas F1 mice contained significantly fewer lymphocyte foci and more diminutive infiltrates. This difference in autoimmune severity reflects the rapid onset and accelerated disease of MRL/lpr mice (9,10). However, as demonstrated in figure 1, the extent of this lymphocyte infiltration increased significantly in placebo-treated controls of both strains during the experimental time course. In contrast, testosterone therapy induced a precipitous decrease in the magnitude of lymphocyte infiltration in lacrimal tissue (figure 1). After 34 days of androgen administration (10 mg pellet), the percentage infiltrate had undergone a 14-fold reduction in glands of MRL/lpr mice, compared to those of placebo-treated controls. Similarly, testosterone treatment (10 mg pellet) in F1 mice resulted in a 25-fold decrease in the extent of lymphocyte infiltration in lacrimal tissue. These physiological hormone effects, which were duplicated by exposure to supraphysiological amounts of testosterone, involved a significant decline in both infiltrate size and number. Moreover, no evidence of fibrosis or disruption of acinar and ductal epithelium was detectable in glands of testosterone-treated mice. Androgen therapy also stimulated a significant 2-4 fold rise in lacrimal gland weight and/or acinar area and a 2-fold decrease in acinar density/field, compared to values in placebo-treated controls. Testosterone action on tissue weight could not account for the parallel reduction in percentage lymphocyte infiltration.

Androgen influence on lymphocytes in lacrimal glands of MRL/lpr mice appeared to be exerted primarily on T cells. Preliminary analysis (4-6 tissues/group) of placebo tissues indicated that infiltrates were composed principally of T cells (75-95% Thy 1.2 +) of the helper subclass (40-60% L3T4 +), that were positive for Ia antigen (40-60% of cells). Suppressor/cytotoxic T cells (Lyt 2 +) and B (surface IgM +) cells represented between 1-5% and 5-10% of lymphocytes, respectively. Testosterone treatment significantly decreased the total number, but not the apparent subclass distribution, of infiltrate cells.

As concerns the submandibular gland, physiological and supraphysiological androgen exposure significantly reduced the magnitude of lymphocyte infiltration in both MRL/lpr and F1 mice, as compared to that observed in placebo-treated controls (figure 1). This action also involved a decrease in the quantity and area of individual infiltrates.

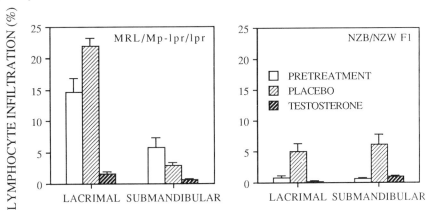

Figure 1. Mice (n = 6-11/group) were treated with placebo- or testosterone (10 mg)-containing pellets and lacrimal and submandibular glands were obtained 34 (MRL/lpr) or 51 (F1) days after androgen exposure. Bars and vertical lines equal the mean ± SE. Data from (6,7).

DISCUSSION

Our findings demonstrated that testosterone administration caused a marked suppression of autoimmune disease in MRL/lpr and F1 mice. Androgen therapy induced a dramatic reduction in the density and area of lymphocyte infiltrates, as well as the total magnitude of lymphocyte infiltration, in both lacrimal and submandibular glands. In addition, no evidence of fibrosis or glandular destruction was observed in lacrimal or submandibular tissue following testosterone treatment.

Considering the known dissimilarites between MRL/lpr and F1 mice in autoimmune pathology and tissue lymphocyte populations (10-12), the similar impact of testosterone in glands of both strains is intriguing. Our preliminary results indicated that hormonal influence appeared directed primarily towards T cells in MRL/lpr lacrimal tissue, but F1 glands contain a significant B cell infiltrate (11). One possible mechanism to explain testosterone action may involve androgen modulation of Ia expression in the glandular epithelium; this class II expression is enhanced in exocrine glands during autoimmune disease and may be susceptible to testosterone control (1).

Overall, our findings show that androgens reverse autoimmune sequelae in lacrimal and submandibular glands in mouse models of Sjögren's syndrome.

ACKNOWLEDGEMENTS

This research was supported by NIH grant EY05612 (DAS), a postdoctoral fellowship grant PD88-046 from the Association for Research in Vision and Ophthalmology and funded through Alcon Laboratories, Inc. (HA) and scholarships from CNPq-Brazil (ACV, EHS).

REFERENCES

1.   Talal N, Ahmed A (1987) Int J Immunotherapy 3:65-70

2.   Adamson TC, Fox RI, Frisman DM, Howell FV (1983) J Immunol 130:203-208

3.   Tabbara KF (1983) In Smolin G, Thoft RA (eds) Cornea. Scientific
     Foundations and Clinical Practice. Little, Brown and Co, Boston, pp 309-314

4.   Michalski JP, McCombs CC, Roubinian JR, Talal N (1983) Clin exp Immunol
     52:229-233

5.   Sullivan DA (1990) In Freier S (ed) The Neuroendocrine Immune Network.
     CRC Press, Boca Raton, FL, pp 199-238

6.   Ariga H, Edwards JA, Sullivan DA (1989) Clin Immunol Immunopathol
     53:499-508

7.   Vendramini AC, Soo C, Sullivan DA (1990) submitted.

8.   Sato EH, Ariga H, Vendramini AC, Sullivan DA (1990) Invest Ophthalmol Vis
     Sci Suppl 31: in press

9.   Hoffman RW, Alspaugh MA, Waggie KS, Durham JB, Walker SE (1984)
     Arthritis Rheum 27:157-165

10. Theofilopoulos AN, Dixon FJ (1985) Adv Immunol 37:269-390

11. Jabs DA, Prendergast RA (1988) Invest Ophthalmol Vis Sci 29:1437- 1443

12. Steinberg AD, Roths JB, Murphy ED, Steinberg RT, Raveche ES (1980) J
     Immunol 125:871-873

© 1990 Elsevier Science Publishers (Biomedical Division)
Ocular Immunology Today. M. Usui, S. Ohno and K. Aoki, editors.

AN IMMUNOHISTOCHEMICAL STUDY OF REJECTION PROCESS IN A RAT PENETRATING KERATOPLASTY MODEL

MAURO NISHI [*], MASAO MATSUBARA[*], ISAMU SUGAWARA[†], SHIGEO MORI[†], MANABU MOCHIZUKI [§]

* Dept. of Ophthalmology, Facult. of Med.; [†] Dept. of Pathol., Inst. Med. Sci.; [§]Dept. of Opthalmol., Branch Hospital, The University of Tokyo, Tokyo, Japan.

INTRODUCTION

The main cause of late corneal failure resides in allograft rejection[1]. For the better understanding of the immunological process of allograft rejection, we performed an immunohistochemical study using a rat model of orthotopic penetrating keratoplasty. We also studied the effects of two immunosuppressants FK506 and Cyclosprorine (CsA) on the cell infiltration of corneal allografts.

MATERIALS AND METHODS

Animals. Male inbred Lewis rats (Rt1[l]) and male inbred Fisher rats (Rt1[lv1]) weighting 200-250 g (8-12 week old), purchased from Charles River Japan (Atsugi, Kanagawa), were used in the study. Forty eight recipients were used. They were divided into three groups as described in the following paragraphs. They were sacrificed at four different periods, as also described below.

Surgical Technic. The surgical procedure followed our methods described in our previous study[2]. Briefly, full thickness donor corneas from Fisher rats were prepared excentrically using a 3.0 mm trephine. The grafts were transplanted onto 2.5 mm recipient beds of Lewis rats. Eight sutures were placed using 10-0 monofilament nylon. Anterior chamber was reformed by air at the end of the procedure. Postoperative care consisted of daily application of atropine 1% ointment and gentamycin eye drops once daily for 7 days, together with intramuscular gentamycin (5mg/kg) for 4 days.

Drug Treatment Schedule. Three groups were placed in accordance with immunosuppressive treatment: FK506 treated rats, CsA treated rats and non treated control rats. FK506 (a gift from Fujisawa Pharmaceutical, Osaka, Japan) was suspended in physiological saline and a dose of 1 mg/kg/day was administered intraperitoneally for 15 days, initiating on the day of surgery. CsA (a gift from Sandoz, Basel, Switzerland) was administered intramuscularly for 15 days.

Periods of Sacrifice. Animals were sacrificed and examined immuno-histochemically at four different stages of postoperation: 1)pre-rejection stage, 2) rejection stage, 3) 1 week after rejection and 4) 2 weeks after rejection. Since the onset of acute rejection in allograft usually occurs on days 12-14 postoperation[2], the control rats were sacrificed on day 10, 14, 21 and 28 postoperation. For the treated groups, the pre-rejection time were chosen as the 14th day of postoperation, since the grafts were still clear but control corneas were rejected. The treated rats were observed under an operating microscope every other day, starting from 14th day, to determine the rejection time. The cornea evaluation was based on parameters for opacity, edema and neovessels in the graft, as described previously[2]. Rejection was diagnosed when there was important deterioration of these parameters. Following the observation, rats were sacrificed at the time of rejection, 1 week after rejection, and 2 weeks after rejection. The eyeballs were enucleated, embedded in OCT compound (Miles Lab, Neperville, Ill, US), snap-frozen with dry ice and acetone, and stored in -80 C until use.

Immunohistochemistry. The frozen tissues were cut at 5 μm thick, fixed with 4% paraformaldehyde, and stained immunohistochemically by the use of avidin-biotin-peroxidase complex method[3]. The primary monoclonal antibodies used consisted of: OX6 that reacts specifically against rat Ia antigen, W3/25 for rat T helper/inducer lymphocytes (Th/i cells), OX8 for rat T suppressor/cytotoxic lymphocytes (T s/c cells) (Sera-lab, Sussex, UK), OX42 for rat macrophage (Serotec, Kidington Oxford, UK), ART18 for interleukin-2 receptor (IL-2R) (provided by Dr. T.D., Immun. Res. Unit, Berlin, Germany[4]). The secondary antibody (biotin labelled horse anti-mouse IgG) and reagents for third phase reaction (avidin-biotin-peroxidase complex) were purchased from Vector Lab. (Burlingame, CA, US). 3-3' diaminobenzidine was used as the staining substrate of peroxidase. After the staining procedure were completed, the positive cells in the central part of the cornea were counted using a grid mounted in contact lens of the microscope (0.015 mm^2), at 100x magnification. Also the cornea sections were stained using hematoxylin and eosin solutions.

RESULTS

The allografts of the control rats at the rejection time (14th day of postoperation) presented a heavy infiltration of mononuclear cells in all layers of the grafts. The treated allograft and taken on day 14 did not present such mononuclear cell infiltration.

The types of infiltrating cells at the different stages of rejection are summarized in table 1. In control corneas, such mononuclear cells as Th/i cells, macrophages, Ia antigen bearing cells and IL-2R bearing cells exhibited highest number at the time of rejection. However, much more Ts/c cells were observed lately, i.e., 1 week after the rejection has begun. Macrophages and Ia antigen-expressing cells were presented in the graft even before the clinical rejection became evident. FK506 and CsA suppressed the infiltration of the immune cells. The immunosuppressive effects of the drugs were most remarkable at the time when cell infiltration became highest in control group.

TABLE 1
IMMUNOHISTOCHEMICAL STUDY
Number of positive cells/0.015mm^2

Markers	Pre-Rejection			Rejection			1 week Rejection			2 week Rejection		
	Ctl	CsA	FK	Ctl	CsA	FK	Ctl	CsA	FK	Ctl	CsA	FK
Th/i cells	2*	0	6	60	40	32	39	38	31	12	3	4
Ts/c cells	2	0	0	29	35	13	47	22	6	13	17	5
macrophage	10	0	4	58	53	35	39	41	24	22	28	3
Ia antigen	17	1	3	90	71	19	68	56	44	42	15	13
IL-2R	0	0	0	21	8	8	1	2	2	2	4	0

Ctl=control group, CsA=cyclosporine treated group, FK=FK506 treated group
*=average of positive cells/0.015mm^2

DISCUSSION

The present study demonstrated heavy infiltration of T lymphocytes subsets, Ia antigen- and IL-2R-presenting cells at the time of acute rejection. The presence of macrophage and Ia antigen expressing cells at the pre-rejection time may be related to their function as antigen presenting cells, triggering the rejection process. These data may suggests the role of T-cell mediated immune reaction in the present cornea rejection. OX8 positive cells (Ts/c cells) exhibited its highest peak at the first week after rejection. Our previous study analizing clinical parameters have shown that the rejection process already began to decrease at the first week after rejection[2]. Therfore, the OX8 positive cells infiltrating in late stage may be involved in the mechanisms of down-regulation of the immune reaction.

Pepose et alli[5] showed the presence of T lymphocyte subsets as well as macrophages in human rejected cornea. They suggested that the influx of macrophages in the rejected cornea might be secondary to the lymphokynes released by T helper cells. Studies of heart rejection in rats have shown a critical role of macrophages in the graft destruction[6]. The present study also demonstrated that macrophages were significantly present at the time of the acute rejection . In addition, the rejected corneas exhibited the highest scores with severe opacity, edema and neovascularization in the grafts. On the other hand, cytotoxic T cells which are known to have effector function on tissue damage, exhibited its highest expression 1 week later. This finding suggests that the macrophage play important

102

roles as the effector cells in allograft cornea desctruction.

The immunosuppressive efects of FK506 and CsA persited even after the cessation of drug administration. Previous study has demonstrated that FK506 has much higher potency of immunosuppression than CsA in experimental transplantation[7]. Similarly, the present study demonstrated that FK506 exhibited the immunosuppressive effect at a dose 1/10 of the CsA.

The present experimental model is useful for recognizing the cell lineages that are involved in the rejection process and for understanding of the role of immunosuppressant treatments. Further studies should performed to clarify the functional aspects of cells involved in the rejected cornea.

REFERENCES
1.   Council on Scientific Affairs (1988): Report of the Organ Transplant Panel; Corneal Transplantation. JAMA 259: 719-722.
2.   Herbort C, Matsubara M, Nishi M, Mochizuki M (1989): Penetrating Keratoplasty in the rat: A Model for the study of Immunosuppressive treatments on Graft Rejection.   Jpn J Ophthalmol 33(2): 212-220.
3.   Hsu SM, Raine L, Fanger H (1981): A Comparative study of the Peroxidase-Anti-Peroxidase Method and an Avidin-Biotin-Complex Method for Studing Polypeptide Hormones with Radioimmunoassay Antibodies. Am J Clin Pathol 75: 734-738.
4.   Osawa H and Diamantstein (1983): The characteristics of a Monoclonal Antibody that binds specifically to Rat T Lymphoblasts and inhibits IL 2 Receptor functions. J Immunol 30(1): 51-55.
5.   Pepose JS, Nestor KM, Gardner KM, Foos RY, Pettit TH (1985): Composition of cellular infiltrates in rejected human corneal allografts. Graefe's Arch Clin Exp Ophthalmol 222: 128-133.
6.   Chistmas SE, Macpherson GG (1982): The role of mononuclear phagocytes in cardiac allograft rejection in the rat. II. Characterization of Mononuclear Phagocytes Extracted from Rat Cardiac Allografts. Cell Immunol 69: 271-80.
7.   Ochiai T, Nakajima K, Nagata M, Suzuki T, Asano T, Uematsu T, Goto T, Hori S, Kenmochi T, Nakagori T, and Isono K (1987): Effects of a New Immunosuppressive Agent , FK506, on Heterothopic Cardiac Allotransplantation in the Rat. Transplant Proc 19: 1284-86.

© 1990 Elsevier Science Publishers (Biomedical Division)
Ocular Immunology Today. M. Usui, S. Ohno and K. Aoki, editors.

PROLONGATION OF RABBIT CORNEAL GRAFT SURVIVAL FOLLOWING SYSTEMIC ADMINISTRATION OF UROCANIC ACID

KA WILLIAMS, D LUBECK, FP NOONAN* and DJ COSTER

Department of Ophthalmology, Flinders University of South Australia, Flinders Medical Centre, Bedford Park, SA 5042, Australia and *Department of Dermatology, GWU Medical Centre, Ross Hall, 2300 I Street NW, Washington DC 20037 USA

INTRODUCTION

Ultraviolet (UV) radiation has profound effects on the immune system, including the generation of a state of transient systemic immune suppression (1). The mechanisms involved remain uncertain, but treatment of rodents with UV-B radiation has been shown to generate T suppressor cells and to depress antigen-presenting cell function (2,3). The target photoreceptor for UV radiation in the epidermis has variously been suggested to be urocanic acid (deaminated histidine), present in mammalian stratum corneum (4,5), or (in marsupials) the pyrimidine dimer of DNA(6).

Under some circumstances, UV irradiation can modulate the immune response to a graft (7). Direct UV irradiation, prior to graft, has been shown to prolong the survival of heterotopic mouse corneal allografts (8). Further, modest prolongation of orthotopic rabbit corneal allograft survival can be achieved by UV irradiation of either host and donor (9) or donor alone (10). We were interested to determine whether urocanic acid (UCA) would also prolong rabbit corneal allograft survival.

MATERIALS AND METHODS

Animals

Adult female New Zealand White rabbits were used as recipients of corneal grafts from adult female coloured strain donors to minimize chance histocompatibility. Animals were allowed unlimited access to water and rabbit chow and were caged individually under a twelve-hour light-dark illumination cycle.

Corneal transplantation

High risk model. Recipient rabbit corneas were vascularized and anterior segment inflammation induced prior to transplantation, to mimic the situation occurring in patients with a history of anterior segment inflammation and/or evidence of corneal neovascularization at graft. Such patients have a greater chance of rejecting a corneal graft than do patients without these risk factors (11). Five interrupted 8-0 braided silk sutures were inserted into the cornea under general anaesthetic, several weeks before transplantation. Suture ends were cut short but the knots were deliberately left exposed. The degree of neovascularization was scored regularly at the slit-lamp. Vessel growth into each of four quadrants was assessed on a scale of 0-4, with 0 being little growth, 1 being a leash extending at least one-quarter of the way from limbus to central cornea, 2 being growth at least half-way to the centre, 3 being growth three-quarters of the way in and 4 being a vessel leash extending from the limbus to the central cornea. Scores for each quadrant of a cornea were summed and a rabbit was grafted when the sum was greater than or equal to 8. Experimental groups were made as similar as possible with respect to the degree of vascularization of individual animals. Once the cornea was suitably vascularized and was inflamed, the sutures were removed under local anaesthetic and the animal grafted.

Post-operative assessment. Animals were examined daily at the slit-lamp. Topic 1% atropine sulphate and 0.5% chloramphenicol were applied once daily for 14 days, at which time the graft sutures were removed under local anaesthesia. Grafts were scored daily for the degree of graft clarity, oedema, fibrin and cells in the anterior chamber, graft neovascularization and inflammation, and for signs of rejection.

Diagnosis of rejection. The day of rejection was diagnosed as the first day on which an epithelial and/or an endothelial rejection line was observed, or the first day on which spreading stromal oedema was present (in the absence of a line) in a graft which previously had been clear and thin. Animals which reached 100 days post-graft without signs of rejection were deemed to be long-survivors. Animals with rejected grafts or long-surviving grafts were killed and the cornea removed for end-point histology.

Urocanic acid

Urocanic acid (4 imidazoleacrylic acid) was obtained from the Sigma Chemical Company (cat. no. U7500, St Louis, MO, USA) and was stored dessicated at 4°C, shielded from light.

Preparation of isomers. A solution of mixed cis and trans isomers of UCA was prepared from the trans material by UV irradiation of the latter. UV irradiation was accomplished using a bank of Westinghouse FS40 sunlamps, emitting broad-band UV radiation with a peak at 313 nm (in the UV-B range). The dose-rate, measured with a UVX radiometer and a UVX-31 sensor (Ultraviolet Products Inc, San Gabriel, CA, USA), was 15 $J/m^2/s$. Trans-UCA was prepared by dissolving the powder to 4 mg/ml in 10% v/v dimethyl sulphoxide in normal saline (12). This solution was split into two. Half was exposed to the FS40 sunlamps for two hours at room temperature, in shallow containers (1 cm deep). The total dose was 108 kJ/m^2. Evaporative losses were made good and the solution of mixed isomers passed through a 0.22 micron millipore filter. The remainder was treated identically, except that the solution was enveloped in aluminium foil during the irradiation procedure, so that isomerization would not occur. Both the trans-UCA and the mixed isomers solutions were aliquotted and stored frozen at -20°C, shielded from light. The composition of isomers in the two solutions, determined by HPLC analysis, was 100% trans-UCA (sham-irradiated) and 60:40% cis:trans-UCA (irradiated), respectively.

Experimental protocol

Animals were grafted in pairs, with one animals being given trans isomer (control) and the other being given mixed isomers (test). UCA was administered on two occasions to each animal: on day minus 3 with respect to the graft and on day 0, at a dose of 20 mg/kg by intraperitoneal injection. No further immunosuppressive treatment was given post-operatively.

Statistical analysis

Graft outcome in the experimental groups was analysed by comparing survival times, using the Mann-Whitney U-test, corrected for ties.

RESULTS

Graft outcome in the two experimental groups is shown in Table 1. The median time to rejection was prolonged in the animals given mixed isomers, compared with the controls, and there were more long survivors in the former group. The two groups differ significantly at the 5% level ($p < 0.05$, two-tailed).

TABLE 1

CORNEAL GRAFT OUTCOME IN RABBITS GIVEN UCA ISOMERS

Group	No.	Day of Rejection	Median
Trans-UCA	21	14 14 14 14 16 15 17 17 17 20 20 20 22 23 24 30 >100 >100 >100 >100 >100	20
Cis-UCA and trans-UCA (60:40)	19	12 15 16 17 18 19 30 38 40 48 >100 >100 >100 >100 >100 >100 >100 >100 >100	48

No ill effects were attributable to the administration of UCA, despite the relatively large volume of the intraperitoneal injections (20 ml for a 4 kg rabbit). Furthermore, end-point histology on all grafted corneas was unremarkable.

DISCUSSION

Our data indicate that systemic administration of mixed isomers of urocanic acid (containing predominantly the cis isomer) to rabbits, can produce a modest but significant prolongation of corneal graft survival. The regimen used was similar to those previously shown to suppress delayed-type hypersensitivity in the mouse (5, 12) but not otherwise optimized for the rabbit. No toxicity was evident, but it should be stressed that the experimental animals were not followed for more than four months. Reeve and her colleagues have recently demonstrated that topical cis-urocanic acid can enhance the early survival of UV-initiated tumours in hairless mice and have noted that urocanic acid shows some structural similarities to azathioprine (13). Urocanic acid may thus warrant further examination as a potentially useful immunosuppressive drug.

ACKNOWLEDGEMENTS

We acknowledge the support of the NH&MRC and the ORIA. KAW was supported by the Wellcome Trust. We thank Susan Rosewarne for expert secretarial assistance and Graham Aldous for kindly performing the HPLC analyses.

REFERENCES

1.   Kripke ML (1984) Immunol Rev 80:87

2.   Fisher MS, Kripke ML (1978) J Immunol 121:1139

3.   Greene MI, Sy MS, Kripke ML, Benacerraf B (1979) Proc Natl Acad Sci (USA) 76:6592

4.   De Fabo EC, Noonan FP (1983) J Exp Med 158:84

5.   Noonan FP, De Fabo EC, Morrison H (1988) 90:92

6.   Applegate LA, Ley RD, Alcalay J, Kripke ML (1989) 170:1117

7.   Deeg HJ (1988) Transplantation 45:845

8   Ray-Kiel L, Chandler JW (1986) Transplantation 42:403

9.   Williams KA, Ash JK, Mann TS, Noonan FP, Coster DJ (1987) Transplant Proc 19:2889

10.   Young E, Olkowski ST, Dana M, Mallete RA, Stark WJ (1989) Transplant Proc 21:3145

11.   Coster DJ (1989) Eye 3:251

12.   Ross JA, Howie SEM, Norval M, Maingay J, Simpson TJ (1986) 87:630

13.   Reeve VE, Greenoak GE, Canfield PJ, Boehm-Wilcox C, Gallagher CH (1989) Photochem Photobiol 49:459.

© 1990 Elsevier Science Publishers (Biomedical Division)
Ocular Immunology Today. M. Usui, S. Ohno and K. Aoki, editors.

LOCAL INJECTION OF MONOCLONAL ANTIBODIES INTO THE ANTERIOR CHAMBER OF RABBITS WITH CORNEAL GRAFT REJECTION

KA WILLIAMS and DJ COSTER

Department of Ophthalmology, Flinders University of South Australia, Flinders Medical Centre, Bedford Park, SA 5042, Australia

INTRODUCTION

The use of antibody as an immunosuppressant for experimental corneal transplantation is not new. Systemically-administered anti-lymphocyte serum (ALS) or globulin (ALG) can prolong rabbit corneal graft survival (1,2,3), although rejection tends to occur once treatment is stopped (3). Antibody given topically or by subconjunctival injection, in contrast, has essentially no immunosuppressive effect (4,3,5). Recent reports (6,7) have suggested that local injection of one or more mouse anti-human T cell monoclonal antibodies into the anterior chambers of patients with ongoing corneal graft rejection, can favourably modify the course of these rejection episodes, although the long-term efficacy of the monoclonal antibody therapy was difficult to assess because systemic steroids were subsequently administered. We were interested to determine whether local injection of monoclonal antibody could reverse rabbit corneal graft rejection, in the absence of any other immunosuppression.

MATERIALS AND METHODS

Animals

Adult female New Zealand White rabbits were used as recipients of corneal grafts from adult female coloured strain donors. Animals were allowed unrestricted access to water and rabbit chow.

Corneal transplantation

Graft. Eight mm diameter penetrating corneal grafts were inserted into prevascularized, inflamed eyes, using a running 10-0 nylon suture. Vascularization and inflammation were induced in the recipient eye as described in a companion paper in this volume.

Post-operative assessment. Rabbits were examined daily at the slit-lamp. Topical 1% atropine sulphate and 0.5% chloramphenicol were applied daily to the graft for the first 14 days, at which time the graft suture was removed under local anaesthetic. Grafts were scored each day for the degree of graft clarity, oedema, presence of cells and fibrin in the anterior chamber, neovascularization of the graft, anterior segment inflammation and signs of corneal graft rejection. Animals were generally followed for 100 days following transplantation, at which time the rabbit was killed and the graft taken for end-point histology.

Diagnosis of rejection. The day of rejection was defined as the first day that an epithelial or endothelial rejection line (or both) was observed in a previously thin, clear graft. Forewarning of impending rejection was usually given by a slight kick-up of inflammation in the anterior segment in the 24 hours preceding the appearance of the rejection line.

Monoclonal antibodies

Four mouse anti-rabbit monoclonal antibodies were used: L11/135, an IgG1 antibody detecting a 120 kd glycoprotein determinant present on thymocytes, peripheral T cells and on some neutrophils and monocytes (8); LION 2, an IgM antibody detecting a myeloid antigen present on rabbit neutrophils, platelets and 65% of monocytes; LION 3A, an IgM antibody detecting a subset of rabbit lymphocytes (35% of spleen lymphocytes and 45% of peripheral blood lymphocytes, PBL); and LION 4, an IgG1 antibody detecting rabbit platelets. The hybridoma producing L11/135 was obtained from the American Type Culture Collection (Rockville, MD USA; catalogue no. TIB 188). The hybridomas producing LION 2, 3A and 4 were produced by fusion of mouse spleen cells (prepared from BALB/c mice immunized with rabbit leucocytes), with the aminopterin-sensitive mouse myeloma line P3-X63-Ag8.653, using standard methods (9). The lines were cloned twice by limiting dilution.

Preparation of antibodies for injection. Hybridoma culture supernatants were dialysed extensively against Dulbecco's A phosphate buffered saline and filter-sterilised by passage through a 0.22 micron membrane. They were then re-tested for activity by indirect immunofluorescence assays on rabbit peripheral blood leucocytes, aliquotted and stored frozen at -20°C.

Administration of monoclonal antibodies. On the first day that a rejection line was observed at the slit-lamp, the animal was anaesthetised. Under the operating microscope, a limbal paracentesis was made using a 27 gauge needle attached to a tuberculin syringe, and approximately 100 microlitres of anterior chamber fluid was withdrawn. Using the same paracentesis, 100 microlitres of monoclonal antibody was injected into the anterior chamber. A further 50 microlitres was used to saturate the tear film. Chloramphenicol ointment 1% was then applied to the graft. The procedure was repeated three to four days later. No other immunosuppression was given and the animals continued to be examined daily at the slit-lamp by an observer who was unaware of the identity of the monoclonal antibody given.

RESULTS

The effect of monoclonal antibody injection on rejection was categorised in one of three ways: firstly, no observable effect, with rejection proceeding in the usual way until the graft was thick and opaque; secondly, apparent reversal of rejection as evinced by the temporary disappearance of the rejection line (and in several instances, a reduction in anterior segment inflammation) but later recurrence of the line, followed by thickening and opacification of the graft; and finally, longer term reversal of rejection, marked by disappearance of the rejection line with a gradual reduction in inflammation and a slow settling down of the graft until it appeared clear and thin with no further signs of rejection to at least 100 days after graft. The graft outcome in each of the four experimental groups is shown in Table 1.

TABLE 1
EFFECT OF LOCAL ADMINISTRATION OF MONOCLONAL ANTIBODY ON ONGOING CORNEAL GRAFT REJECTION EPISODES IN THE RABBIT

Antibody	Specificity	No.	Nil	Effect on Rejection Reversal, Re-rejection	Reversal
LION 2	anti-myeloid	6	5	1	0
LION 3A	anti-PBL subset	6	6	0	0
LION 4	anti-platelet	6	5	1	0
L11/135	anti-T cell	14	7	3	4

Three of the antibodies, LION 2, 3A and 4, had no lasting effect on rejection, although it was interesting that the rejection line was reported to disappear temporarily in two instances. Only L11/135 was able to induce what appeared to be reversal of corneal graft rejection, in 4/14 cases.

In the four animals in which rejection was reversed, there were two cases of epithelial rejection, one case of endothelial rejection and one case of mixed epithelial and endothelial rejection, a not unusual pattern of rejection lines in this model. Vessel leashes within the graft regressed in three of the four cases; the fourth graft remained heavily vascularized. The grafts took 14, 26, 39 and 53 days following the second injection of antibody to become completely clear, thin and quiet. Closer inspection of the records in these four animals showed that rejection first occurred at days 26, 27, 31 and 31 post-graft, compared with rejection occurring at a median of day 18.5 in the cohort as a whole, suggesting that these animals were not representative of the total pool of rabbits.

Administration of antibody into the anterior chamber was tolerated surprisingly well, considering that purified antibody was not used. No cases of sympathetic ophthalmia were observed. However, a substantial fibrinous reaction was noted in the anterior chamber of the grafted eye in 16/32 animals during the 48 hours following injection of antibody. Such a response is occasionally seen during

110

unmodified rejection in this model, but is nonetheless rare. A sterile hypopyon developed in two animals but quickly cleared.

DISCUSSION

Administration of the monoclonal antibody L11/135 into the anterior chamber of rabbits with ongoing corneal graft rejection was able to reverse rejection in a small number of animals, in the absence of other, intercurrent immunosuppression. Interestingly, disappearance of the rejection line did not necessarily signal reversal of rejection, which tended to be a somewhat drawn-out process. Antibodies against other, extraneous cell-surface antigens were ineffective.

Our data indicate that local injection of L11/135 is not a panacea for the treatment of rejection, in that relatively few animals responded, and those that did respond appeared to be a subgroup in which rejection was in any event delayed. On the other hand, no attempt was made to inject purified antibody into our animals and more animals may have responded, had more antibody been given. We conclude that there may be a place for local administration of anti-T cell monoclonal antibodies in the treatment of corneal graft rejection, but the procedure is not without risk.

ACKNOWLEDGEMENTS

Supported by the NH&MRC and the ORIA. KAW was supported by the Wellcome Trust. We thank Susan Erickson for technical assistance and Susan Rosewarne for preparing the manuscript.

REFERENCES
1. Smolin G (1968) Arch Ophth 79:603

2. Waltman SR, Faulkner HW, Burde RM (1969) Invest Ophthalmol 8:196

3. Polack FM, Townsend WM, Waltman S (1972) Am J Ophth 73:52

4. Smolin G (1969) Am J Ophth 67:137

5. Shirao E, Deschênes J, Char DH (1986) Current Eye Res 5:817

6. Ippoliti G, Fronterrè A (1987) Transplant Proc 19:2579

7. Ippoliti G, Fronterrè A (1989) Transplant Proc 21:3133

8. Jackson S, Chused TM, Wilkinson JM, Leiserson WM, Kindt TJ (1982) J Exp Med 157:34

9. Köhler G, Milstein C (1975) Nature 256:495.

© 1990 Elsevier Science Publishers (Biomedical Division)
Ocular Immunology Today. M. Usui, S. Ohno and K. Aoki, editors.

ROLE OF ANTIBODY IN PREVENTION OF HERPES SIMPLEX STROMAL KERATITIS

C. STEPHEN FOSTER, M.D., THOMAS M. IHLEY, B.S., RAMZI HEMADY, M.D., RICHARD R. TAMESIS, M.D., BEVERLY A. RICE, B.A., AND PETER A. WELLS, PH.D.. From the Hilles Immunology Laboratory, Harvard Medical School, Massachusetts Eye and Ear Infirmary, Boston, MA.

INTRODUCTION

The possible role the humoral response may have in preventing destructive inflammation in the eye after ocular encounter with HSV-1 is relatively under-investigated. Metcalf (1) demonstrates the efficacy of monoclonal AB (antibody) recognizing HSV-1 specific glycoproteins, in preventing HSK development. We have shown that subcutaneous immunization with active HSV (2), u.v. inactivated HSV (3), HSV glycoprotein D (4), or with a defined peptide sequence from one of the epitopes of glycoprotein D (5) provides protection against HSK following corneal inoculation with HSV-1. We have also shown that passive transfer of anti-HSV AB can confer pronounced protection from HSK (6). To further investigate the role of AB in HSK we used mu chain specific AB's to deplete IgM bearing B-cells from C.B-17 mice, which are normally resistant to development of HSK. Mice so treated uniformly developed severe HSK. In addition, anti-HSV-1 AB transfer techniques were performed in HSK susceptible, athymic, immune T-cell adoptively-enriched Balb/c mice. These AB treated mice, in contrast to their immune T-cell adoptively-enriched littermates not receiving AB, were completely protected from destructive stromal HSK.

EXPERIMENTAL DESIGN

To investigate the possible role of AB in HSK protection we exploited previous findings which demonstrated HSK resistance in C.B-17 mice. These mice express the Igh-1^b gene which encodes for products that are correlated with HSK protection. Neonatal C.B-17 mice were thus treated with mu chain specific AB's daily for the first week of life and then administered 3 times weekly for the remainder of the experiment.

Corneal inoculation was performed at 5 weeks of age. The right cornea of these anti-mu treated and untreated mice were needle scarified and HSV-1 strain KOS was applied topically. HSK severity and incidence was monitered on various days post corneal challenge. HSK severity was then graded on a 0 to 4+ scale and disease patterns were compared between anti-mu treated and untreated (control) groups of C.B-17 mice.

Individual serum samples were collected from anti-mu treated and untreated mice on various days post corneal challenge. The HSV-1 specific AB titers were then determined utilizing an Indirect ELISA technique. Monitorization of HSV-1 specific humoral and cellular mechanisms were observed by measuring HSV-1 AB titers, DTH and CTL responses in the anti-mu treated and untreated groups of C.B-17 mice.

In addition to the B-cell depletion experiment a passive AB transfer experiment was performed. HSV-1 AB transfer techniques were employed in HSK susceptible, athymic, immune T-cell adoptively-enriched Balb/c mice which were corneally challenged with HSV-1. HSK was graded as described above, and disease patterns were compared between the T-cell reconstituted mice receiving anti-HSV serum and that group which did not.

RESULTS

<u>Keratopathy</u> The incidence of early HSK development after corneal inoculation (Table 1) was significantly different between anti-mu treated and untreated C.B-17 mice (p< 0.0001) on day 11 post corneal challenge. In addition to this striking difference in keratopathy incidence, Figure 1 demonstrates that there was also a marked difference in HSK severity between treated and untreated mice. By day 18 post corneal inoculation all anti-mu treated mice had developed a severe (4$^+$) stromal infiltrate; and all were accompanied by corneal ulceration and perforation. In contrast, only three of 10 mice in the untreated group developed HSK; none perforated and only one reached severe (4$^+$) keratopathy by day 18 post corneal challenge.

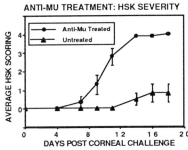

Figure 1. Graph demonstrating the difference in mean HSK scores between both treated and untreated groups at different times post HSV-1 corneal challenge.

Table 1. Incidence of stromal keratitis (1^+ or >) in C.B-17 mice (anti-mu treated and untreated) on various days post corneal challenge.

Group	Days post corneal challenge						e
	4	7	9	11	15	17	18
Anti-mu treated	0/10	2/10	5/10	9/10	10/10	10/10	10/10
Untreated	0/10	0/10	0/10	0/10	2/10	3/10	3/10
P values	---	---	---	<.0001	---	---	<.001

<u>HSV-1 AB Titers</u> Figure 2 illustrates the effectiveness of anti-mu treatment on B-cell depletion as documented by an impaired ability of anti-mu treated C.B-17 mice to produce HSV-1 specific AB after HSV-1 corneal inoculation. Antibody titers were as much as 10^2 times greater for untreated C.B-17 mice compared with anti-mu treated ones on days 14 and 18 post corneal challenge as documented by indirect ELISA technique. Complete inhibition of HSV-1 specific AB production was induced in 44% of the anti-mu treated mice on day 18 (Table 2).

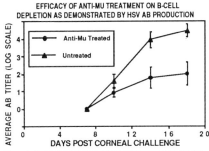

Figure 2. Comparison of mean HSV-1 AB titers between treated and untreated groups on four different days post corneal challenge.

Table 2. Incidence of C.B-17 mice (anti-mu treated and untreated) exhibiting detectable (>1/12.5) HSV-AB titers on various days post corneal challenge.

Group	Days post corneal challenge			e
	7	10	14	18
Anti-mu treated	0/10	2/9	5/9	5/9
Untreated	0/10	7/10	10/10	10/10

<u>DTH and CTL Responses</u> The HSV-1 specific DTH responses in immunized C.B-17 mice (anti-mu treated and untreated) were strikingly greater than in unimmunized (control) mice of the same murine strain (Figure 3). The DTH indices were, however, quite similar between anti-mu treated and untreated groups. HSV-1 specific CTL responses were also quite similar when comparing anti-mu treated and untreated groups of C.B-17 mice (Figure 4). These results are important since it has been suggested that B-cell depletion may induce T-cell mediated enhancement (8) and T-cells (helper-inducer and cytotoxic) have been implicated in HSK pathogenesis (9-11). These results demonstrate that anti-mu induced HSK enhancement is independent of any compromization (i.e. enhancement of) in T-cell mediated DTH and CTL responses.

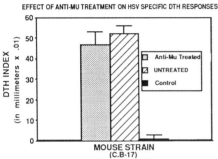

Figure 3. Graph demonstrating similar DTH responses between treated and untreated groups. T bars denote S.E.M..

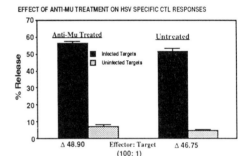

Figure 4. Graph demonstrating similar CTL responses between treated and untreated groups. T bars denote S.E.M..

<u>T-cell and AB Transfers</u> Athymic mice of Balb/c origin inoculated with HSV-1 did not develop HSK (data not shown). When HSV-1 immune T-cells were adoptively transferred from appropriate donor mice to athymic Balb/c mice which were then corneally challenged with HSV-1; keratopathy developed (Figure 5) and attained levels consistent with those seen in normal (thymus+) Balb/c mice. These findings confirmed previous reports that T-cells are essential participants in HSK development (9). Passive transfer of HSV-1 specific AB prior to and after corneal challenge abrogated this phenomenon (Figure 5).

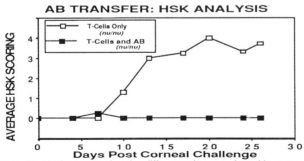

Figure 5. Graph demonstrating the difference in mean keratitis scores between the T-cell reconstituted athymic mice receiving anti-HSV serum and that group which did not.

DISCUSSION

Recurrent herpes simplex keratitis is a major contributor to the production of morbidity from corneal blindness around the world. This blindness results from loss of corneal clarity, secondary to the damage produced by the individual's immune/inflammatory response to HSV-1 encounter. An important goal, therefore, is to better understand the immunologic details of the cornea after ocular HSV-1 encounter in the hope of minimizing corneal damage.

One of the immunologic details which has been under-investigated is HSV-1 antibody. Our original effort (6) in this area disclosed the profound protection conferred upon ordinarily HSK susceptible mice by adoptively transferred anti-HSV immunoglobulins; similarly, the passive antibody transfer studies in nude mice reported herein confirm the efficacy of anti-HSV serum in providing protection against necrotizing stromal keratitis.

We also exhibit further evidence that anti-HSV antibody is an extremely important ingredient to the immunlogic recipe for protection against HSK through HSV-1 AB depletion methods. Treatment with anti-mu serum enhanced HSK and decreased anti-HSV-1 AB titers in HSV-1 corneally inoculated C.B-17 mice. These results coupled with those in athymic mice suggest that anti-HSV-1 AB not only can provide protection against destructive inflammation of the cornea after HSV-1 corneal challenge but is also a critical element for protection in mice which typically enjoy an innate resistance to HSK.

REFERENCES
1. Metcalf JF, Chatterjee S, Koga J, and Whitley RJ (1988) Protection against herpetic ocular disease by immunotherapy with monoclonal antibodies to herpes simplex virus glycoproteins. Intervirology 29(1):39.
2. Sandstrom IK, Foster CS, Wells PA, Knipe D, Caron L, and Greene MI (1986) Previous immunization of mice with herpes simplex virus type-1 strain MP protects against secondary corneal infection. Clin Immunol Immunopathol 40:326.
3. Thompson P, Wells PA, Sandstrom IK, Opremcak EM, Millin JA, Daigle JA, and Foster CS (1988) Immunomodulation of experimental murine herpes simplex keratitis: I. UV-HSV protection. Curr Eye Res 7:1043.
4. Foster CS, Sandstrom IK, Wells PA, Thompson P, Daigle J and Opremcak EM (1988) Immunomodulation of experimental murine herpes simplex keratitis: II. Glycoprotein D protection. Curr Eye Res 7:1051.
5. Wells PA, Ihley TM, and Foster CS (1988) Immunization with a synthetic HSV-1 glycoprotein D peptide protects mice from herpes simplex keratitis. ARVO abstracts. Invest Ophthalmol Vis Sci 29(suppl.):153.
6. Raizman MB, and Foster CS (1988) Passive transfer of anti-HSV-1 IgG protects against stromal keratitis in mice. Curr Eye Res 7:823.
7. Foster CS, Opremcak EM, Rice B, Wells P, Chung H, Thompson P, Fong LP, and Raizman M (1987) Clinical, pathologic, and immunopathologic characteristics of experimental murine herpes simplex virus stromal keratitis and uveitis is controlled by gene products from the Igh-1 locus on chromosome 12. Tr Am Ophth Soc 35:293.
8. Jordan C, Baron S, Dianzani F, Barber J, and Stanton GJ (1983) Ocular herpes simplex virus infection is diminished by depletion of B lymphocytes. J of Immunol 131:1554.
9. Russel RG, Naisse MP, Larsen LS and Rouse BT (1984) Role of T-lymphocytes in the pathogenesis of herpetic stromal keratitis. Invest Ophthalmol Vis Sci 25:938.
10. Newell CK, Martin S, Sendele D, Mercadal CM, and Rouse BT (1989) Herpes simplex virus induced stromal keratitis: role of T-lymphocyte subsets in immunopathology. J Virol 63:769.
11. Hendricks RL, Epstein RJ, and Tumpey T (1989) The effect of cellular immune tolerance to HSV-1 antigens on the immunopathology of HSV-1 keratitis. Invest Ophthalmol Vis Sci 30:105.

© 1990 Elsevier Science Publishers (Biomedical Division)
Ocular Immunology Today. M. Usui, S. Ohno and K. Aoki, editors.

ANTI-IDIOTYPIC VACCINATION AGAINST HSV-1 KERATITIS

T HOANG-XUAN, M.D., JC BAER, M.D., TM IHLEY, BA RICE, PA WELLS,
CS FOSTER, M.D.

Hilles Immunology Laboratory, Massachusetts Eye and Ear Infirmary, Harvard
Medical School, Boston, U.S.A.

INTRODUCTION

In 1963 Kunkel (1) and Oudin (2) independently described antibodies which bind
to antigenic determinants on the immunoglobin variable region (idiotypes, Id).
These molecules were called anti-idiotypic antibodies (anti-Id). Anti-Ids can be used
as vaccines if they represent the internal image of the viral antigen that served to
produce the immunoglobulin bearing the Id. Anti-idiotypic vaccination has already
been shown to induce protective immunity to various infectious diseases (3, 4). The
purpose of this study was to produce an anti-Id behaving like the mirror image of
HSV glycoprotein D (gD) which is known to protect mice from stromal keratitis after
corneal HSV-1 challenge (5). Passive immunization with anti-gD monoclonal
antibody with high *in vitro* virus neutralizing activity has also been shown to protect
mice against HSV keratitis (6, 7).

MATERIAL AND METHODS

Animals

BALB/c inbred female mice, 6-8 -week old, were obtained from Jackson
Laboratories, Bar Harbor, ME, and 4-5 pound N-Z white rabbits (NZW) were obtained
from Pine Acre Rabbitry, Norton, MA.. The use of animals in this investigation
conformed to NIH guidelines.

Virus

HSV-1, strain KOS, was obtained from Dr. David Knipe (Harvard Medical School,
Boston, MA) and was passed in Vero cells (ATCC, OCL 81) in our laboratory.

Production of anti-Id

Monoclonal anti-gD antibody (McAb) #4 was selected because of its high virus
neutralizing titer (>1/800). 300 µg of McAb #4 emulsified in same volume of
complete Freund's adjuvant (CFA) was injected subcutaneously (SC) in two NZW
rabbits. Three intramuscular boosts of 200 µg of monoclonal antibodies emulsified
in incomplete Freund's adjuvant (IFA) were performed every other week. Serum
was harvested from the marginal ear vein one week after the last boost.

Anti-idiotype purification

Rabbit serum was lipocleaned and absorbed by two passages over a CNBr Sepharose 4B column coupled with normal mouse sera. The effluent from the second passage was passaged over a second column coupled with normal mouse IgG until anti-normal mouse IgG antibodies had disappeared from the eluent. Effluent from this column was then passaged over a third column coupled with McAb#4. The anti-Id #4 was eluted with glycine pH 2.5, dialyzed against PBS, and concentrated.

Inhibition ELISA

We used the method described by Hampar et al. (8) with some modifications. Briefly, McAb#4 was incubated for one hour at 37°C with four-fold dilutions of either anti-Id #4 or rabbit preimmune IgG. The mixture was then added to 96-well flat-bottomed microtiter plates (Flow Labs) the wells of which had been coated with 0.2 µg of HSV-1 gD. Rabbit anti-mouse IgG-alkaline phosphatase conjugate (ICN Immunobiologicals) was used as secondary antibody. The substrate was p-nitrophenyl phosphate diluted in diethanolamine buffer (Kirkegaard and Perry Lab.). The reaction was stopped by 3M NaOH. The absorbance was read at 405 nm in a Titertek Multiscan spectrophotometer (Flow Laboratories). A preliminary checkerboard ELISA had determined the optimal concentrations of McAb #4 alone and secondary antibody (giving an absorbance of 1.0). to be used.

DTH study

Four groups of 8 BALB/c mice were immunized SC with live HSV-1 KOS strain (2.5 x 10^4 pfu), gD (3 µg), anti-Id #4 (6 µg), or rabbit preimmune IgG (6 µg). Anti-Id #4, rabbit preimmune IgG, and gD were emulsified in equal volume of CFA. Five days later, each mice received an intradermal injection of 50 µl of UV-inactivated HSV-1 (3×10^8 pfu/ml) into the right footpad. Footpad swelling was measured the following day with a micrometer, the left footpad serving as a control.

Keratitis study

Five groups of 6 BALB/c mice were immunized SC with live HSV-1 (2.5 x 10^4 pfu), gD (3 µg), rabbit preimmune IgG (6 µg), anti-Id#4 at two different doses (6µg and 12µg). A control group included 6 naive mice. Three SC boosts with half the original dose were given every other week. Corneal inoculation with KOS strain HSV-1 (1.75×10^4 pfu/ml) was performed one week after the last boost. Inoculation technique and grading system of the keratitis were detailed in a previous study (9).

RESULTS

Anti-Id #4 behaves like the mirror image of HSV gD

The inhibition ELISA showed that preincubation of anti-gD #4 with anti-Id #4 (at a concentration of 5 µg/ml) prevented anti-gD #4 from binding to gD (no absorbance), whereas preincubation with rabbit preimmune IgG did not. This signifies that anti-Id #4 binds to the same paratope of anti-gD #4 as gD does.

DTH study

Table 1 shows that immunization with anti-Id #4 is capable of inducing a DTH reaction to UV-inactivated HSV, similar to that produced by live HSV or gD.

TABLE 1

Immunizing agents	preimmune IgG	HSV	gD	anti-Id4
differential swelling R-L footpad (mm x 10^{-1})	3	21	0	8
	4	17	7	13
	7	8	7	7
	0	0	14	5
	5	26	0	5
	0	4	10	7
	6	8	13	10
	died	27	died	1
mean	3.57	13.87	7.28	7
standard deviation	2.55	9.61	5.23	3.35

Comparison of groups by Chi squared statistic:

	preimmune IgG	HSV	gD
anti-Id4	t=2.201 (p<0.05)	t=-1.911 (NS)	t=-1.300 (NS)

Active immunization with anti-Id #4 failed to protect mice against HSV keratitis
Figure 1

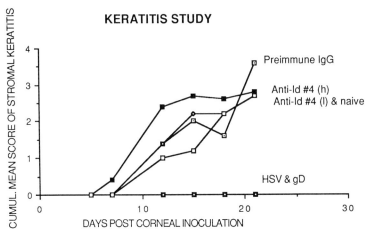

Immunization with either low-dose or high-dose anti-Id#4 did not protect against HSV keratitis when compared to the naive group and the preimmune IgG group (in these groups, 4/6 or more mice developed severe keratitis). Conversely, HSV and gD offered complete protection against HSV-1 keratitis.

DISCUSSION

Our results demonstrate that anti-Id #4 represents the "internal image" of gD as demonstrated by inhibition ELISA. We also showed that UV-inactivated HSV-1 induced a DTH response in anti-Id #4 -primed mice, similar to the response seen in HSV and gD-primed mice. Gell and Moss (10) found also that anti-Ids could mimic gD in eliciting DTH, and Lathey et al. (11) showed that immunization of mice with anti-Id to gD could prime splenocytes *in vivo* to proliferate in response to HSV antigen stimulation *in vitro*. However, active immunization with anti-Id #4 failed to protect mice against stromal keratitis following corneal HSV-1 inoculation. We expected more protection from anti-Id #4, since it was generated from McAb #4 which produces a high virus neutralizing titer. Actually Kennedy et al. (12) showed that anti-Ids to anti-HSV-2 McAbs shortened survival time of HSV-2 intraperitoneally-infected mice.

The reasons for the failure of anti-Id #4 to protect mice against keratitis are unclear. Subsequent experiments performed in our laboratory demonstrated that anti-Id #4 failed to induce virus neutralizing anti-anti-Id antibodies and cytotoxic activity against 3T3-infected target cells. Failure to induce virus neutralizing anti-anti-Id antibodies and/or generation of T-suppressor cells may play a significant role in the absence of protection against keratitis by the anti-Id.

REFERENCES

1- Kunkel HG, Mannick M, Williams RC (1963) Science 140:1218

2- Oudin J, Michel M (1963) C. R. Acad. Sci. (Paris) 257:805

3- Kennedy RC, Eichberg JW, Lanford RE, Dreesman GR (1986) Science, 232:220

4- Ertl HCJ, Homans E, Tournas S, Finberg RW (1984) J. Exp. Med. 159:1778

5- Foster CS, Sandstrom IK, Wells PA, Thompson P, Daigle J, Opremcak EM (1987) Current Eye Res. 7:1051

6- Metcalf JF, Koga J, Chatterjee S., Whitley R (1987) Current Eye Res. 6:173

7- Hoang-Xuan T, Wells PA, Raizman MB, Ihley TM, Foster CS (1988) Proc. ARVO Meeting, Invest. Ophthalmol. Vis. Sci., 29 Suppl.:152

8- Hampar B, Zweig M, Showalter SD, Bladen SV, Riggs CW (1985) J. Clin. Microbiol. 21:496

9- Thompson P, Wells PA, Sandstrom IK, Opremcak EM, Millin JA, Daigle J, Foster CS (1988) Curr. Eye Res. 7:1043

10- Gell GH and Moss PAH (1985) J. Gen. Virol. 66:1801

11- Lathey JL, Rouse BT, Wiley DE, Courtney RJ (1986) Immunology 57:29

12- Kennedy RC, Adler-Stortzh K, Burns JW, Henkel RD, Dreesman GR (1984) J.Virol. 50:951

© 1990 Elsevier Science Publishers (Biomedical Division)
Ocular Immunology Today. M. Usui, S. Ohno and K. Aoki, editors.

Igh-1 INFLUENCE ON DEVELOPMENT OF HSV-1 RETINITIS IN A MOUSE MODEL

RAMZI K. HEMADY, E. MITCHEL OPREMCAK, MANDI ZALTAS, JOE TAUBER,
C. STEPHEN FOSTER.
From the Hilles Immunology Laboratory, Massachusetts Eye and Ear
Infirmary, Harvard Medical School, Boston, MA.

INTRODUCTION

Inoculation of HSV-1 into the anterior chamber (AC) of susceptible mice results in a distinctive ocular disease pattern whereby the inoculated eye develops severe iridocyclitis and relative sparing of the retina, while the uninoculated contralateral eye develops necrotizing chorioretinitis (1). This model of HSV-1 retinitis is commonly referred to as the von-Szily model. We previously demonstrated a profound influence of the Igh-1 gene locus on development of the von-Szily model: 5% C.B-17 (Igh-1[b]) and 75% of BALB/c (Igh-1[a]) congenic mice developed contralateral retinal necrosis (2). We wished to determine the mechanism of Igh-1 influence on the development of the von-Szily model by studying the spread of HSV-1 to the uninoculated eye, systemic immune responses, and ocular immune cell populations, in the resistant C.B-17 and susceptible BALB/cByJ congenic mice. We also determined retinal pigment epithelial cell (RPE) permissivity to HSV-1 replication in vitro. The most pertinent results; virus isolation, neutralizing antibody levels, and delayed type hypersensitivity responses, are presented here.

MATERIALS AND METHODS

Under ether anesthesia, the right eyes of C.B-17 and BALB/cByJ mice (congenic mouse strains) were inoculated with 2.0×10^4 plaque forming units (PFU) of HSV-1. Ten days post inoculation (pi), mice were bled via the tail vein and serum was obtained and processed for virus neutralizing antibody (VNA) levels. The mice were then killed using ether overdose and the contralateral eyes were enucleated. Virus isolation by a standard plaque assay was performed on the enucleated eyes. In other mice, a footpad assay was used to asses delayed type hypersensitivity reactions (DTH) 5 or 10 days after HSV-1 challenge. These two time points were chosen in order to better understand the kinetics of DTH responses after AC challenge. Eight days pi, spleens were removed from additional mice and processed for lymphocyte proliferation assays (LPA) or cytotoxic T-lymphocyte assays (CTL). Permissivity of the RPE to HSV-1 was studied by incubating cultured

RPE cells with HSV-1 before washing. Samples were then assayed for infectious virus at different time intervals. All experiments were performed in duplicate or triplicate and conformed to the ARVO resolution on the use of animals in research.

RESULTS

Virus isolation . Ten days pi, HSV-1 was cultured from 5/7 (mean titer $2.7 \times 10^3 \pm 1.5 \times 10^3$ PFU) and 6/7 (mean titer $5.3 \times 10^3 \pm 1.3 \times 10^3$ PFU) contralateral, uninoculated eyes of C.B-17 and BALB/cByJ mice respectively. The difference between the means was not significant ($0.1 < p < 0.2$).

Virus neutralizing antibody. Neutralizing antibody levels were determined 10 days after inoculation with HSV-1 in the AC. Five mice of each mouse strain were used. Virus neutralizing antibody titers were higher in C.B-17 mice (mean titer 20.0 ± 3.0) than in BALB/cByJ mice (mean titer 12.5 ± 4.0). The difference between the means approached significance ($0.05 < p < 0.1$).

Suppression of delayed type hypersensitivity. Delayed type hypersensitivity responses and suppression of DTH responses were determined in C.B-17 and BALB/cByJ mice 5 or 10 days after HSV-1 challenge (8 - 14 mice were used in each group). Both mouse strains developed vigorous DTH responses 5 and 10 days after subcutaneous (SC) challenge (comparing the middle and bottom columns in figures 1 - 4). Simultaneous SC and AC inoculations with HSV-1 resulted in suppressed DTH responses in both mouse strains 5 days pi ($p \leq 0.005$ for either mouse strain) (comparing the middle and top columns in Figures 1 and 2). In contrast, DTH responses 10 days later were not suppressed in CB-17 mice ($p < 0.1$) (middle and top columns in figure 3) and were hyperactive in BALB/cByJ mice ($0.1 < p < 0.05$) (middle and top columns in figure 4).

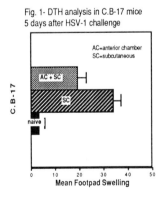

Fig. 1- DTH analysis in C.B-17 mice 5 days after HSV-1 challenge

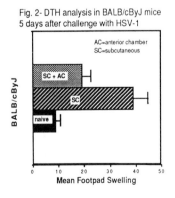

Fig. 2- DTH analysis in BALB/cByJ mice 5 days after challenge with HSV-1

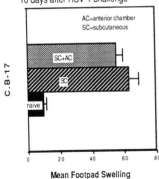

Fig. 3- DTH analysis in C.B-17 mice
10 days after HSV-1 challenge

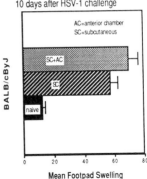

Fig. 4- DTH analysis in BALB/cByJ mice
10 days after HSV-1 challenge

DISCUSSION

The pathogenesis of contralateral retinitis in the von-Szily model is unclear. Some investigators believe that viral cytopathic effects play a dominant role while others attribute the destructive retinitis to a rampant immune response following viral infection.

Previous studies demonstrated two temporally distinct waves of virus reaching the uninoculated eyes of retinitis-susceptible BALB/c mice after uniocular HSV-1 inoculation (3). Our data demonstrate the ability of HSV-1 to spread to the contralateral normal eyes of C.B-17 mice in amounts equivilant to those achieved in the contralateral eyes of retinitis susceptible BALB/cByJ mice. We conclude, therefore, that the mere presence of replicating virus in uninoculated eyes is insufficient for the development of destructive retinitis in susceptible mice. Other investigators reached similar conclusions by demonstrating the presence of infectious virus in histologically intact contralateral eyes after ipsilateral inoculation of HSV-2 in BALB/c mice, or HSV-1 in athymic mice (4,5).

The role of DTH responses in the evolution of the von-Szily model is controversial. Some authors postulated that contralateral retinitis in susceptible mice was a function of suppressed HSV specific DTH responses; those mice that did not develop DTH suppression after AC inoculation were protected from retinitis (6,7). In addition, mice developed neither retinitis nor suppressed DTH responses after AC inoculation of HSV-2 (4). Others demonstrated that development of retinitis did not correlate with systemic immune responses, specifically suppressed DTH (8,9). We now demonstrate significantly suppressed DTH responses 5 days after AC inoculation in both congenic mouse strains. In contrast, BALB/cByJ mice demonstrated a reversal of DTH suppression ten days pi: vigorous DTH responses were measured. This might reflect a saturation of the DTH suppression capabilities of these mice secondary to intense viral immunogenicity or to destruction of the local ocular immunosuppressive mechanisms, and suggest a role for hyperactive DTH responses in the development of retinitis in susceptible mice.

The protective role of antibody in herpetic diseases of the eye remains underestimated. We previously demonstrated a protective effect of antibodies against herpes keratitis (10) and now demonstrate higher neutralizing antibody levels in resistant C.B-17 mice. Transfer of hyperimmune serum conferred (VNA titer dependant) protection from retinitis in BALB/c mice, and depletion of B-cells in C.B-17 mice neonatally rendered them retinitis susceptible (Hilles laboratory, unpublished data). These data suggest an important protective role for neutralizing antibody against HSV-1 retinitis in resistant mice even though neutralizing antibodies do not appear to prevent the spread of HSV to the contralateral eye.

ACKNOWLEDGEMENTS

Supported by the Fogarty International Program of the NIH (RKH), the Heed/Knapp Foundation (JT), and NIH grant EY06008 (CSF).

REFERENCES

1. Whittum JA, McCulley JP, Niederkorn JY, Streilein JW (1984) Invest Ophthalmol Vis Sci 25: 1065.
2. Opremcak EM, Foster CS, Hemady R, Rice BA, Daigle JA, Raizman MB, Chung H, Zaltas M (1989) Invest Ophthalmol Vis Sci 30: 1041.
3. Atherton SS, Streilein JW (1987) Invest Ophthalmol Vis Sci 28: 571.
4. Atherton SS, Streilein JW (1987) Curr Eye Res 6: 133.
5. Atherton SS, Altman NH, Streilein JW (1989) Curr Eye Res 8: 1179.
6. Kielty D, Cousins SW, Atherton SA (1987) Invest Ophthalmol Vis Sci 28: 1994.
7. Streilein JW, Atherton S, Vann V (1987) Curr Eye Res 6: 127.
8. Metzger EE, Whittum-Hudson JA (1987) Invest Ophthalmol Vis Sci 28: 1533.
9. Whittum-Hudson JA, Pepose JS (1988) Curr Eye Res 7: 125.
10. Raizman MB, Foster CS (1988) Curr Eye Res 7: 823.

© 1990 Elsevier Science Publishers (Biomedical Division)
Ocular Immunology Today. M. Usui, S. Ohno and K. Aoki, editors.

EXPERIMENTAL AUTOIMMUNE UVEITIS (EAU) IN THE MOUSE : H-2 RESTRICTION OF
EAU INDUCTION

KO IWASE[1], MUTSUHIKO MINAMI[2], IZUMI NAKASHIMA[3], YASUAKI FUJII[4], NOBUO
KATO[4] and MANABU MOCHIZUKI[5]
[1]Department of Ophthalmology and [2]Department of Blood Transfusion, School
of Medicine Tokyo University, [3]Department of Immunology and [4]Department of
Bacteriology, Nagoya University School of Medicine, and [5]Department of
Ophthalmology, Kurume University, School of Medicine.

INTRODUCTION

Experimental autoimmune uveitis (EAU) can be readily induced by
immunization with retinal specific antigens in the rat, the guinea pig and
the monkey. However, EAU was hardly induced in the mouse, which is the
most well-defined spieces for its immunogenetic background. We have
recently established a EAU model in the mouse(1).

It has been reported that genes within the major histocompatibility
complex (MHC) in the mouse control the susceptibility to various
autoimmune diseases, e.g. thyroiditis(2), encephalomyelitis(3), myasthenia
gravis(4), hemolytic anaemia(5) and diabetes(6). However, it has not been
determined which genes within MHC are important for the induction of EAU.
The present study was aimed at analysing the genetic control for the
induction of EAU using the mouse EAU model.

MATERIALS AND METHODS

Animals

Five strains of B10 congenic mice, B10.BR, B10.A, B10.A(4R), B10.MBR,
B10.A(5R) were used. Also, F1(B10.BR x C57BL/6), C57BL/6 and AKR/J were
used. The H-2 haplotype of the mice are summarized in Table 1. All mice
were purchased from Charles River Japan (Atsugi, Kanagawa, Japan). Mice
were used at their age of between 6 and 8 weeks old.

Antigen

S-antigen was prepared from fresh bovine retinas according to the method
of Dorey et al.(7).

Adjuvant

Klebsiella O3 lipopolysaccharide (KO3 LPS) was used as an adjuvant. KO3
LPS was prepared from Klebsiella pneumoniae strain LEN-1(O3:K1-) as
described previously(8).

Immunization

The best immunization protocol to induce EAU in the SMA mouse
demonstrated in our previous study(1) was used. The KO3 LPS was dissolved
in 0.01M phosphate buffered saline (PBS) and mixed with antigen solution
(1:1 v/v). The mixture containing 100 _g of KO3 LPS and 20 µg of S-
antigen was given by a subcutaneous injection at the inguinal region 4
times at intervals of 4 weeks.

Evaluation of EAU induction in mice

Animals were killed 3 weeks after the last immunization and all eyes
were examined histologically. Immediately after enucleation, eyes were
placed in 2.5% glutaraldehyde 2% formalin and fixed. Then, the eyes were
embedded in glycol methacrylate, cut at 3 µm and stained with hematoxylin
and eosin.

Evaluation of immune responses to S-antigen

Immediately after the sacrifice of mice, the blood and the spleen were
obtained. The antibody titers to S-antigen in the serum was measured by
the enzyme linked immunosorbent assay (ELISA), and proliferative responses
of lymphocytes to S-antigen were examined using nonadherent splenocytes,
as described previously(1). The proliferative responses were expressed as
a stimulation index (S.I., mean cpm in cultures with S-antigen (2
µg/ml)/mean cpm in cultures without S-antigen).

TABLE I

H-2 RESTRICTION OF EAU IN THE MOUSE

Strain	H-2 haplotype				Induction rate of EAU
	K	A	E	D	
B10. BR	k	k	k	k	10/12 (83.3%)
B10. A	k	k	k	d	7/10 (70.0%)
B10. A (4R)	k	k	b	b	7/11 (63.6%)
B10. MBR	b	k	k	a	4/7 (57.1%)
B10. A (5R)	b	b	k	d	0/11 (0.0%)
F$_1$ (B10. BR x C57BL/6)	k,b	k,b	k,b	k,b	13/19 (68.4%)
C57BL/6	b	b	b	b	2/8 (25.0%)
AKR/J	k	k	k	k	2/6 (33.3%)

(S-antigen; 20µg, 4 weeks interval, 4 times)

RESULTS

EAU susceptibility in various strains of mice

The evaluation for the development of EAU was determined by histopathological examination of the eyes. When histopathology of the eye exhibited cell infiltration in the intraocular tissue, particularly in the retina and the choroid, retinal vasculitis, and destruction of the photoreceptor cell layer, the eye was considered to develop EAU. Table 1 shows EAU susceptibility in various strains of mice used in this study. Among the five strains of B10 congenic mice, B10.A(5R) was not susceptible to EAU, whereas other 4 strains, B10.BR, B10.A, B10.A(4R) and B10.MBR, were highly susceptible. Also, C57BL/6 and AKR/J were considered to be low susceptible mice. However, F1(B10.BR x C57BL/6) was highly susceptible to EAU.

Immune responses to S-antigen

Table 2 summarized the antibody levels and the mitotic responses to S-antigen in each strains of mice. Antibody titers were similar in almost all strains of mice. There was no correlation between the antibody levels and the induction rates of EAU.

The proliferative responses to S-antigen as indicated by stimulation index were over 2.0 in all strains except for B10.A(5R), which exhibited no susceptibility to EAU.

DISCUSSION

It has been reported that genes within MHC influence the susceptibility to certain experimental autoimmune diseases in mice e.g. thyroiditis, encephalomyelitis, myasthenia gravis, hemolytic anaemia and diabetes. The

TABLE 2

IMMUNE RESPONSES TO S-ANTIGEN

Strain	Antibody* level	Proliferative responses of lymphocytes		
		None	S-antigen (2 μg/ml)	S.I.
B10. BR	1.59 ± 0.14	9829 ± 124**	28504 ± 5526**	2.90 ± 0.58
B10. A	1.39 ± 0.10	9376 ± 243	27471 ± 1312	2.93 ± 0.14
B10. A(4R)	1.61 ± 0.07	9124 ± 313	27007 ± 3740	2.96 ± 0.41
B10. MBR	1.22 ± 0.33	8754 ± 516	24423 ± 1925	2.79 ± 0.22
B10. A(5R)	1.21 ± 0.33	7321 ± 743	10322 ± 2562	1.41 ± 0.35
F1 (B10.BR x C57BL/6)	1.22 ± 0.22	9247 ± 354	25151 ± 2034	2.72 ± 0.22
C57BL/6	1.25 ± 0.08	8213 ± 943	18725 ± 328	2.28 ± 0.04
AKR/J	1.18 ± 0.13	8143 ± 754	16774 ± 3501	2.06 ± 0.43

* The values indicate OD values at 410 nm of a serum dilution at 1:320 ELISA assay (mean$\pm$SE)

** CPM (mean$\pm$SE)

data recorded here clearly demonstrated that genes within H-2 have significant role in controlling the susceptibility of EAU induction in the mouse. As demonstrated in Table 1, among the five strains of B10 congenics, all the high susceptible strains, B10.BR, B10.A, B10.A(4R), B10.MBR, are I-A^k, whereas B10.A(5R), which is non-susceptible strain, is I-A^b. It was, therefore, suggested that EAU susceptibility in the mouse is controlled by genes in I-A subregion. F1(B10.BR x C57BL/6) is also the high susceptible strain to EAU. This suggested that the high responder genes within H-2 are dominant. The H-2 haplotypes of the AKR/J mouse were exactly the same as those of B10.BR. And yet, the AKR/J mouse was low responder for EAU development while B10.BR mouse was high responder (Table 1). Therefore, non-MHC genes may have some role for the susceptibility to EAU.

Serum antibody titers showed similar levels in almost all tested strains of mice. There was no correlation between the antibody levels and the susceptibility to EAU (Table 2). The finding suggested the possibility of separate or additional genetic control of antibody production. In contrast, the proliferative responses of lymphocytes to S-antigen was paralleled with the disease susceptibility among the tested strains of mice (Table 2).

In conclusion, susceptibility for EAU induction in the mouse is under multigenic control. The susceptibility is regulated by genes in the I-A subregion of H-2 complex. Also, the non H-2 genetic background may play a certain role in influencing susceptibility to EAU.

CORRESPONDING AUTHOR

Manabu Mochizuki, MD., Department of Ophthalmology, Kurume University, School of Medicine, 67 Asahi-machi, Kurume, Fukuoka, JAPAN

REFERENCES
1. Iwase, K., Fujii, Y., Nakashima, I., Kato, N., Fujino, Y., Kawashima, H., and Mochizuki, M. Current Eye Research (in press).
2. Tomazic, V., Rose, N.R., and Shreffler, D.C. (1974) J. Immunology, 112: 965-969.
3. Bernard, C.C.A. (1976) J. Immunogenet., 3: 263-274.
4. Berman, P.W., and Patrick, J. (1980) J. Exp. Med., 152: 507-520.
5. Warner, N.L. (1973) Clin. Immunol. Immunopathol., 1: 353-363.
6. Kromann, H., Lernmark, A., Vestergaard, B.F., Egeberg, J., and Nerup, J. (1979) Diabetologia, 16: 107-114.
7. Dorey, C., Cozette, J., and Faure, J.P. (1982) Ophthalmic Res., 14: 249-255.
8. Ohta, M., Mori, M., Hasegawa, T., Nagase, F., Nakashima, I., and Kato, N. (1981) Microbial. Immunol. 25: 939-948.

© 1990 Elsevier Science Publishers (Biomedical Division)
Ocular Immunology Today. M. Usui, S. Ohno and K. Aoki, editors.

EXPERIMENTAL AUTOIMMUNE UVEORETINITIS (EAU) IN THE MOUSE MODEL

R. R. CASPI, C.C. CHAN, B. WIGGERT, G. J. CHADER AND R. B. NUSSENBLATT.
National Eye Institute, Bethesda, USA.

INTRODUCTION

A number of human posterior uveitic diseases of a putative autoimmune nature are characterized by a chronic, relapsing clinical course and tight HLA associations (1) . Experimental autoimmune uveoretinitis (EAU) in animals, induced by immunization with one of several ocular antigens in complete Freund's adjuvant (CFA), serves as a model for these conditions (2-4). Rodent models of EAU exist in the rat, guinea pig and rabbit, but none of these species fully reproduces the complete spectrum of human disease, and there is insufficient knowledge of their immunogenetics. EAU in nonhuman primates closely resembles the human disease, but immunogenetic analysis is again not feasible, due to the outbred nature of the species.

Recently, we have reported the development of a murine model of EAU , which is characterized by a focal pathology and a relatively chronic course (5). To further develop this promising model, we have concentrated our work on the quantitation of the uveitogenic response and on its dependence on immunogenetic parameters.

MATERIALS AND METHODS

Animals. Mice of various strains were purchased from commercial breeders or obtained from non-commercial sources, and used between 2 and 5 months of age (5). Animals were treated in accordance with the NIH Guidelines and the ARVO Resolution for Use of Animals in Research.

Retinal antigens. The retinal Soluble antigen (SAg) and the Interphotoreceptor retinoid binding protein (IRBP) were used. Antigens were purified from bovine retinas as described (6,7)

Immunization procedure. Animals were immunized by the split-dose protocol, or by the single-dose protocol, as previously described (5,8).

Evaluation of disease. Enucleated eyes were processed for histopathology as described (8). Incidence and severity of EAU were scored by an independent observer on a scale of 0 to 4, using a semiquantitative grading system (5). Fundoscopy was performed after pupil dilatation under systemic anesthesia, under a dissecting microscope.

RESULTS AND DISCUSSION

A large number of independent haplotypes, as well as H-2-recombinant and H-2 congenic strains, were screened for susceptibility to SAg- and IRBP-induced EAU, using the split-dose immunization protocol. The results indicated that the ability to mount a uveitogenic response is controlled by the major histocompatibility (H-2) complex (MHC). EAU was inducible in strains of the H-2^k haplotype (and their I-A-identical congenics) and in representative strains of the H-2^r and H-2^b haplotypes. Haplotypes which tested negative for EAU susceptibility were s, d, q, u, v and f (5, and Caspi, unpublished). IRBP was a more potent uveitogen than SAg under the immunization conditions used, with respect to the number of susceptible strains, as well as intensity of the resulting disease. Interestingly, susceptibility to the two uveitogens did not correlate. For example, the AKR strain appeared to be susceptible to SAg, but not to IRBP, while other strains of the same haplotype showed susceptibility to IRBP (5). The reason for this is unclear, but may imply the presence of extra-H-2 regulation of EAU in the mouse. Recent results obtained in H-2 congenic strains (see ahead) are in line with this interpretation. Lymphocyte and antibody responses to SAg and to IRBP were present in all the haplotypes which were tested for these parameters, and were not predictive of their ability to develop EAU (5).

In experiments using a series of H-2^k-based recombinant strains (5), we were able to tentatively map the control of EAU susceptibility to the I-A region of MHC class II, and to show that there is no requirement for I-E expression. This latter conclusion is based on the finding that the strain B10.S(8R), which carries a null allele at the E$_\alpha$ locus and consequently does not express the I-E gene product, is able to develop EAU (Table I). The possibility that I-E expression can have a quantitative influence on disease is currently being explored using additional class II recombinants and larger group sizes. We are not yet able to definitively exclude a possible participation of the MHC class I gene K^k, for lack of a suitable recombinant in the region between A$_\beta$ and K (5). This point is also being addressed in current experiments.

TABLE I

EAU SUSCEPTIBILITY DOES NOT REQUIRE EXPRESSION OF THE I-E GENE PRODUCT

Strain	H-2	(KA$_\beta$A$_\alpha$E$_\beta$E$_\alpha$SD)	EAU index ($\pm$SD)*
B10.A	a	(kkkkkdd)	1.8 ($\pm$ 1.1)
B10.S(8R)	as1	(kkkksss)	0.4 ($\pm$ 0.4)
B10.S(7R)	t2	(sssssd)	0

* Composite rating, combining EAU severity and incidence. Calculated as the average score of all animals (positive as well as negative) in a given group.
Animals (groups of 4) were immunized with IRBP by the split-dose protocol.

Recent data indicate that non-MHC genes may also contribute to the regulation of EAU. We compared the incidence and severity of disease in congenic strains sharing the same H-2 on a different background, to strains sharing the same background in the context of a different H-2. The results show that in susceptible strains, a permissive background such as B10 results in an enhanced expression of disease, while a non-permissive background results in a reduced expression of disease (Table II). However, the presence of a permissive background cannot overcome MHC-determined nonresponsiveness, since the B10.S(7R) strain is still a nonresponder to EAU (Table I). Susceptibility is inherited as a dominant or a co-dominant trait, as indicated by the finding that an F1 hybrid of susceptible x nonsusceptible haplotype (AKR x SJL) can develop disease (5).

TABLE II

NON-MHC GENES DETERMINE THE INTENSITY OF THE UVEITOGENIC RESPONSE TO IRBP IN EAU-SUSCEPTIBLE HAPLOTYPES

Strain	H-2	Background	EAU index ($\pm$SD)*
A	a	A	1.2 ($\pm$ 1.5)
B10.A	a	B10	2.6 ($\pm$ 1.2)
B10.RIII	r	B10	2.7 ($\pm$ 1.0)
LP.RIII	r	LP	0.6 ($\pm$ 0.9)

* See previous table for explanation.
 At least 16 animals were averaged for each group.

Dependence of disease induction on qualitative and quantitative parameters of immunization was studied in B10.A mice (I-A^k) immunized with IRBP in CFA (5,8). It was found that Bordetella pertussis adjuvant, as well as its mode of preparation, is of critical importance for disease induction. No disease was induced if the pertussis adjuvant was omitted. When the vaccine form of pertussis adjuvant was used, the minimal effective protocol for EAU induction consisted of pretreatment with cyclophosphamide, 100 µg of IRBP in complete Freund's adjuvant (CFA) divided into two weekly doses, and two doses of B. pertussis vaccine. Any reduction in this immunization scheme resulted in a drastically reduced incidence of disease. In contrast, substituting purified B. pertussis toxin (PTX) for the vaccine allowed reduction of the immunization protocol to a single dose of IRBP in CFA and omission of the cyclophosphamide pretreatment (8). Severity and incidence of disease, as well as its clinical course, could be quantitatively controlled by varying the respective doses of

130

IRBP and PTX. High-dose immunization induced an acute form of EAU, characterized by a rapid onset, short duration and widespread photoreceptor destruction, which was similar to the disease obtained in the Lewis rat. Low-dose immunization resulted in a milder, more chronic form of EAU, with a later onset, prolonged duration and focal photoreceptor damage, similar to the disease observed previously in the presence of pertussis vaccine (8,9). Kinetics experiments and long-term followup of individual animals by fundoscopy revealed that in the chronic (but not the acute) type of EAU the disease tends to relapse, with lesions reappearing after a brief period of essential quiescence (9,10). The time of recurrence may vary in individual experiments, and usually occurs between 8 and 12 weeks after immunization. The relapsing model of EAU should facilitate studies of therapeutic intervention in established disease, by better approximating the clinical situation.

The extensive knowledge of the immunological parameters of the mouse and the availability of genetically defined strains offers important advantages for the study of cellular mechanisms and immunogenetics of ocular autoimmune disease. Establishment of a single dose induction protocol and the quantitation of the immunopathogenic response as a function of the variables of immunization lay the foundation for the further development and utilization of the mouse model of ocular autoimmunity. The ability to control the clinical course of the disease by adjusting the intensity of the immunological stimulus, makes the mouse EAU a versatile model that can be adapted to the needs of the particular experimental system.

REFERENCES

1.   Nussenblatt RB, Palestine AG (1989) Year Book Medical Publishers, Inc.

2.   Faure JP (1980) Current Topics in Eye Res. 2:215-301

3.   Gery I, Mochizuki M, Nussenblatt RB (1986) Prog. Retinal Res. 5:75-109

4.   Caspi RR (1989) In: Immunology of Eye Disease (S.L. Lightman, Ed.), MTP Press Ltd., London. Ch. 5, pp. 61-86

5.   Caspi RR, Roberge FG, Chan CC, Wiggert B, Chader GJ, Rozenszajn LA, Lando Z, Nussenblatt RB (1988) J. Immunol. 140:1490-1495

6.   Dorey C, Cozette J, Faure JP (1982) Ophthalmic Res. 14:249-255

7.   Redmond TM, Wiggert B, Robey FA, Nguyen NY, Lewis MS, Lee L, Chader GJ (1985) Biochemistry 24:787-793

8.   Caspi RR, Chan CC, Leake WC, Higuchi M, Wiggert B, Chader GJ (1990) J. Autoimmun. (in press)

9.   Chan CC, Caspi RR, Ni M, Leake WC, Wiggert B, Chader GJ. Nussenblatt RB (1990) J. Autoimmun. (in press)

10.   Caspi RR, Chan CC, Wiggert B, Chader GJ (1990) Curr. Eye Res. (in press)

© 1990 Elsevier Science Publishers (Biomedical Division)
Ocular Immunology Today. M. Usui, S. Ohno and K. Aoki, editors.

EXPERIMENTAL AUTOIMMUNE UVEORETINITIS (EAU) INDUCED IN
NEONATAL THYMECTOMIZED A/J MICE WITH BOVINE S-ANTIGEN AND
INTERPHOTORECEPTOR RETINOID-BINDING PROTEIN (IRBP)

TAKAO TANAKA, M.D., NAOYUKI YAMAKAWA, Ph.D.,

TOSHIHIRO ICHIKAWA, M.D., MICHIKO HASEMI, Ph.D.,

OSAMU TAGUCHI, M.D*., MASAHIKO USUI, M.D.

Dept. of Ophthalmology, Tokyo Medical College Hospital,

6-7-1, Nishishinjuku, Shinjuku, Tokyo 160. (Japan)

*Aichi Cancer Center Research Institute, Chikusa-ku, Nagoya 464

(Japan)

INTRODUCTION

The distinctive features of neonatal thymectomized A/J mice have
already been reported[1]. Neonatal thymectomized A/J mice develop
autoimmune diseases, for example, oophoritis, orchitis, thyroiditis,
gastritis, and prostatitis. These diseases always develop
spontaneously. Investigators[2] have suspected that the diseases
might be caused by an inadequate lymphocyte population and
by lymphocyte recognition of autoantigen, brought about by neonatal
thymectomy. This report discusses the induction of experimental
autoimmune uveoretinitis (EAU) in neonatal thymectomized A/J mice
through inoculation with retinal S-antigen[3] and IRBP[4].

MATERIAL AND METHODS

I. Preparation of Thymectomized A/J Mice and Innoculation with a
Total of 60μg of S-antigen or 60μg of IRBP with Complete Freund's
Adjuvant.

Thymectomy was done on the 3rd day after birth.
When the mice became adults, between 2 months and 4 months of

age, mice were innoculated twice with 30µg of antigens with Complete Freund's Adjuvants (CFA, GIBCO, Grand Island, NY).
Eight thymectomized mice were immunized with S-antigen, and another eight with IRBP Others were used for control groups.

II. Determination of the Features of Pathology found by Microscopic Examination.

The progress of the consequent ocular inflammatory change was determined by microscopic examination.

RESULTS

Half of the thymectomized mice which were immunized with S-antigen developed EAU at an average of 27.0 days after the first immunization and half of thymectomized IRBP immunized mice also developed EAU at an average of 22.5 days after the first immunization. No disease was observed in the control groups (Table I).

TABLE I. INDUCTION OF THE DISEASE

Treatment	Antigen	Incidence	Days to Onset*
TX	S-Ag+CFA	4/8	27.0±5.78
	IRBP+CFA	4/8	22.5±5.51
	PBS+CFA	0/5	n.d.
	none	0/5	n.d.
NON-TX	S-Ag+CFA	0/6	n.d.
	IRBP+CFA	0/5	n.d.
	PBS+CFA	0/5	n.d.
	none	0/5	n.d.

* Mean ± Standard Deviation

Figure 1 shows some pathological features which developed in an IRBP immunized thymectomized mouse. Inflammatory cell infiltration of the iris , ciliary body and vitreous body was observed.

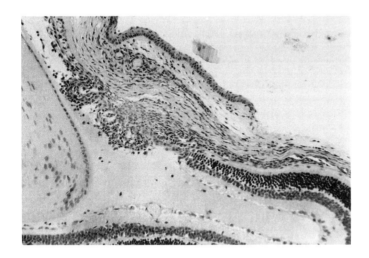

Fig.1. IRBP immunized thymectomized mouse. (X40)

Figure 2 shows the posterior portion of the eye of an S-antigen immunized thymectomized mouse. In this case, the main feature was retinal vasculitis.

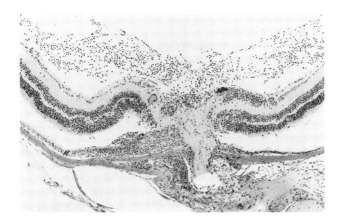

Fig. 2. S-antigen immunized thymectomized mouse. (X20)

134

DISCUSSION

Ordinal A/J mice were not susceptible to the induction of EAU through immunization with antigens. Yet, EAU could be induced when thymectomy was used as a pretreatment. Neonatal thymectomy might play a very important role in the induction of EAU. The day of thymectomy is critical for the induction of autoimmune diseases. Thymectomy at 3 days after birth is effective in eliminating the peripherization of autoreactive suppressor T-lymphocytes[2]. But, thymectomy at Day 0 and Day 7 is not effective. Therefore, it was considered that autoreactive T-lymphocytes which recognized S-antigen and IRBP might be activated by sensitization with retinal antigens. Therefore, neonatal thymectomy could alter the immune system to permit the induction of EAU.

REFFERENCES

1. Kojima A , Prehn RT (1981) Immunogenetics 14:15-27

2. Taguchi O , Nishizuka Y (1987) J. Exp. Med. 165:146-156

3. Wacker WB, Donoso LA, Kalsow CM,Yankeelov JA Jr, Organisciak DT (1977) J . Immunolo. 119 :1949-1958

4. Redmond TM, Wiggert B, Robey FA, Ngoyen NY, Lewis MS, Lee L, Chader GJ (1985) Biochemistry 24:787-793

© 1990 Elsevier Science Publishers (Biomedical Division)
Ocular Immunology Today. M. Usui, S. Ohno and K. Aoki, editors.

GENETIC CONTROL OF EXPERIMENTAL AUTOIMMUNE UVEITIS IN RATS: SEPARATION OF THE MHC AND NON-MHC GENE EFFECTS

SHIGETO HIROSE, YOICH SASAMOTO, KAZUMASA OGASAWARA*,
TAKASHI NATORI[†], KAZUNORI ONOE*, SHIGEAKI OHNO,
AND HIDEHIKO MATSUDA

Dept. of Ophthalmol. Hokkaido Univ. Sch. of Med, *Dept. of pathology, Inst.
of Immunol. Sci., Hokkaido Univ., Sapporo, †CIEA & Tokushima Res. Inst.,
Otsuca Pharma. Co., Ltd., Kawasaki, Japan.

INTRODUCTION

The differences of susceptibility to Experimental autoimmune uveitis
(EAU) among rats of various strains have been reported[1,2], However,
immunogenetic studies on susceptibility to EAU in rats has not been
completed. The present study was aimed at separating the effects of the
MHC and non-MHC genes on the development of EAU.

MATERIALS AND METHODS

Animals. Male rats, 10-14 weeks old, maintained at the Institute for Animal
Experiments, Hokkaido University School of Medicine, were used
throughout this study.

Antigens. S-Ag was prepared from bovine retinas as described by Dorey et
al[3]. Peptide M(18 amino acids in length which corresponds to the peptide
303-320 of bovine S-Ag, D T N L A S S T I I K E G I D K T V, molecular
weight 1903) was synthesized by an automated peptide synthesizer (430A,
Applied Biosystems, Inc., Foster City, CA), as described by Ogasawara et al[4].
Induction of EAU. Antigens were emulsified in a 1:1 (v/v) CFA containing
2.5 mg/ml of Mycobacterium tuberculosis H37Ra and were injected one-
footpad in a total volume of 0.1 ml. An additional adjuvant, Bordetella
pertussis (BP) (Wako pure chemical Ind, Ltd., Osaka, Japan) organisms
(10^{10}) was injected i.v. as indicated.

RESULTS

Induction of S-Ag EAU with or without BP

LEW (RT1^l), WKAH (RT1^k), and WKAH.1L congenic rats (RT1^l), were
tested for development of EAU by injecting 50 ug of bovine S-Ag emulsified
in CFA, with or without an additional i.v. administration of BP. All eight LEW
rats developed clinical and histologic EAU without BP. However, none of the

8 WKAH or 6 WKAH. 1L rats which were immunized without BP developed any clinical or histologic EAU, In contrast, all rats which had been injected BP, 8 LEW, 8 WKAH, and 6 WKAH 1L, developed clinical and histologic EAU.

Induction of EAU by peptide M in LEW, WKAH, and WKAH. 1L rats

Three strains of rats, LEW, WKAH, and WKAH. 1L, were immunized with peptide M with administration of BP. All eight LEW and B WKAH.1L rats, which have $RT1^l$, developed EAU by peptide M with BP. None of the 8 WKAH rats ($RT1^K$) developed EAU by peptied M, although the BP was injected in the same conditions. These findings revealed that development of EAU induced by peptide M was strongly correlated with MHC. Although the ocular inflammation induced by peptide M was distinctively milder than that induced by native S-Ag in both, LEW and WKAH. 1L, strains and largely confined to the posterior part of the eye, with mild anterior chamber involvement, typical histopathologic findjngs of EAU were seen in both strains.

Induction of EAU in different inbred strains of rats by peptide M or S-Ag with administration of BP.

To further clarify the influence of MHC on the development of EAU Induced by peptide M, another nine inbred strains representing different RT1 haplotypes were tested for EAU induction by the immunization of 100 μg of peptide M or 50 μg of S-Ag with an additional administration of BP. LEW, F344 ($RT1^{lvl}$), and NIG-III ($RT1^q$) developed EAU by peptide M with BP. These three strains of rats have 1 specificity in the $RT1-B$ and D subregions which are class II loci of the rats MHC. None of the other strains developed EAU by peptide M and none of them have 1 specificity in the class II loci. On the other hand, all tested rats ACI ($RT1^{avl}$), BUF ($RT1^b$), LEJ ($RT1^j$), W ($RT1^k$), WKAH, LEW, F344, BN ($RT1^n$), NIG-III ($RT1^q$), TO ($RT1^t$), and SDJ ($RT1^u$) developed EAU by native S-Ag with BP. Although the intensity of the inflammation in the F344 and NIG-III rats immunized with peptide M were milder than that of LEW, typical histopathologic changes of EAU were also seen.

DISCUSSION

The present study showed that both MHC and non-MHC genes were involved in the development of EAU in rats. The effect of non-MHC gene(s) was clearly shown by the finding that none of the WKAH. 1L RT1 congenic rats developed EAU, although this strain has the same MHC as LEW which is highly susceptible to EAU. Experimental autoimmune models undoubtedly involve a complex series of immunologic steps. Following sensitization with antigen, lymphocytes are driven into proliferation, differentiation, and recirculation to the target organ. Both LEW and refractory strains developed same range of lymphocyte proliferation and humoral immune responses against S-Ag. Nontheless, only LEW rats showed substantial DTH response (data not shown here). Furthermore, refractory strains of rats could develop disease when given BP. The lymphocytes migrate into the tissue through the vascular endothelium in most organs to develop pathological lesions. Thus, resistance to disease in the refractory strains may be due to the failure of lymphocyte-endothelium interaction which results in inefficient migration of the commited lymphocytes into the target tissues. Thus, we consider that the lymphocyte-endothelium interactions may be under the control of non-MHC gene(s).

EAU has been considered to be a model of Sympathetic Ophthalmia and Vogt-Koyanagi-Harada disease. These diseases belong to the same clinical entity of ocular inflammation and have been reported to have a high, almost 100%, association with HLA-DR54 and DQW4 (=DQWa) antigens[6]. However, since the native S-Ag, 404 amino acid, it has been difficult to precisely analyze the influence of MHC genes on the development of S-Ag EAU. Thus, in the present study, peptide M was used concurrently with BP to investigate the role of MHC on the development of EAU. Rat strains which have the specificity 1 at B and D loci of the class II MHC, LEW and WKAH.1L, F344 and NIG-III, developed EAU. On the other hand, none of the other strains which do not have the specificity 1 at class II loci developed EAU by peptide M with BP. However, the strains of rats failed to develop EAU with peptide M could develop EAU when these were immunized with native S-Ag concurrently with BP. These findings clearly show that the restriction of MHC class II exists on the development of EAU induced by peptide M and suggested that different determinants on S-Ag are uveitogenic for different inbred strains of rats.

The antigen appears to existed in situ as a whole protein (multideterminant antigen) but not as a form of small peptide (single determinant). Thus, if not all, lymphocytes in rats of majority of MHC class II haplotypes seem to recognize the target antigen as it was shown by immunization with S-Ag in this study. How could we interpret the mechanism of HLA class II association with human disease as shown in the Vogt-Koyanagi-Harada disease? In EAU model, Sigh et al[7]. found that an Escherichia coli protein has six consecutive amino acids identical to the sequence of peptide M and that immunization of a synthetic peptide derived from E. coli protein could induce EAU in LEW rats. Thus, it may be possible that infection with E. coli triggers the immune response that cross-react with ocular antigen. The cross-reaction may result in ocular inflammation by a mechanism termed molecular mimicry. If this is the case in human disease, cross reactivity may occur at the level of small determinant and be under the specific MHC class II restriction. Consequently, it is possible to detect association of some disease and particular MHC class II alle. Thus, our findings support the molecular mimicry hypothesis on the organ specific autoimmune disease as one of the mechanisms which cause association between MHC class II antigen and disease.

The conclusions we drawed from the present data is that both MHC and non-MHC genes are involved in the development of EAU in rats. Thus, MHC class II (RT1^1) restricted the susceptibility to EAU induced by peptide M. However, this restriction could not be observed when multideterminant S-Ag was used as immunogen. The eventual development of EAU was under the influence of non-MHC gene(s). BP could break this effect of non-MHC gene, probably, by affecting the lymphocyte-endothelial interaction.

ACKNOWLEDGEMENTS

This study was supported in part by The Special Grant in Aid for Promotion of Education and Science in Hokkaido University Provided by the Ministry of Education, Science and Culture.

REFERENCES

1. Gery I (1984) In : Chandler JW, O'Connor GR (eds) Proceedings of the third international symposium on immunology and immunopathology of the eye. Masson Publishing, New York, pp 242-245.

2. Mochizuki M, Kuwabara T, Chan CC, Nussenblatt RB, Detcalfe DD, Gery I (1984) J Immunol 133:1699-1701.

3. Dorey C, Cozette J, de Kozak Y, Faure JP (1982) Ophthalmic Res 14:249-255.

4. Ogasawara, K., P.P. Wambua, T. Gotohda, and K, Onoe, (1990) International Immunol (in press).

5. de Kozak Y, Sainte-Laudy J, Benveniste J, Faure JP (1981) Eur J Immunol 11:612-617.

6. Kunikane, H. 1986. Hokkaido J. Med. Sci. 61:672-681.

7. Singh VK, Yamakik, Abe T, Shinohara T (1989) Cell Immunol 122:262-273.

© 1990 Elsevier Science Publishers (Biomedical Division)
Ocular Immunology Today. M. Usui, S. Ohno and K. Aoki, editors.

PINEAL AND RETINAL RELATIONSHIPS IN THE IMMUNOPATHOLOGY OF EXPERIMENTAL AUTOIMMUNE UVEITIS

CAROLYN M. KALSOW

Department of Ophthalmology, University of Rochester, Rochester, New York 14642 (U.S.A.).

INTRODUCTION

Although the strong structural and functional homology between pineal and retinal photoreceptor cells of lower vertebrates is obscured in higher vertebrates, there is a strong biochemical homology between retinal photoreceptor cells and pinealocytes of mammals. Some of these proteins such as S-antigen and interphotoreceptor retinoid binding protein (IRBP) can be used to induce an experimental autoimmune response that involves both retina and pineal gland. Immunopathology of the retina is different than that of pineal gland. Pineal infiltrate occurs before retinal or even ocular infiltrate. Although infiltrate into the pineal gland is strictly lymphocytic, retinal infiltrate is mixed. In the pineal gland there are many normal appearing pinealocytes adjacent to lymphocytic infiltrate, while in the retina there is loss of the photoreceptor cell layer. Such differences in immunopathology present a unique opportunity to compare two distinct, local, organ specific immune responses induced by systemic sensitization to a single autoantigen. (See ref. 1 for a review.)

In these experiments, immunohistochemistry was used to monitor changes in pineal and retinal cells for Class II MHC antigen and glial fibrillary acidic protein (GFAP) expression, and to characterize infiltrating lymphocytes in rats sensitized to a uveitopathogenic synthetic peptide of IRBP (2).

MATERIAL AND METHOD

Female, Lewis rats were given a single footpad injection of 0.1 ml of 50 ug of IRBP peptide emulsified in Freund's Adjuvant complete. This peptide, a gift from Dr. Larry A. Donoso, Wills Eye Hospital, Philadelphia, was synthesized to correspond to amino acid residues 521-540 of human IRBP (2). At 7, 12, 17, and 21 days postinjection (dpi), eyes and brains were obtained from 4 or 5 sensitized rats. Tissues were fixed in 95% cold ethanol and embedded in paraffin. Immunopathology was evaluated by light microscopy of hematoxylin and eosin stained sections and peroxidase-anti-peroxidase immunohistochemistry with monoclonal antibodies (MAb): OX6 to rat Ia antigen, OX22 to B cells and some T cells, OX33 to B cells (Accurate Chemical & Scientific Corp., Westbury, NY.), and a cocktail of 3 MAb to human GFAP (Biomedical Technologies Inc., Stoughton, MA).

RESULTS

In pineal glands of control rats, vascular pericytes were reactive with MAb OX6, and cells in the proximal portion of the gland near the stalk were reactive with GFAP MAb. Neither lymphocytic infiltrate nor OX22 or OX33 MAb reactive cells were observed in pineal glands of control rats. There were no overt changes in GFAP reactivity in the pineal glands of sensitized rats. At 7 dpi, there was an increase in OX6 MAb reactivity for Ia antigen on cells of vascular areas and on infiltrating lymphocytes. Many of these infiltrating cells were also reactive with OX22 MAb for B and some T lymphocytes, and many of these, in turn, were reactive with OX33 MAb for B lymphocytes. At 12, 17, and 21 dpi, increased lymphocytic infiltration of the pineal gland was observed with similar proportions of cells reactive with OX6, OX22 and OX33 MAb as those seen at 7 dpi (Fig. 1).

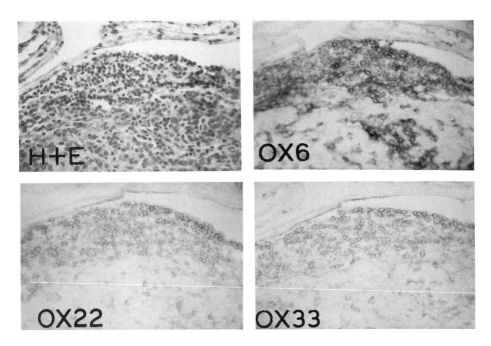

Figure 1. Immunopathology of pineal gland of a rat 12 dpi with IRBP peptide, as demonstrated by hematoxylin and eosin stain, and immunohistochemistry using OX6 MAb to Ia antigen, OX22 MAb to B lymphocytes and some T lymphocytes, and OX33 MAb to B lymphocytes.

The retinas of control rats did not show reactivity with OX6, OX22, or OX33 MAb. Only the retinal astrocytes were reactive with MAb for GFAP. At 7 dpi the retinas of sensitized rats showed no histopathology nor changes in immunoreactivity. At 12, 17, and 21 dpi immunoreactivity with OX6 MAb for Ia antigen was observed on retinal vascular endothelial cells and on infiltrating cells. Just as in the pineal glands, many of the infiltrating lymphocytes were reactive with OX22 MAb and with OX33 MAb (Fig 2). There was also detectable GFAP reactivity on retinal Muller cells.

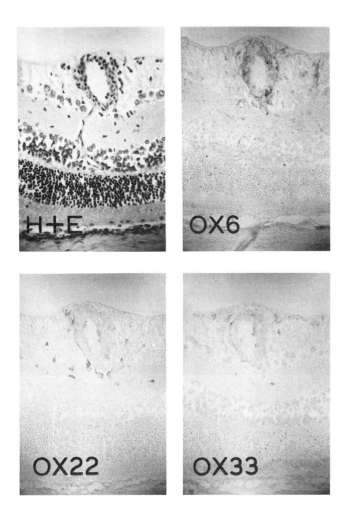

Figure 2. Immunopathology of retina of a rat 17 dpi with IRBP peptide, as demonstrated by hematoxylin and eosin stain, and immunohistochemistry using OX6 MAb to Ia antigen, OX22 MAb to B lymphocytes and some T lymphocytes, and OX33 MAb to B lymphocytes.

DISCUSSION

Results of these experiments are consistent with those of previous investigations as to: Ia antigen expression in normal rat pineal gland (3) and GFAP expression in normal rat pineal gland and retina (4,5), clinical and histopathologic response of rats to this IRBP peptide (2), and Ia antigen expression accompanying immunopathology in experimental autoimmune uveoretinitis (EAU) (6-8). The use of ethanol fixed/paraffin embedded tissue to demonstrate OX22 and OX33 MAb reactive lymphocytes in retina and pineal gland stands in contrast to previous studies of EAU in which cryopreserved tissue was examined for other lymphocyte markers (6-11).

142

These experiments show that rats sensitized with a synthetic, uveitogenic peptide of IRBP develop significant changes in their pineal glands prior to changes observed in retina. At 7 dpi, there was increased Ia antigen expression and a lymphocytic infiltrate including T and B lymphocytes. These changes were more pronounced at later time periods. Similar immunopathology was seen in retinas, but not until 12 dpi and thereafter. Immunoreactive GFAP was also found in Muller cells of affected retinas. Such changes in GFAP immunoreactivity were not seen in pineal gland.

Early participation of pineal gland in IRBP peptide-induced EAU is consistent with similar findings in S-antigen-induced EAU (12). The existence of the pineal gland outside of the blood-brain barrier along with its already expressed Ia antigen in vascular areas and the availability of the inciting autoantigen, sets the stage for interaction with passing lymphocytes that were recently sensitized by footpad injection. In addition, interaction between infiltrating T and B lymphocytes could also affect expression of immunopathology. Such events in pineal gland *i.e.,* interaction of sensitized cells and target tissue or between sensitized cells, could modulate that which is later observed as retinal immunopathology, thereby explaining the differences in immunopathology observed in pineal gland and retina.

ACKNOWLEDGEMENTS

The author gratefully acknowledges the expert technical assistance of Loel Turpin and Mary Morgenstern. This work was supported by NIH grant EY06866.

REFERENCES
1. Gery I, Mochizuki M, Nussenblatt RB (1986) Prog Retinal Res 5:75
2. Donoso LA, Merryman CF, Sery TW, Vrabec T, Arbizo V, Fong S-L (1988) Curr Eye Res 7:1087
3. Kalsow CM, Searl SS (1989) Invest Ophthalmol Vis Sci Suppl 30:277
4. Moller M, Ingild A, Bock E (1978) Brain Res 140:1
5. Bignami A, Dahl D (1979) Exp Eye Res 28:63
6. Chan C-C, Nussenblatt RB, Wiggert B, Redmond TM, Fujikawa LS, Chader GJ, Gery I (1987) Immunol Invest 16:63
7. Fujikawa LS, Chan C-C, McAllister C, Gery I, Hooks JJ, Detrick B, Nussenblatt RB (1987) Cell Immunol 106:139
8. Usui M, Takamura K, Shima Y, Mitsuhashi M, Matsushima T (1989) In: Secchi AG Fregpma IA (eds) Proc 4th Int Symp Immunol & Immunopathol of the Eye. Masson, Milano, pp 320
9. Chan C-C, Mochizuki M, Nussenblatt RB, Palestine AG, McAllister C, Gery I, BenEzra D (1985) Clin Immunol Immunopathol 35:103
10. Dua HS, Sewell HF, Forrester JV (1989) Clin Exp Immunol 75:100
11. Brown EC, Kasp E, Dumonde DC (1989) Clin Exp Immunol 77:422
12. Kalsow CM, Wacker WB (1986) In: O'Brien PJ Klein DC (eds) Pineal and Retinal Relationships. Academic Press, Inc., Orlando, pp 315

© 1990 Elsevier Science Publishers (Biomedical Division)
Ocular Immunology Today. M. Usui, S. Ohno and K. Aoki, editors.

ANTERIOR CHAMBER INJECTION OF S ANTIGEN PREVENTS THE DEVELOPMENT OF EXPERIMENTAL AUTOIMMUNE UVEITIS (EAU)

KAORU MIZUNO[1] AND J. WAYNE STREILEIN[2]

[1]Department of Ophthalmology, Osaka Railway Hospital, Osaka, Japan and
[2]Departments of Microbilogy, Immunology and Ophthalmology, University of Miami School of Medicine, Miami, USA

INTRODUCTION

Certain antigens injected into anterior chamber of the eye elicit uniquely a deviant form of immune responses[1]. This spectrum of immunity has been termed Anterior Chamber Associated Immune Deviation (ACAID)[2], characterized by (a) impairmant of antigen-specific delayed hypersensitivity(DH), (b) suppression of complement-fixing antibodies production and (c) intact generation of non-complement fixing antibodies and cytotoxic T cells. To date ACAID has been induced by using insoluble---histoincompatible tumor cells[3] and herpes siplex virus, type 1[4] or soluble antigens---hapten-derivatized spleen cells[5], BSA and S antigen in mice.[6] Currently we tested the possibility that intracameral injection of S antigen can prevent Lewis rats from development of EAU. The purpose of this study is to confirm whether ACAID mechanism can be induced during the course of clinically detectable EAU.

MATERIALS AND METHODS

Animals: Ten weeks old, 150-200gm female Lewis rats were used.

Antigens: Bovine retinal S antigen was purified by our method described elsewhere.[7]

Assay for immune responses: DH was determined by measuring ear swelling at 24 hours after ear challenge with antigens. Anti S antigen antibodies were determined by ELISA described elsewhere[7].

Clinical examination: Clinical observation was performed by a binocular fundoscope and a slitlamp.

RESULTS

Immune responses

Immune response to intracameral injection of S Ag in CFA. S antigen in Complete Freund's Adjuvant (S Ag-CFA) was inoculated into the anterior chamber of one eye of Lewis rats on day 0. Seven days later their immune responses were measured. As shown in Figure 1, rats receiving anterior chamber injection of S Ag revealed no immune response (Figure 1).

144

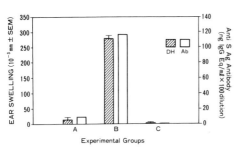

Fig.1. IMMUNE RESPONSE TO INTRACAMERAL INJECTION OF
S AG IN CFA

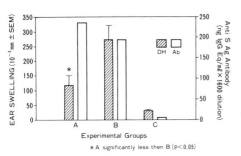

* A significantly less then B (p<0.05)

Fig. 2. EFFECT OF INTRACAMERAL S AG INJECTION ON SUBSEQUENT
IMMUNIZATION WITH SUBCUTANEOUS S AG INJECTION

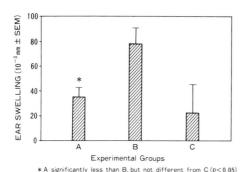

* A significantly less than B. but not different from C (p<0.05)

Fig.3. ADOPTIVE TRANSFER OF S AG-SPECIFIC ACAID

Effect of intracameral S Ag injection
on subsequent immunization with
subcutaneous S Ag injection. To test
whether specific suppression exists,
animals received intracameral injection
of S Ag in CFA on day 0, then followed
by footpad injections of S Ag in CFA
on day 4. These rats showed remarkable
suppression of DH, whereas the production of S Ag specific antibodies was
intact (Figure 2).

Adoptive transfer of S Ag-specific
ACATD. In order to confirm the above
suppression of DH we performed adoptive
transfer. Rats received intracameral
injection of S Ag in CFA. Seven days
later spleen cells from these rats were
injected intravenously into naive rats
(100 million/rat). DH was assayed seven
days later. In experimental group, they
showed significantly lower DH compared
to positive control group (Figure 3).

Clinical evaluation for induction of
EAU. We clinically tested the possibility that the above suppression of
DH would impair the development of EAU
in rats. On day 0 rats received
intracameral injections of S Ag in CFA
into one eye. Four days later all rats
including positive control rats received
injections of S Ag in CFA into footpads,
then followed by clinical observation.
See Table 1. As expected, almost all
rats developed severe EAU in positive
control (Group 1). Interestingly, in
the rats pretreated with intracameral
injection of S Ag with or without CFA,
then followed by footpad injection of
S Ag in CFA, only few animals developed
EAU (one out of eight in Group 2, three

out of eight in group 3 developed EAU). In addition, three rats in Group 3
showed mild EAU.

Histopathological examination

After the termination of EAU on day 30 post-inoculation, all rats were killed
and their eyes were examined hitologically. The results confirmed the clinical
assessment of uveitis.

TABLE I

CLINICAL EVALUATION FOR INDUCTION OF EAU

| Groups | Inoculation routes | | Clinical findings |
	Day 0	Day 4	Number of positive EAU
1	—	S Ag in CFA FP	8/9
2	S Ag AC	S Ag in CFA FP	1/8
3	S Ag in CFA AC	S Ag in CFA FP	3/8

DISCUSSION

ACAID is the predictable, if poorly understood, consequence of antigenic en-
counters via the anterior chamber of the eye. In the studies reported here, we
have explored the possibility that antigen-specific suppression, which is typical
of ACAID, can be used to thwart the expression of an autoimmune disease. Retinal
S protein is a soluble antigen from the retina that, when mixed with adjuvant
and injected subcutaneously into susceptible Lewis rats, induces autoimmune
uveoretinitis. Our experimental results indicate that prior inoculation of S
antigen into the anterior chamber of one eye inhibits the eventual development
of EAU in rats receiving a uveitogenic regimen. Since similarly treated rats
and mice[6] dispaly S antigen-specific ACAID, and since their spleens contain
specific suppressor T cells, we conclude that anterior chamber pretreatment with
S antigen inhibits uveitis by virtue of the suppressor cells that are induced.

Other antigen-specific strategies have been employed by other investigators
to prevent EAU, including intravenous injections of S antigen, and administration
of anti idiotype antibodies. In general, repeated administrations were necessary
in order to achieve amelioration of uveoretinitis. The advantage of a treatment
regimen based of ACAID is that only a single injection of antigen is required,
and the protection of the uveal tract is virtually complete.

It has been reported that S antigen never escapes the uveal tract under normal circumstances, and is not present in the aqueous humor. If this is true, then S antigen would represent a truly "sequestered" antigen, one to which self-tolerance had never been attained. Perhaps that is why it is possible to immunize adult Lewis rats with this antigen and create an autoimmune uveoretinitis. Moreover, the capacity of intracamerally injected S antigen to induce ACAID in adult rats and therefore protect against autoimmune uveoretinitis also makes sense. However, Faure[8] has recently reported that S antigen-immunoreactivity can be detected in various non-ocular tissues, implying that this antigen may not be sequestered. Therefore, explanations of the immunopathogenesis of S antigen-induced uveitis, and for protection by intracamerally-injected S angigen may be considerably more complicated.

The success with which EAU can be abrogated by AC injection of S antigen suggests a potential avenue of therapy for ocular autoimmune disorders. Our results lead us to suggest that intraocular injections of autoantigens might be considered as a means of preventing ocular disease, especially if the molecular nature of the antigen(s) is known.

REFERENCES

1. Streilein JW (1987) FASEB J 1:199

2. Streilein JW, Niederkorn JY (1981) J Exp Med 153:1058

3. Streilein JW, Niederkorn JY, Shadduck JA (1980) J Exp Med 152:1121

4. Whittum JA, Niederkorn JY, Streilein JW (1983) Curr Eye Res 2:691

5. Waldrap JC, Kaplan HJ (1983) Invest Ophthalmol Vis Sci 24:1086

6. Mizuno K, Clark AF, Streilein JW (1989) Invest Ophthalmol Vis Sci 30:1112

7. Mizuno K, Clark AF, Streilein JW (1989) Invest Ophthalmol Vis Sci 30:772

8. Faure JP (1989) Recent development in the immunopathology of intraocular inflammation, Amsterdam

© 1990 Elsevier Science Publishers (Biomedical Division)
Ocular Immunology Today. M. Usui, S. Ohno and K. Aoki, editors.

IMMUNOHISTOCHEMICAL STUDY OF CORNEAL ALLOGRAFT REJECTION IN INBRED RATS

H. OTSUKA, R. MURAMATSU AND M. USUI
Tokyo Medical College, Tokyo, Japan

INTRODUCTION

There have been few immunohistochemical studies concerning rejection in penetrating keratoplasty. We devised a corneal graft rejection model by performing keratoplasty in rats and analyzed the pattern of infiltration of helper T(Th) cells, suppressor-cytotoxic T(Ts-c) cells, Ia-antigen positive cells, and macrophages into the grafts by the use of anti-rat monoclonal antibodies. Furthermore, the Th/Ts-c ratio in the peripheral blood was compared with that in the grafts. The Ia antigen plays an important role in rejection as a histocompatibility antigen (MHC class $\parallel$), but its extent of expression in the corneal endothelium is not well known. Therefore, Ia antigen expression during rejection was studied using endothelial flat preparations.

MATERIALS AND METHODS

Penetrating keratoplasty was performed using inbred DA (Dark Agouti) rats (RT 1^a) as the donors and Lewis rats (RT 1^ℓ) as the recipients in this experiment (allogeneic model), and the same procedure was performed between Lewis rats only, as the control group (syngeneic model). Full-thickness grafts in 3 mm diameter were transplanted using 8 interrupted sutures of 10-0 nylon. Postoperatively, only topical antibiotics and mydriatics were adoministered. The transparency and vascularization of the graft observed sequentially by a slit lamp, and rats with early opacification or other complications within 7 days were excluded from this study.

6 μm frozen section
↓
fixed in cold acetone   15min.
↓
0.3% H_2O_2 solution   30min.
↓
normal goat serum   20min.
↓
murine monoclonal anti-rat antibody   30min.
↓
goat anti-mouse Ig G
with rat immunogloburin   30min.
↓
peroxidase-conjugated murine IgG   30min.
↓
substrate solution
(3-amino-9-ethyl carbazole)
↓
counterstained with hematoxylin
↓
examined by a light miroscopy

Fig. 1. Peroxidase-antiperoxidase Method.

Blood samples were collected on postoperative days 2, 4, 7, on the day rejection occured (12 ± 2 days, mean ± S.D.), and on day 21. The eyeballs were enucleated and freeze-embedded, then stained immunohistochemically by the peroxidase-antiperoxidase method using the anti-rat monoclonal antibodies (W3/25; Th, OX8; Ts-c, OX6; rat Ia of all strains, OX42; macrophages, granulocytes, Sera-Lab Ltd.) (Fig. 1). The Th/Ts-c ratio in the peripheral blood was examined by flow cytometry.

Ia antigen expression in the endothelium after the occurrence of rejection was observed using flat preparations.

RESULTS

Clinical Findings

On postoperative day 7, the vessels reached the periphery of the graft from all around the limbus, and from day 10 rejection was first noted. By day 14, rejection was recognized in all the rats of the experiment group. In the control group, all the grafts remained transparent.

Histological Findings

The intensity of cell infiltration was devided into five grades and was assesed for both the central and the peripheral parts of the grafts (Fig. 2). All the subsets of cells investigated could be identified in the grafts on day 4. Infiltration was more marked in the peripheral regions than in the central regions of the grafts, and was especially prominent in the sutured portions.

Rejection model group (DA→LEW)

Days after transplantation		2	4	7	Time of Intense Rejection (12±2)	21
W3/25	g.p	±	+	++	+++	++ ~ +++
	g.c	−	±	+	+	+ ~ ++
O X 8	g.p	−	+	+	+++ ~ ++++	+
	g.c	−	±	±	+++ ~ ++++	+
O X 6	g.p	±	+	++	+++	+++
	g.c	−	+	+	++	++
O X 42	g.p	++	++	+++	+++ ~ ++++	+ ~ ++
	g.c	++	+	+	+++ ~ ++++	+

Control group (LEW→LEW)

Days after transplantation		2	4	7	14	21
W3/25	g.p	±	+	+	+	±
	g.c	−	±	+	+	±
O X 8	g.p	−	+	+	+	±
	g.c	−	+	+	±	−
O X 6	g.p	+	+	++	++	+
	g.c	−	+	±	++	±
O X 42	g.p	++	++	+	++	±
	g.c	++	+	±	++	±

Fig. 2. The intensity of cell infiltration

g.p : graft periphery   − : absent   ++ : moderate

g.c : graft center   ± : very light   +++ : heavy

       + : light   ++++ : very heavy

W3/25-positive cells were slightly predominant to OX8-positive cells before the occurrence of rejection, and both cells increased with rejection, with the increase in OX8-positive cells being particularly remarkable(Fig.3)

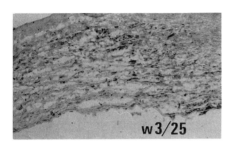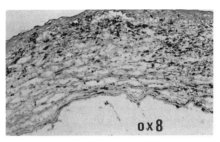

Fig. 3.   14 days postgraft.   Ts-c cells were predominant over Th cells.

OX42-positive cells showed diffuse infiltration on day 2, and diminished sharply in numbers after rejection occurred.   OX6-positive cells were increased in number during rejection, and also showed a persistent marked infiltration of the periphery of the grafts until day 21.   When we observed OX6-positive cells in the endothelium using flat preparations, the normal endothelium was OX6-negative, but changed to OX6-positive after rejection (Fig. 4)

The Th/Ts-c ratio in the peripheral blood showed no marked changes before and after occurrence of rejection(Fig.5).

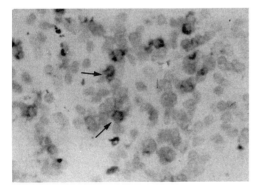

Days after transplantation	W3/25 (%)	OX8 (%)	W3/25/OX8 ratio
2	62.7	27.8	2.26
	62.4	27.9	2.24
4	56.3	27.4	2.05
	55.1	27.8	1.98
7	55.7	27.3	2.04
	57.8	24.8	2.33
12±2	54.3	26.2	2.07
	59.7	25.0	2.39
	61.7	32.3	1.91
21	51.1	29.9	1.71
normal (before transplantation)	54.3± 3.2	27.6± 1.6	1.97± 0.14

Fig. 4.   The endothelium exhibited Ia antigen positivity during rejection.

Fig. 5.   Changes in lymphocyte subsets in the peripheral blood in the rejection model group.

DISCUSSION

There have been many reports[1,2] suggesting that T cell-mediated immunity was related keratoplasty rejection, but this subject has not yet been studied in detail immunohistochemically using monoclonal antibodies. One of the reasons is the technical problems in dealing with rats or mice, although they have the advantage of beeing inbred and posessing antigenic purity.

We found that before rejection occurred "Th" cells were predominant in the cornea, while after rejection Ts-c cells increased markedly and became predominant. These findings which were also seen in other organs[3,4], suggests that the dynamic changes of the lymphocyte subsets are likely to represent the induction phase and effector phase of cell-mediated immunity. On the other hand, in studies of experimental heart or lung transplantation in rats[3,4], the Th/Ts-c ratio in the peripheral blood was reported useful to monitor rejection, but it was of no value to monitor corneal rejection in this model, which agrees with previous reports on human cases[5]. It may be due to the fact that the cornea is a very small organ.

Since OX6-positive cells were prominent in the infiltrates after rejection, it may be considered that they played an important role in the rejection reaction. Infiltration around wound persisted for a long period of time in the syngeneic model also, and this may have been a reaction to the suture threads, as we have previously mentioned.

The expression of Ia antigen has been reported previously in cultured endothelium[6], endothelium after uveitis[7], and in human corneal graft rejection[8], but there have been few reports concerning experimental corneal rejection models. It was difficult to judge Ia positivity of the rejeted endothelium using traditional transverse sections because Ia positive cells were observed also in the anterior chamber which was in contact with endothelial cells. So we utilized flat preparations of the rejected endothelium. The Ia antigen expresstion that was noted suggested that the endothelium may act as a "target" during the occurrence of rejection.

REFERENCES

1) Khodadoust AA and Silverstein AM: Induction of corneal graft rejection by passive cell transfer. Invest Ophthalmol 15:89, 1976.
2) Pepose JS, Nestor MS, Gardner KM, Foos RY, and Pettit TH: Composition of cellular infiltrates in rejected human corneal allografts. Graefe's Arch Ophthalmol 222:128, 1985.
3) Imura M: Analysis of Leucocyte Subsets in Rats with Cardiac Transplantation. Mie Igaku 31:243-250, 1987.
4) Higashi K et al: Experimental Lung Transplantation in The Rat. Igakuno-

ayumi 20:653-661, 1985.

5) Young E, Stark WJ : Ophthalmology Immunology of Corneal Alloglaft Rejection 92:223-227, 1985.

6) Young E, Stark WJ, and Prendergast RA : Immunology of Corneal Allograft on Human Corneal Cells. Invest Ophthalmol Vis Sci 26:571-574, 1985.

7) Donnelly JJ, Li W, Rockey JH, and Prendergast RA : Induction of Class Ⅱ (Ia) Alloantigen Expression on Corneal endothelium In Vivo and In Vitro. Invest ophthalmol Vis Sci 26:575-580, 1985.

8) Pepose JS, Gardner KM, Nestor MS, Foos RY, Pettit TH : Detection of HLA Class Ⅰ and Ⅱ Antrgen in Rejected Human Corneal Allografts. Ophthalmology 92:1480-1484, 1985.

© 1990 Elsevier Science Publishers (Biomedical Division)
Ocular Immunology Today. M. Usui, S. Ohno and K. Aoki, editors.

INFLAMMATION AFTER INTRAOCULAR SURGERY AND IOL IMPLANT IN INBRED RATS

GERD NEUBAUER, ELLEN KRAUS-MACKIW

Department of Orthoptics, Pleoptics and Motility Disturbances, Eye Hospital, Ruprecht-Karl University, D-6900 Heidelberg 1 (FRG)

INTRODUCTION

Phacogenic reactions in animal experiments by lens discision alone are equivalent to lens-induced cellular reactions in humans. They are caused by mechanical rupture of the lens capsule due to trauma and/or surgery and by spontaneous release of lens material with advancing age or in complicated cataract. The various types of morphological changes observed in human lenses and reproduced experimentally in inbred rats have been classified as reaction types 1-6 (1). The incidence of the different reaction types observed in humans is also to be seen in animal experiments (Fig. 1).

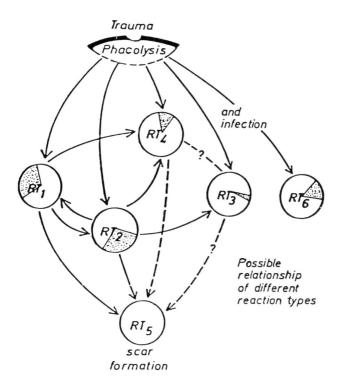

Fig. 1. Incidence of the different reaction types on the basis of all eyes enucleated at the Heidelberg University Eye Hospital from 1935 to 1981.

Progressive intraocular inflammation in animal experiments is characterized clinically by vascularization in cornea, iris and lens material. This suggests increased accessibility of the lens to induction of sensitization and its target function in terms of attracting specific attention. Transfer experiments in isogenic and "autogenic" systems from the results of Rusek and Kostrzewa following a simple method for continuous cross transfusion of blood between unrestrained rats by Müller-Ruchholtz and Sonntag occasioned investigations of the following questions: the influence of possible microbial factors in inbred rats which have so far remained undetected and the clinicomorphological reactions in pseudophakic rat eyes (2 -6).

RESULTS

Transfer experiments

Despite the use of inbred rats and the induction of extensive lens damage, progressive inflammation (RT 3 = epitheloid cell granulomas focussed primarily around lens capsule residue, iris and ciliary body) also occurred in 5% or less of the rats after continuous cross-transfusion of blood between CAP (RtH-1^c) inbred rats. This was confirmed by Kostrzewa after reevaluation of the results of blood cross-transfusion following experimental lens discision and - as a second procedure after an interval of 14 days - lens discision in the partner eye: RT 1 (macrophages and foreign-body giant cells in the vicinity of exposed lens material) in 13 out of 17, RT 2 in 02 out of 17, RT 3 in 01 out of 17, and RT 6 in 01 out of 17 "partner" eyes (Fig. 2).

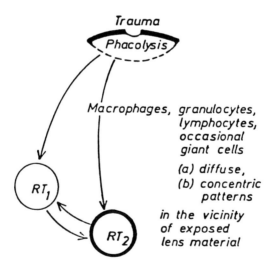

Fig. 2. Reaction type 2: clinical manifestation of phacogenic endophthalmitis.

Therefore, factors other than lens injury may be important in the production of lens-induced uveitis in both rats and man.

Experimental intraocular infections

The investigation of concomitant local infections (lens discision combined with a single injection of 2×10^8 Staphylococcus aureus in the anterior chamber of Lewis (RtH-1[1]) inbred rats) by Adams showed that RT 2, which has features in common with RT 6 (secondary involvement of the lens due to infection), occurred in 15 out of 16 eyes ten days later. Since there is no definite proof of microorganisms following intraocularly induced infection of less recent origin, it can be conjectured that very slight contamination with microorganisms accompanying exposure of lens material is involved in the triggering of type 2 reactions, which may result in progressive lens-induced uveitis (7).

Skin tests

Only two out of 48 rats tested with 6 mg of sygeneic lens material 70, 100 or 140 days after simple lens discisions showed positive skin-test reactions. The latter, on biopsy, consisted of severe lymphocytic infiltrations with some giant cells. The eyes of these two animals showed type 3 reactions, which are clinically known to have sympathogenic potential.

Intraocular lens implantation

A modified Binkhorst lens was implanted in Lewis inbred rats following opening of the anterior chamber and enlargement of the corneal incision 1. after total lens extirpation (ICCE) in the anterior chamber, 2. after lens extirpation leaving behind the capsule (ECCE) in the posterior chamber. The tissue reaction was analyzed histologically after clinical observations in each of the two experimental series, after ten days (n(1) = 7, n(2) = 5) and after 40 days (n(1) = 42, n(2) = 42). A specially developed histological technique was used which enabled positive imaging of pseudophakos in histological sections.

Postoperative success is endangered by secondary glaucoma and neovascularization with corneal damage and with cellular reactions in the remaining lens material and synechias in the pupil region in conjunction with mechanical effects of the implanted IOL on the iris epithelium and ciliary body.

CONCLUSION

Intraocular inflammation of exogenous origin, which may lead to the loss of visual function in both eyes, i.e. sympathetic ophthalmia, is much less rare than might be expected, especially following secondary surgical operations on predamaged eyes with fresh intraocular hemorrhages, vascular neoplasia and secondary glaucoma (8).

Recently, Apple has pointed to the importance of intraocular occult infections because of their significance for the success or failure of modern lens surgery (9). Ronald Smith, who reported on animal experimental studies also emphasizes this aspect with regard to the adjuvant effect of occult infections in progressive cases of endophthalmitis after cataract surgery (10).

Questions with regard to the pathogenicity and efficacy of therapy can only be solved by means of long-term observations and animal experiments. Epidemiological as well as erg-ophthalmological studies in collaboration with immunologists make it evident that detection and evaluation of the underlying "immunopathological" processes will be possible on the basis of clinical findings in postsurgical intraocular inflammation correlated with the histo-logical picture to be encountered at a specific time (11, 12).

The role of various clinico-pathological factors which are prerequisites for exogenous progressive lens-induced uveitis can be specifically investigated in the experimental model presented, i.e. IOL material and design, intraoperative microbial contaminations, genetic effects of the recipient animals, e.g albino-Lewis versus black-hooded-CAP, and prior dam-age to the eyes owing to injuries - using modern immunopathological followup techniques and evaluation of medication measures with regard to the time and duration of postopera-tive application in this experimental model.

ACKNOWLEDGEMENTS
For careful preparation of the manuscript we are grateful to Ingrid Blaszkewicz and Editori-al Consultant David John Williams, B.Sc., Heidelberg, and to Anja Jung for photographs.

REFERENCES

1. Daus W, Adams H, Müller-Hermelink HK (1984) Fortschr Ophthalmol 81: 54-58

2. Rusek A (1980) Thesis. Ruprecht-Karl University, Heidelberg

3. Kostrzewa L (1990) Thesis in preparation. Ruprecht-Karl University, Heidelberg

4. Müller-Ruchholtz W, Sonntag HG (1970) J Applied Physiology 28:383-386

5. Adams H, Daus W, Neubauer G (1984) In: Saari KM (ed) Uveitis update. Elsevier, Amster-dam, pp 391-394

6. Neubauer G (1989) Thesis. Ruprecht-Karl University, Heidelberg

7. Adams H (1990) Thesis in preparation. Ruprecht-Karl University, Heidelberg

8. Kraus-Mackiw E (1990) In: Kijlstra A (ed) Recent developments in the immunopathology of intraocular inflammation. Current Eye Research, Oxford, in press

9. Apple DJ, Tetz M, Hunold W (1988) In: Jacobi KW, Schott K, Gloor B (eds) 1. Kongress der Deutschen Gesellschaft für Intraokularlinsenimplantation. Springer, Berlin - Heidel-berg - New York - London - Paris - Tokyo, pp 6-14

10. Smith RE (1989) Intraocular inflammation after surgery. 10th Anniversary International Uveitis Study Group, Paris, June 29-30

11. De Jong P (1989) Epidemiology and prevention of ocular trauma in The Netherlands. 5th World Congress of Ergophthalmology, Beograd, September 24-29

12. Kraus-Mackiw E, Mayer H, Manthey KF (1990) Sympathetic ophthalmia as a late com-plication of occupational eye damage: examination and correction of a forecast algo-rithm. 13th International Ergophthalmological Symposium, Singapore, March 14-16

© 1990 Elsevier Science Publishers (Biomedical Division)
Ocular Immunology Today. M. Usui, S. Ohno and K. Aoki, editors.

NATURAL KILLING OF HSV-1 INFECTED AND NONINFECTED TARGET CELLS IN IGH-1 DISPARATE MICE

RICHARD R. TAMESIS, M.D. AND C. STEPHEN FOSTER, M.D.. From the Hilles Immunology Laboratory, Harvard Medical School, Massachusetts Eye & Ear Infirmary, Boston,MA

INTRODUCTION

We have previously shown that susceptibility to HSV-1 stromal keratitis in mice is linked to the Igh-1 locus on chromosome 12 (1). CAL-20 (Igh-1 ^{d}) mice develop severe HSK , while C.B-17 (Igh-1^b) mice are resistant(1). BALB/c (Igh-1^a) mice are intermediately susceptible to HSK. Natural killer (NK) cells have been implicated in a number of diverse immunologic functions including cytotoxicity against tumor cells and virus-infected cells(2). An H-2D region gene and two non-H-2 linked genes are involved in regulating NK activity in the mouse (3-4). We studied *in vitro* murine NK activity against HSV-1 infected targets in order to investigate the role of NK cells in resistance to HSK.

MATERIALS AND METHODS

Virus. HSV type1(KOS strain) was propagated on Vero cell monolayers (ATCC CCL 81, Rockville, MD) in our laboratory.

Target cells. YAC-1 (ATCC TIB 160) and PU5-1R (ATCC TIB 61) cells, which are lysed by NK cells, were grown in RPMI 1640 supplemented with 10% fetal calf serum and antibiotics. Cell suspensions were infected with HSV-1 at a multiplicity of infection of 5.0 for 2 hours, labelled with ^{51}Chromium, and suspended to a final concentration of 4×10^5 cells/ml. Uninfected cells were prepared in a similar fashion.

Animals. BALB/c, CAL-20, and C.B-17 adult (6 to 8 weeks old) mice were obtained from Jackson Laboratories, Bar Harbor, Maine. Animals infected with HSV-1 were inoculated intraperitoneally with 10^7 PFU of HSV-1. Splenic lymphocytes were obtained by Lympholyte-M (Cedarlane Laboratories, Hornby, Ontario) buoyant density centrifugation and washed twice in Hanks Balanced Salt Solution before use in the microcytotoxicity assay.

Microcytotoxicity assay. The microcytotoxicity assay was performed in six replicates in 96-well flat bottomed microtiter plates (Becton Dickinson & Company, Lincoln Park, NJ). A 150-ul portion of either effector cells diluted to obtain the desired effector-to-target cell ration, medium alone (for spontaneous release) or 5% Triton X (Sigma Chemical Co., St. Louis, MO)(for total release) were added to 50 ul of target cells (2×10^4) in each well.

After 12 hours of incubation at 37^0 C and 5% CO_2 for 12 hours, 100 ul of supernatant was collected from each well, and the amount of ^{51}Cr released was counted in an LKB Wallac 1272 gamma counter. The percent ^{51}Cr release was determined using the following formula. Percent ^{51}Cr release = 100 x (experimental release-spontaneous release)/(total release-spontaneous release). Spontaneous release was less than 30% of total release. The data was expressed as lytic

158

units (LUs), defined as the number of effector cells required for 10% specific chromium release. LUs were calculated using an exponential fit equation previously described (5).

Statistical analysis. Multifactorial analysis of variance (ANOVA) followed by Fisher's Least Significance Difference Test was used.

RESULTS

NK activity in naive mice. The NK activity of splenic lymphocytes of CAL-20 and BALB/c mice was significantly greater than C.B-17 mice using YAC-1 as cell targets (Figure 1). HSV-1 infected targets were lysed better than uninfected targets. No difference in virus-enhanced lysis, which we will define as the difference between the lysis of infected and uninfected cells [NK(HSV-YAC)-NK(YAC)], was observed among the three strains of mice

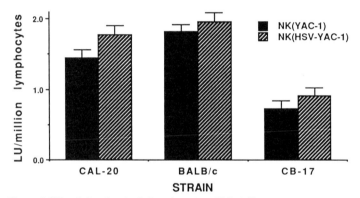

Figure 1. NK activity of splenic lymphocytes of Igh-1 disparate mice using YAC-1 cell targets

NK activity after I.P. infection with HSV-1. Figure 2 illustrates the effect of intraperitoneal infection with 10^7 PFU of HSV-1. Groups of CAL-20 and C.B-17 mice were infected at 6, 12, and 24 hours prior to sacrifice. A rapid augmentation in NK cell activity was observed in both strains of mice during the first 24 hours after infec tion. Splenic lymphocytes from infected C.B-17 mice showed higher NK lytic activity against HSV-1 infected targets than CAL-20 splenocytes 24 hours after I.P. infection with HSV-1. In contrast, uninfected CAL-20 splenocyteshad higher NK activity than splenocytes from uninfected C.B-17 mice.

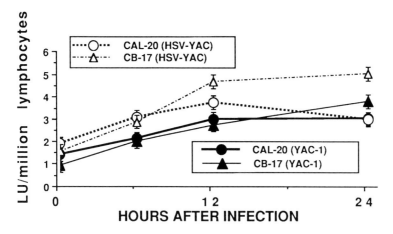

Figure 2. Igh-1 NK activity after I.P. infection with HSV-1
using YAC-1

NK activity using PU5-1R targets. Splenic lymphocytes from the three mouse strains were tested
for their ability to lyse PU5-1R cell targets. As shown on figure 3, no appreciable lytic activity
was seen until 24 hours after I.P. infection with HSV-1. CAL-20 splenocytes showed the highest
cytotoxic activity against infected and uninfected targets while BALB/c and C.B-17 splenocytes had
similar lytic activities. In both time course studies using YAC-1 and PU5-1R cell targets, no
difference in virus-enhanced lysis was seen among the mouse strains tested.

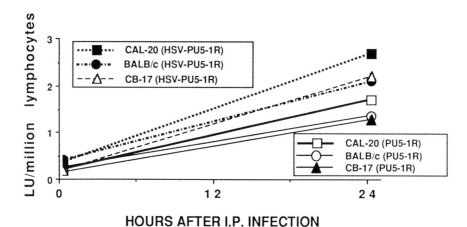

HOURS AFTER I.P. INFECTION

Figure 3. Igh-1 NK activity after I.P. infection with HSV-1
using PU5-1R

DISCUSSION

The role of natural killer cells in resistance to HSV-1 infection is unclear. Correlations between genetically high NK activity in mice and increased resistance to HSV-1 infection have been made previously (6). Depletion of NK cells with antibody to asialo GM1 or with ^{89}Sr enhances susceptibility to HSV-1 induced encephalitis in mice (7). On the other hand, SJL mice, which have low NK activity, are relatively resistant to HSV-1 infection (8).

Our results demonstrate that the Igh-1 locus influences the ability of murine splenic lymphocytes to lyse cell targets recognized by NK cells. The pattern of NK activity observed in our study appears to be dependent on the cell line tested. One report suggests that Igh-1 linked products are expressed on NK cell receptors responsible for recognizing target cell structures (9). It is not presently known whether NK cells recognize viral determinants alone or in combination with some other structure normally present on the surface of an uninfected target cell. No differences in virus-enhanced lysis were observed among the Igh-1 disparate congenics. One report suggests that the increased lysis mediated by NK cells against virus infected targets is due to a nonspecific mechanism involving interferon-dependent self activiation of NK cells upon contact with an infected cell(10). It is therefore unlikely that the Igh-1 locus influences cytotoxicity directed against virus determinants expressed on the cell surface of an infected cell.

In summary, our studies show that the Igh-1 gene locus may be one of the genes which regulate NK cell activity in the mouse. However, the differences in NK cell activity observed among these Igh-1 disparate congenics do not correlate with the resistance pattern to HSK seen in these mice.

REFERENCES

1. Foster CS, Tsai Y, Monroe JG, Campbell R, Wetzig R, Knipe D, Greene MI (1986) Immunol Immunopathol 40:313.

2. Lopez C (1981) In: Haller O (ed) Current Topics in Microbiology and Immunology. Springer-Verlag, New York, pp 15-24.

3. Clark EA, Harmon RC (1980) Adv Cancer Res 31:227.

4. Lopez C (1980) Immunogenetics 11:87-92.

5. Pross HF, Baines MG, Rubin P, Shragge P, Patterson MS (1981) J Clin Immunol 1:51-63.

6. Habu S, Akamatsu K, Tamaoki N, Okumura (1984) J Immunol 133:2743-2747.

7. Lopez C, Ryshke R, Bennet M (1980) Infect Immunol 28:1028-1028-1032.

8. Kirchner H, Engler H, Zawatzky R, Schindler L (1982) Adv Exp Med Biol 155:785-797.

9. Okumura K, Habu S, Kasai M (1982) Adv Exp Med Biol 155:773-784.

10. Colmenares C, Lopez C (1986) J Immunol 136:3473-3479.

© 1990 Elsevier Science Publishers (Biomedical Division)
Ocular Immunology Today. M. Usui, S. Ohno and K. Aoki, editors.

ULTRAMICROSCOPY OF THE LENS IN THE COURSE OF EXPERIMENTAL ALLERGIC UVEITIS

A.G. SECCHI, G. DE CARO, M.S. TOGNON and I.A. FREGONA

Institute of Ophthalmology, University of Padova, School of Medicine, Padova, Italy

INTRODUCTION

The integrity of the lens capsular/epithelial structures is essential for the maintenance of its transparency; a normal function of the membrane Na+/K+ pump counteracts the natural tendency of the lens fibers, which are negatively charged, to attract sodium and, therefore, undergo swelling.

The presence of the junctions among adjacent fibers and among epithelial cells, allowing ionic and electrical coupling, is another mechanism of osmotic regulation of the lens.

Our previous studies (1-7) have demonstrated that significant permeability changes, characterized by intracellular Na+ accumulation and outflow of K+, take place in the lens in the course of ocular inflammation.
The present investigation analyzes the ultramicroscopic changes which may appear in the lens after experimental uveitis.

MATERIALS AND METHODS

Experimental inflammation was induced in 21 New Zealand rabbits by an intravitreal injection of 0.1 ml of EA solution in saline (1mg/ml) followed, 20 days later, by an intravenous administration of 1ml of the same solution.

Twenty-four hours later the rabbits' eyes were observed by slit lamp: aqueous flare, cells, iris hyperemia and fibrinous exudate were graded according to Hogan et al. (8). Several relapses of uveitis were induced in the same way, after complete resolution of each previous clinical episode. The rabbits were then divided into four separate groups (A,B,C,D) and sacrificed after 1,2,3 and 4 relapses of uveal inflammatory episodes. The eyes were enucleated and, after 48 hours' fixation in Karnowsky solution (pH 7.3), each lens was dehydrated and a slice was cut, osmicated and embedded in Epon 812 for T.E.M. evaluation (Elmiscop 101-Simens).
The remaining part of the lens was critical-point dried, then sputter coated with palladium gold and examined in a Cambridge Stereoscan 250.
T.E.M. evaluation was performed and included:

A.Pathology of the epithelial cells:junction loss,enlargement of the intercellular spaces,atrophy of the cytoplasmatic organelles,cellular hypertrophy with
collagen production (pseudometaplasia),rupture of lens cell membranes with production of multilamellar structures (myelin-like bodies),nuclear fragmentation.
B.Pathology of the fiber cells: junction loss,enlargement of the intercellular
spaces, electron-density decrease, swelling, calcium deposits, degeneration.
The ultrastructural changes were recorded as present or absent.
S.E.M. evaluation was also performed in order to investigate the integrity of
the anterior lens capsule; the morphological changes of the lens capsule were
quantified using the following arbitrary score:1=slight, 2=moderate, 3=severe.

RESULTS
    The results are summarized in the following table:

GROUP/n of rabbits				
CLINICAL INFLAMMATION				
Severity of the inflammation				
-allergic uveitis*/n of +ve cases	36/5	29/5	33/5	27/6
-relapses*/n of +ve cases I	56/5	27/5	14/3	10/3
II		41/5	41/5	21/4
III			36/5	32/6
IV				41/6
ULTRASTRUCTURE OF THE LENS				
T.E.M.				
Pathology of epithelial cells				
n of +ve cases				
-junction loss	4	4	4	3
-enlarg. of intercell. spaces	2	4	3	2
-atrophy of cytopl. organell.	2	3	1	0
-hypertrophy	0	0	0	0
-rupture of cell membranes	1	2	1	2
-nuclear fragmentation	0	1	0	1
Pathology of fiber cells				
n of +ve cases				
-junction loss	2	3	2	3
-enlarg of intercell. spaces	1	2	1	2
-electron-density decrease	1	0	0	0
-swelling	0	0	0	0
-calcium deposits	0	0	1	0
-degeneration	0	0	0	0
S.E.M.				
-fibrin **/n of +ve cases	1.5/2	2/3	1.5/4	1.5/4
-holes **/n of +ve cases	3/3	2.5/2	2.5/2	1.5/2

* mean value of inflammation severity according to Hogan et al. (8)
** arbitrary mean value of morphological changes of the lens capsule
   (1=slight; 2=moderate; 3=severe).

T.E.M. :

in all four groups the most frequent observation was the loss of intercellular junctions among fibers and among epithelial cells, particularly along the lateral edges at basal and apical poles (Fig. 1).

The enlargement of intercellular spaces, due to junction loss, was mostly found in groups B and C.

The atrophy of cytoplasmatic organelles of the lenticular epithelial cells was more frequently observed in groups A and B: mitochondria appeared swollen with degenerated christae.

Occasional myelin-like bodies, multilamellar structures made up of masses of concentrically arranged membranes enclosing parts of the cell matrix,were seen (Fig.2). Nuclear fragmentations and ruptures of the lens cell membranes occurred in two cases. Cellular hypertrophy was never demonstrated, whereas pseudometaplasia was observed in one case (Fig. 2).

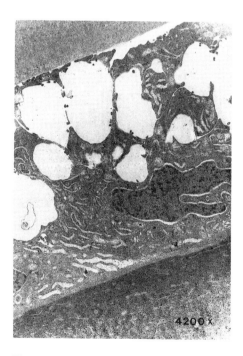

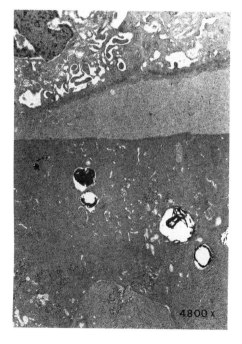

Fig.1.Loss of intercellular junctions, enlargement of intercellular spaces.

Fig.2.Pseudometaplasia and myelin-like bodies.

In one case belonging to group A, the electron microscopical appearance of the lenticular fiber cells was less dense,probably due to the paucity of fibrillar matrix. One case exhibited calcium scattered intracytoplasmatic deposits in the lenticular fibers. Neither swelling nor degeneration of lenticular cell fibers were ever observed.

All control lenses appeared completely intact as far as these parameters were concerned.

S.E.M.:

Thirteen out of 21 uveitic lenses, more often in groups C and D, showed on the anterior capsular surface a fine mesh of fibrin. In several cases, where the inflammation was more severe, a firm adherence of leukocytes and a fibrinous coating on the anterior capsular surface were evident (Fig. 3).

In nine cases "holes", about 1μ in diameter, were seen on the outer surface of the anterior capsule (Fig. 4).

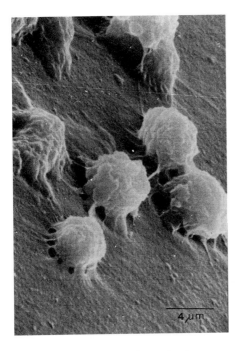 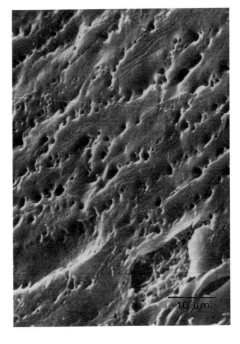

Fig.3.Leukocytes on the anterior capsular surface of the lens.

Fig.4."Holes" on the outer surface of the anterior capsule.

The anterior capsular surface of the control lenses was always intact and smooth, without any fibrin mesh.

CONCLUSIONS

The T.E.M. observation of lenses from eyes which suffered from experimental allergic inflammation showed three chronologically subsequent stages of lesion: 1. an initial stage, characterized by loss of junctions and enlargement of the intercellular spaces; 2. an intermediate stage, with degeneration of cytoplasmic organelles; 3. a stage of lasting (irreversible?) damage, with rupture of the cell membrane and nuclear fragmentation.

Our S.E.M. findings confirm that, after an initial stage characterized by a firm adherence of leukocytes and a fibrinous coating on the anterior capsular surface (related to the acute exudative phase of the uveitis), a more important membrane damage characterized by the appearance of actual "holes" may take place. Such "holes" may appear also after a single inflammatory episode, and correlate with our previous findings concerning the post-inflammatory lens permeability changes (efflux of K+, accumulation of Na+ and H_2O, leakage of soluble proteins), possibly relevant in both development of complicated cataract in uveitis and self-maintenance of certain kinds of uveitis which relapse through an autoimmune pathogenesis.

A close relationship between number of inflammatory relapses and entity of the lens morphological damage could not be identified while a correlation between severity of the relapses and entity of the lens damage was usually clear.

REFERENCES

1. D'Ermo F, Secchi AG, Mancini B, Fregona IA (1978) Immunopathology of the lens. I. 86Rb efflux and protein leakage from normal lenses exposed to unrelated antigen-antibody interactions. Ophthalmologica 176:164-169

2. D'Ermo F, Secchi AG, Mancini B, Segato T, Fregona IA (1978) Immunopathology of the lens. II. 86Rb efflux and protein leakage from normal lenses exposed to antilens and antiuveoretinal antibodies. Ophthalmologica 176:230-234

3. D' Ermo F, Secchi AG, Segato T, Mancini B, Fregona IA (1978) Immunopathology of the lens. III. The effects of experimental allergic uveitis on the cation balance in the lens. Ophthalmologica 176:258-261

4. Secchi AG, Fregona IA, D'Ermo F (1979) Lens Permeability Factors (LPF) in the aqueous humor during ocular inflammation. In: Silverstein AM, O'Connor G (eds) Immunology and Immunopathology of the Eye. Masson, New York, pp 58:61

5. Secchi AG, Fregona IA, D'Ermo F (1979) Lysophosphatidyl choline in the aqueous humor during ocular inflammation. Brit J Ophthal 63:768-770

6. Secchi AG (1982) Cataracts in Uveitis. Trans Ophthal Soc U K 102:390-394

7. Secchi AG, Fregona IA (1986) Lens permeability changes related to uveal "immune" inflammation. Lens Research 3:201-206

8. Hogan MJ, Kimura SJ, Thygeson P (1959) Signs and symptoms of uveitis. Am J Ophthalmol 47:155-170

© 1990 Elsevier Science Publishers (Biomedical Division)
Ocular Immunology Today. M. Usui, S. Ohno and K. Aoki, editors.

EXPERIMENTAL LENS-INDUCED GRANULOMATOUS ENDOPHTHALMITIS IN GUINEA PIGS

SEI-ICHI ISHIMOTO, HIROKI SANUI, TATSURO ISHIBASHI, HAJIME INOMATA
Department of Ophthalmology, Faculty of Medicine, Kyushu University, Fukuoka, Japan

ABSTRACT

We have produced an experimental lens-induced granulomatous endophthalmitis (ELGE) after one intravitreous injection with porcine serum albumin (PSA) and lens disruption in guinea pigs that had previously treated with only one systemic sensitization with PSA in complete Freund's adjuvant. This method is a new and easier way to produce ELGE. Histopathologically, the present animal model showed a typical zonal granulomatous inflammation around the ruptured lens. These findings resemble those in the patients of lens-induced endophthalmitis.

INTRODUCTION

Lens-induced endophthalmitis are seen in the patients with spontaneous rupture of hypermature cataract or traumatic injury of the lens capsule. Histopathologically granulomatous inflammation around the lens is detected in the disease. Experimental model of the disease has been produced previously, but frequent antigen administrations were required[1].

The purpose of this experiment is to establish a new and easier way to produce experimental model of lens-induced endophthalmitis.

MATERIALS AND METHODS

Female Hurtley guinea pigs (300-400g) were injected subcutaneously with 1mg of PSA in complete Freund's adjuvant. One month later, posterior capsule of the lens was disrupted by 27G needle through pars plana and 50 ug of PSA was injected into the vitreous simultaneously. As a control, animals were injected into the vitreous with either 50 ug of egg albumin or saline in stead of PSA. Two weeks later some animals were treated again in the same way. Two weeks after the last treatment, the eyes were enucleated, fixed with 6 % neutral formalin and embedded in paraffin. The sections were stained with hematoxylin and eosin.

RESULTS

The granulomatous inflammation were detected 20% of the 10
animals with lens injured once and 40% of 20 animals with lens
injured twice.   These lesions were not found in the control groups.
Histological examination showed a typical zonal granulomatous
inflammatory lesion around the ruptured lens (Fig.1).   A large
number of polymorphonuclear leukocytes (PMNs) and macrophages
infiltrated in and around the injured lens.   Epithelioid cells and
giant cells were also observed (Fig.2).   The lesions were
surrounded by cyclitic membrane with plasma cells and lymphocytes to
form the outer zone of the inflammation.

DISCUSSION

Marak et al produced ELGE after injury to the lens in rats that
had been previously sensitized to homologous lens protein[1].   But
antigen were injected 6 times at 2-week intervals to induce disease

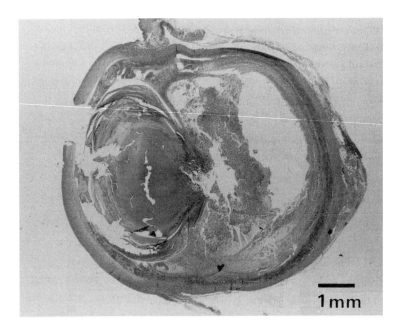

1mm

Fig.1.   A marked inflammatory infiltration is seen in the vitreous
and around the ruptured lens of guinea pig 14 days after disruption
of the lens.   The eye shows iridocyclitis and chorioretinitis.
Hematoxylin and eosin staining.

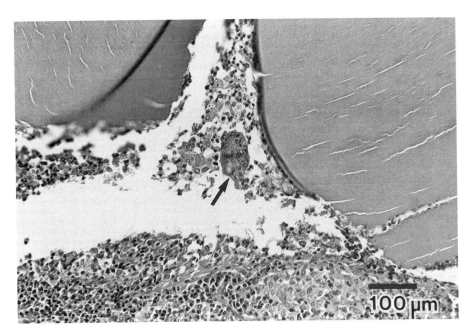

Fig.2.   A light micrography of inflammatory cells infiltrated
around lens.   PMNs and macrophages are seen around the injured
lens.   Epitheloid and giant cells phagocytizing the lens material
are found.   An arrow indicates multinucleated giant cell.
Hematoxylin and eosin staining.

in their experiment.   In the present experimental model, ELGE could
be produced by only one systemic and one local injection and in
shorter time.

Aronson et al reported that the inflammatory activity was
enhanced after accidental lens injury during intraocular injection
of the bovine gamma globulin (BGG) in previously BGG sensitized
rabbits[2].   The histopathologic feature revealed a macrophagic
response around remnants of lens material, but granulomatous
inflammation was not found.   Unlike large rupture of the lens
capsule in our experiment, a small rupture in their experiment may
result in leaking less lens material into the vitreous and inducing
non-granulomatous inflammation.

Lens-induced endophthalmitis in human shows a zonal
granulomatous lesion around the lens with giant cells[3].   A similar

pathological changes to those in human were seen in the present experiment. Thus, this experimental model may be useful to analyze lens-induced endophthalmitis in human.

ACKNOWLEDGEMENTS

We thank for Dr. Taiji Sakamoto for expert technical assistance.

REFERENCES

1. Marak,G E, et al(1974) Experimental lens-induced granulomatous endophthalmitis: Preliminary histopathologic observations. Exp Eye Res 19:311-316

2. Aronson,S B, et al(1971) Altered vascular permeability in ocular inflammatory disease. Arch Ophthalmol 85:455-466

3. Inomata,H, et al(1982) Bilateral lens-induced chronic granulomatous endophthalmitis: A histopathological study. Jap Clinic Ophthalmol 36:241-250

© 1990 Elsevier Science Publishers (Biomedical Division)
Ocular Immunology Today. M. Usui, S. Ohno and K. Aoki, editors.

EXPERIMENTAL CHRONIC UVEITIS IN RATS

HIROKI SANUI[+], IORI MOROOKA[+], HAJIME INOMATA[+] & IGAL GERY[*]
Kyushu University[+], Fukuoka (Japan)
National Eye Institute[*], Bethesda (USA)

ABSTRACT

Lewis rats were immunized with R4, synthetic peptide(23-mer) derived from bovine IRBP, developed mild and chronic EAU (experimental autoimmune uveoretinitis). The inflammation was induced 14 days after immunization and persisted 23 days after the onset. Histologically, the eyes exhibited severe inflammation in the anterior segment and mild inflammation in the posterior segment. Mild retinal detachment with exudates was observed in the early stage, and focal granulomatous lesions are seen in the later stage. The granulomatous lesion was similar to Dalen-Fuch's nodule in sympathetic ophthalmia. It is thought that this experimental animal is a good model for analysis of chronic granulomatous uveitis in human.

INTRODUCTION

Sympathetic ophthalmia and Vogt-Koyanagi-Harada disease (VKH), are chronic and recurrent uveitis characterized by granulomatous inflammation in the choroid. Experimental uveitis has been induced by retinal antigens, S antigen or interphotoreceptor retinoid binding protein (IRBP), in rats[1], guinea-pigs, mice, rabbits or monkeys. However, most of the experimental uveitis exhibit non-granulomatous severe inflammation in the retina and/or choroid. We found that some synthetic peptides, derived from bovine IRBP, induced uveitis in Lewis rat in the experiments to detect uveitogenic sites of bovine IRBP[2]. One of the peptides, named R4, induced mild and late-onset uveitis. In the present study, we studied histologically the uveitis induced by R4.

MATERIALS & METHODS

Male inbred Lewis rats were immunized with 200µg of R4 or 5µg of whole IRBP in complete Freund's adjuvant into hind footpad with Bordetella pertussis intravenously. Rats were monitored daily clinically and eyes were enucleated at various time after the immunization. Eyes were fixed with 4% glutaraldehyde in cacodylate

buffer and 6% neutral formalin, embedded in paraffin.   Sections
were stained with hematoxylin and eosin.

RESULTS

    The rats developed EAU 14 days after immunization with R4,
while 11 days after immunization with whole IRBP.   In the early
stage, one or two days after the onset, the anterior chamber showed
inflammatory cell infiltration with polymorphonuclear leukocytes
(PMNs) and exudates in either rats immunized with R4 or whole IRBP.
Inflammatory cells, mainly mononuclear cells, also infiltrated into
the iris and ciliary body.   In the posterior segment of the eye,
mild exudative retinal detachment and mononuclear cell infiltration
occurred some focal areas of the retina in the rats immunized with
R4 (Fig. 1), while severe retinal detachment was found in the rats
immunized with IRBP.   In the later stage, one or three weeks after
the onset, the anterior chamber became clear but some mononuclear
cells still remained in the iris of the rats immunized with R4.   In

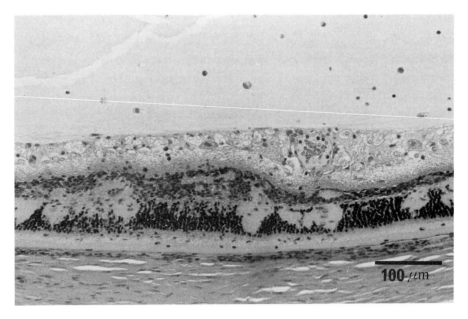

Fig. 1.   Posterior segment of the eye of rats 14 days after
immunization with R4.   Note mild exudative retinal detachment with
inflammatory cell infiltration.   Hematoxylin & eosin staining.

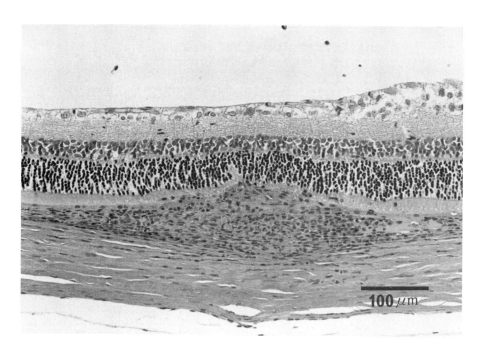

Fig. 2.   Posterior segment of the eye of rats 21 days after
immunization with R4.   A granulomatous lesion, being composed of
epithelioid cells and lymphocytes, is formed in the choroid.   The
lesion protrudes into the photoreceptor cell layer.   Hematoxylin &
eosin staining.

the posterior segment, granulomatous lesions, being composed of

epithelial cells and lymphocytes, were observed in the choroid of

the rats immunized with R4.   The lesion formed a mound with

inflammatory cells and protruded into the retina(Fig. 2).   Some

eyes showed a focal damage of the photoreceptor cells.   The

granulomatous lesions were observed even at 24 days after the onset.

On the other hand, most of photoreceptor cells disappeared in the

rats immunized with whole IRBP.

DISCUSSION

    Most of experimental models of EAU exhibited non-granulomatous

inflammation.   Some experiments, such as immunization with IRBP in

monkeys or that with S antigen in guinea-pigs, induced chronic

inflammation with epithelioid cells in the choroid.   In rats,

inflammation induced by retinal uveitogenic antigens usually showed severe retinal detachment with mononuclear cell infiltration and minimally affected choroid[1]. In this study, we could produce mild, long-lasting inflammation and typical granulomatous nodules, resembling Dalen-Fuch's nodule, in the choroid in rats. There are some reasons why mild EAU could be induced in this experiment. The first, R4 is so small that it may not have enough inflammation-enhancing components which are involved in whole IRBP. The second, R4 may not be able to provoke enough immune responses to produce severe uveitis since R4 induces high cellular immunity but low humoral immunity, while whole IRBP induces high cellular and humoral immunity[3]. This model may be a good system for analysis of chronic granulomatous uveitis in human since it exhibits mild and chronic inflammation with granuloma in the choroid.

REFERENCES

1. Gery I, Wiggert B, et al (1986) Uveoretinitis and pinealitis induced by immunization with interphotoreceptor retinoid binding protein. Invest Ophthalmol Vis Sci 27:1296-1300

2. Sanui H, Redmond, TM, et al (1988) Synthetic peptides derived from IRBP induce EAU and EAP in Lewis rats. Curr Eye Res 7:727-735

3. Redmond TM, Sanui H, et al (1989) Immune responses to peptides derived from the retinal protein IRBP: Immunopatho-genic determinants are not necessarily immunodominant. Clin Immunol Immunopathol 53:212-224

© 1990 Elsevier Science Publishers (Biomedical Division)
Ocular Immunology Today. M. Usui, S. Ohno and K. Aoki, editors.

CELLULAR EVENTS IN THE ADOPTIVE TRANSFER OF EXPERIMENTAL AUTOIMMUNE UVEORETINITIS IN RATS

X. Y. ZHANG, S. KOTAKE, L-H. HU, B. WIGGERT, T.M. REDMOND, G.J. CHADER AND I. GERY.

The National Eye Institute, NIH, Bethesda, MD USA

INTRODUCTION

Adoptive transfer of experimental autoimmune uveoretinitis (EAU) is a useful tool to investigate the immunopathogenesis of this animal disease which is considered a model for certain uveitic conditions in man (1, 2). EAU may be adoptively transferred to naive recipient rats by lymphocytes from donors immunized against uveitogenic antigens, provided the cells are activated in vitro before being injected (3,4). Sensitized spleen cells (SpC) are activated for EAU induction by either the uveitogenic antigen, or by a non-specific mitogen, concanavalin A (Con A). On the other hand, lymph node cells (LNC) become highly uveitogenic by activation with the antigen, but not by Con A (3, 4).

We report here on a study aimed at analyzing the inability of Con A to generate uveitogenicity in LNC sensitized against the interphotoreceptor retinoid-binding protein (IRBP).

MATERIAL AND METHODS

The procedure used for adoptive transfer of EAU was described in detail elsewhere (3, 4), while the method employed to meausre the proliferaiton response of spleen cells from recipient rats was detailed in reference (5).

The skin tests were carried out with recipient rats 2 days after cell transfer. The antigen, IRBP, was injected into the pinna of one ear (20 ug in 20 ul), while PBS was injected into the opposite ear. The data are expressed as net swelling of the ear injected with IRBP, in mm, at 24 hr after injection.

RESULTS

Con A does not stimulate suppressor cells in cultured LNC. The deficient immunological capacity in LNC stimulated with Con A could be attributed to an excessive activation of suppressor cells in these cultures. This hypothesis was tested by injecting recipient rats with mixtures of Con A-stimulated LNC and uveitogenic IRBP- stimulated LNC. The EAU development in recipients of these cell mixtures is summarized in Table 1. Addition of the Con A- stimulated LNC had no effect on the uveitogenicity of the IRBP-stimulated cells, thus indicating that the inactivity of the Con A-stimulated cells is not due to an excessive suppressor cell effect.

TABLE 1

Con A - stimulated LNC   do not suppress uveitogenic lymphocytes

Injected cells*(x10^{-6})		EAU in recipients		
IRBP-stim	Con A -stim.†	Positive/total	Severity (mean±SEM)	Onset day (mean±SEM)
20	0	3 / 5	1.3±0.3	5.0±0.0
100	0	5 / 6	1.4±0.2	4.2±0.2
20	20	3 / 6	1.0±0.0	6.3±0.3
20	100	4 / 5	0.8±0.1	6.5±0.5
100	100	5 / 6	1.4±0.2	4.8±0.8

* LNC from donors immunized against IRBP were cultured with either IRBP or Con A and mixed, as indicated, before being injected into recipients.
† LNC cultured with Con A did not cause disease at the numbers tested here.

Con A generates uveitogencity in LNC in the presence of naive SpC.
Another hypothesis to explain the inactivity of Con A-stimulated LNC attributes this phenomenon to a lack of a cellular component in the LNC, which is essential for the activation of uveitogenic lymphocytes. This hypothesis was tested by adding SpC from naive rats to cultures of IRBP-sensitized LNC during the incubation with Con A. Fig. 1 summarizes the data of repeated experiments and shows that, indeed, the addition of naive SpC facilitated the generation of uveitogenicity in these cultures. In addition, the recipeint rats of these mixed cultures exhibited cellular immune responses with levels similar to those measured in recipients of IRBP-stimulated LNC. The facilitating effect of SpC was obtained with either fresh or irradiated cells, thus underscoring the accessory role of the SpC in this system.

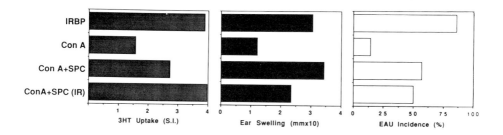

Fig. 1. Development of EAU and immune responses to IRBP in recipient rats. The recipients were injected with 10^8 LNC from IRBP-immunized donors, following incubation in vitro with IRBP (3µg/ml), Con A (2µg/ml), or with Con A in the presence of naive SpC. The LNC were cultured at 2×10^6/ml, while the naive SpC, untreated or irradiated (3000 R) ("IR"), were added to a concentration of 1×10^6/ml.

DISCUSSION

The main issue addressed here has been the inability of Con A-stimulated LNC to adoptively transfer EAU. Two hypothetical explanations for this finding have been examined. The first, attributing the finding to an excessive activation of suppressor cells by Con A, was ruled out by the cell mixing experiments: Con A-stimulated LNC did not affect the uveitogenic activity of IRBP- stimulated LNC (Table 1). On the other hand, our data are in line with the second hypothesis, that Con A fails to generate uveitogenicity in LNC because of a deficiency in an essential accessory cell in these cultures: addition of naive SpC to the LNC cultures significantly increased the uveitogenic activity of these cultures (Fig 1).

The putative accessory cell which is assumed to be lacking in the LNC cultures is still unknown. In preliminary studies, not recorded here, we did not find any significant effect by cytokines produced by macrophages (interleukin 1) or T-lymphocytes (interleukin 2). More studies are underway, to identify the putative accessory cell and its mode of action.

Another noteworthy finding in this study is the correlaiton between the development of EAU and cellular immune responses in the recipient rats (Fig 1). This suggests that the same cell population mediates the disease and the immune responses, or, if different populations are involved, that the activation mechanisms are the same.

178

SUMMARY

We have investigated the inability of Con A to generate uveitogenicity in LNC sensitized against IRBP. The data do not support the hypothesis that Con A stimulates excessive activity of suppressor cells, but are in accord with the notion that LNC cultures are deficient of an accessory cell which is essential for the Con A effect. A correlation was observed in recipient rats between development of EAU and cellular immune responses toward IRBP.

REFERENCES

1. Faure JP (1980) Curr Top Eye Res 2:215.
2. Gery I. Mochizuki M, Nussenblatt RB (1986) Prog Retinal Res 5:75.
3. Mochizuki M, Kuwabara T, McAllister C, Nussenblatt RB, Gery I (1985) Invest Ophthalmol Vis Sci 26:1
4. McAllister CG, wiggert B, Chader GJ, Kuwabara T, Gery I (1987) J. Immunol 138:1416.
5. Hu LH, Redmond TM, Sanui H, Kuwabara T, McAllister CG, Wiggert B, Chader GJ, Gery I (1989) Cell Immunol 122:251.

© 1990 Elsevier Science Publishers (Biomedical Division)
Ocular Immunology Today. M. Usui, S. Ohno and K. Aoki, editors.

Regulation of Experimental Autoimmune Uveoretinitis and Class II Antigen Expression by Interferon-γ

Leslie S. Fujikawa, MD, Chris A. Larson, BA, Alexander Holmes, MD

Experimental autoimmune uveoretinitis (EAU) is a T-cell mediated disease in which class II major histocompatibility complex (MHC) antigens and interferon-γ (IFN-γ) may be expected to play a major role (1-3). Retinal antigen-specific CD4+ T cells are required for the induction of EAU (3), and in susceptible strains of rats, the onset of EAU is associated with the expression of class II antigens by retinal vascular endothelium (1,3). This may allow T cells to act locally in the induction of EAU. We have also demonstrated the induction of class II antigens on the retinal vascular endothelium in retinochoroidal biopsy specimens from patients with uveitis, upon systemic administration of IFN-γ, and *in vitro* upon addition of IFN-γ (4,5). Furthermore, it is likely that T-cell derived lymphokines such as IFN-γ are involved in the inflammatory processes that result in uveoretinitis.

In the present study, we investigated the hypothesis that local IFN-γ and the expression of class II antigens are important in the induction of EAU. Our results are consistent with a critical role for IFN-γ and the class II positive retinal vascular endothelium in the development of retinal inflammation during EAU.

Ocular Immunology Laboratory, Smith-Kettlewell Eye Research Institute, San Francisco, CA

Materials & Methods

Animals and induction of EAU. Lewis rats 195-230 gm were immunized with purified bovine interphotoreceptor retinoid binding protein (IRBP) 150 μg in complete Freund's adjuvant containing 2 mg/ml *Mycobacterium tuberculosis* (H37Ra) (Difco, Detroit, MI) without pertussis adjuvant (6). This was followed at 1 week by an intravitreal injection OD of between 10^2-10^4 U of recombinant rat IFN-γ (AM-Gen, Thousand Oaks, CA). Severity of EAU was assessed by biomicroscopy (6).

Animals were sacrificed at various times for up to 2 months post immunization, and eyes were removed for assay.

Monoclonal antibodies. Antibodies against class II antigens included OX6 (anti-I-A) and OX17 (anti-I-E), specific for the respective class II molecules of the rat; OX18 for class I antigen; OX19 - T cells; W3/25 - CD4+ cells, including T helper cells; OX8 - T suppressor/cytotoxic cells; OX42 - rat macrophages (Bioproducts for Science, Indianapolis, IN).

Immunohistochemistry. Frozen sections of eyes (4μm) were stained using an immunoperoxidase technique. Sections were incubated with primary antibody (monoclonal), followed by biotinylated rat anti-mouse IgG (Accurate, Westbury, NY), each

Table I.
Clinical Grading of Uveitis

Day of evaluation	Anterior chamber		Vitreous	
	O.D.	O.S.	O.D.	O.S.
0-7	0	0	0	0
8-11	3.2 + 0.4*	0.5 + 0.3	2.2 + 1.2	0.1 + 0.2
12-16	2.8 + 0.8	2.5 + 0.5	4.0 + 0.1	2.5 + 0.5
17-20	2.7 + 0.6	2.5 + 0.4	3.2 + 0.2	3.0 + 0.1

*Mean ± standard deviation. Each value represents the gradings of cellular activity on a scale from 0 to 4 in the anterior chamber or vitreous (6) from duplicate or triplicate experiments. Injected eyes (OD) demonstrated more severe inflammation than noninjected eyes (OS) at all time points after intravitreal injection of IFN-γ.

for 10 minutes at 37° Centigrade. This was followed by a 10-minute incubation with avidin plus biotinylated horse radish peroxidase (Vector, Burlingame, CA). Staining was done with 3,3'-diaminobenzidine, nickel sulfate, and hydrogen peroxide. Slides were counterstained with 1% methyl green.

OX6-^{125}I binding assay. Selected retinas were assayed using an OX6-^{125}I binding assay developed in our laboratory to quantitate class II antigen expression in the retina *in situ*. OX6 was labelled with ^{125}I (chloramine T) with specific activities of between 15 and 30 μCuries per μg of protein. Retinas were minced in balanced salt solution, followed by incubation with ^{125}I-OX6 for 30 minutes at 37° C. Retinas were washed to remove unreacted antibody, counted in a gamma counter (Beckman, Palo Alto, CA), and results expressed as counts per minute (cpm) per mg of retina.

Results

Clinical grading of uveitis. Injected eyes (OD) consistently demonstrated inflammation of earlier onset and greater severity than non-injected eyes (OS) (Table I). The mean day of development of both anterior and posterior uveitis was 10.8 days ± 0.8 for eyes injected with IFN-γ, versus 13.5 days ± 2.3 for noninjected eyes. In contrast, rats which did not receive IFN-γ developed panuveitis at 15.3 days ± 2.4.

Immunohistochemistry. *Retinal vascular endothelium.* Upon intravitreal injection of IFN-γ, the retinal vascular endothelium became positive for class II antigens within 3 days (Figure 1a). This class II antigen induction appeared at a time when there was no significant retinal inflammation by T cells. Inflammation around class II positive retinal vascular endothelium appeared sooner in the eye injected with IFN-γ (Figure 1b). Intense retinal vasculitis developed in both eyes (Figure 1c), and by 2 to 3 weeks after immunization, both injected and noninjected eyes demonstrated severe retinal inflammation (Figure 1d).

Overall inflammatory activity. OD: day 10 - moderate anterior uveitis and slight to moderate inflammation of the retina; day 14 - all eyes showed moderate to severe panuveitis; by day 17-20, severe retinal inflammation persisted, but anterior uveitis diminished. OS: day 10 - slight inflammation of iris and ciliary body; none in the retina; day 14 - iris and ciliary body had increased inflammation with the retina showing slight to moderate inflammation; by day 17-20, the retina showed severe inflammation.

Quantitation of class II antigen in the retina *in situ*. More class II antigen was expressed in the retina of injected eyes than in noninjected eyes at all time points observed post intravitreal injection of IFN-γ (days 10 to 21 post immunization with IRBP) (Figure 2).

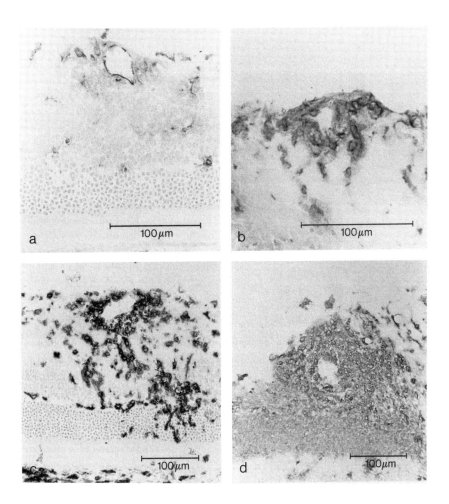

Figure 1. Intravitreal injection of IFN-γ and EAU. (a) By 3 days after intravitreal injection of IFN-γ, the retinal vascular endothelium became positive for class II antigens (OD). (b) Inflammation appeared around class II positive retinal vascular endothelium sooner in the eye injected with IFN-γ (OD). (c) Intense retinal vasculitis developed in both injected and noninjected eyes. (d) By 2 to 3 weeks after immunization, both eyes demonstrated severe retinal inflammation with much of the retina staining positively for class II antigens. (OX6, I-A).

Discussion

The present study clearly demonstrates the induction of class II antigens on the retinal vascular endothelium by the intravitreal injection of IFN-γ, which accelerated the onset and enhanced the severity of EAU in Lewis rats.

These results support our previous studies which indicate a critical role for the class II positive retinal vascular endothelium in the development of retinal inflammation during uveoretinitis (1,2,4,5). Because the capability of accessory cells to present antigen to T helper cells is dependent on the expression of class II antigens, expression of class II antigens on the retinal vascular endothelium is crucial in allowing these cells to participate in local antigen presentation, leading to activation and

182

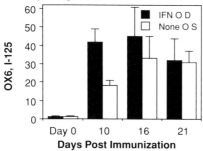

CPM per mg retina X 10-3

Figure 2. OX6-¹²⁵I binding assay revealed more class II antigen expression in the retina of injected eyes (OD) than noninjected eyes (OS).

recruitment of T cells into the site of a developing cell-mediated immune response in the retina. Furthermore, if cytotoxicity is effected by class II-restricted T cells in EAU, as has been suggested for experimental allergic encephalomyelitis (7), then the retinal vascular endothelium expressing class II antigens may serve as important targets for this immune response during uveitis.

Our results also indicate an important role for IFN-γ, a T-cell lymphokine which exerts potent biologic effects. For example, IFN-γ has been reported to augment the production of IL-1 by LPS-stimulated endothelial cells, which may partially underlie the ability of endothelial cells to act as antigen-presenting cells. In the present studies, IFN-γ demonstrated potent ocular inflammatory effects, accelerating and accentuating the natural course of ocular inflammation following systemic immunization with IRBP.

It is clear that IFN-γ led to significant class II antigen expression on the retinal vascular endothelium which preceded inflammation by T cells in the retina, and that this early expression of class II antigens in the retina was unique to the retinal vascular endothelium. This is consistent with our previous *in vitro* results (5) in which the retinal vascular endothelium expressed

much higher levels of class II antigen than retinal pericytes upon exposure to identical amounts of IFN-γ. Thus upon exposure to IFN-γ, the retinal vascular endothelium is most likely to become class II antigen positive and most likely to contribute to the immune response in the retina.

Other work in our laboratory indicates that immune recognition involves the direct binding of class II molecules to specific peptide fragments of retinal antigens and that this binding may correlate with MHC restriction in uveitis (8). Thus, the configuration of the class II molecule may determine its ability to bind retinal antigens thereby creating the bimolecular complex needed to trigger the T cell. These results may help explain immune regulation on a molecular basis, stressing the essential role of the class II molecule in determining immune responsiveness in uveitis.

These studies indicate a critical role for the class II positive retinal vascular endothelium in the development of retinal inflammation during uveitis, and serve as a basis for current *in vitro* studies on the capabilities of Lewis vs Brown Norway retinal vascular endothelial cells to present retinal antigen to syngeneic T cells.

Acknowledgments
Supported by NIH grant EY06948, Research to Prevent Blindness, Inc., NY, Smith-Kettlewell Eye Research Institute, and Pacific Presbyterian Medical Center, San Francisco, California.

References

1. Fujikawa LS (1989) *Ophthalmol* **96**:1115
2. Fujikawa LS et al (1987) *Cellular Immunology* **106**:139
3. Mochizuki M et al (1985) *Invest Ophthalmol Vis Sci* **26**:1
4. Fujikawa LS and Haugen J-P (1987) *Ophthalmol* **94**:136
5. Fujikawa LS et al (1989) *Invest Ophthalmol Vis Sci* **30**:66
6. Broekhuyse RM et al (1986) *Curr Eye Res* **5**:231
7. Fallis RJ et al (1989) *J Immunol* **143**:2160
8. Fujikawa LS (1990) *Invest Ophthalmol Vis Sci*, in press

© 1990 Elsevier Science Publishers (Biomedical Division)
Ocular Immunology Today. M. Usui, S. Ohno and K. Aoki, editors.

A NEW MODEL OF AUTOIMMUNE UVEO-RETINITIS IN NUDE MICE GRAFTED WITH EMBRYONIC RAT THYMUSES

T. ICHIKAWA[#$], T. TANAKA[$], J. SAKAI[$], M. USUI[$], O. TAGUCHI[#], H. IKEDA[&], T. TAKAHASHI[#], Y. NISHIZUKA[#]

[#]Aichi Cancer Center Research Institute, Chikusa-ku, Nagoya 464; [$]Department of Ophthalmology, Tokyo Medical College Tokyo 160; [&]First Department of Pathology, Aichi Medical University, Nagakute-cho, Aichi-ken 480-11 (Japan)

INTRODUCTION

Experimental uveo-retinitis can be induced in laboratory animals by active immunization with retinal S-antigen (1,2) or interphotoreceptor retinoid-binding protein (IRBP) (3,4), suggesting that autoimmune phenomena may play a significant role in the development of uveo-retinitis. Previously we reported that T cell function of congenitally athymic nude (nu/nu) mice can be recovered by implantation of embryonic rat thymic rudiments (TG nude). In the TG nude mice, however, multiple organ-localized autoimmune diseases, such as thyroiditis and gastritis, were observed to develop spontaneously (5). Recently we became to notice autoimmune lesions in the eyes that probably evoked by endogenous IRBP.

MATERIALS AND METHODS

Animals. Two lobes of thymuses harvested from 15-day-old embryonic F344 rats were grafted under renal subcapsule of 4-week-old BALB/c female nu/nu mice. The TG nude mice thus prepared were housed in a specific pathogen-free room.

Indirect immunofluorescence. Cryostat tissue sections of eyeballs from normal adult BALB/c mice and from bovines were fixed with acetone, incubated with sera of TG nude, normal BALB/c or normal BALB/c nu/nu mice, and followed by FITC-labeled anti-mouse IgG.

Immunoblot assay. Crude protein preparations from bovine retinae fractionated with ammonium sulfate solution were used for the target antigen. Proteins separated on 8 % SDS-polyacrylamide gel were transferred to nitrocellulose membranes. After incubation with 100-fold diluted sera, the membranes were stained with horse-radish peroxidase-labeled antisera. The sera used were rabbit anti-S antigen antiserum, rabbit anti-IRBP antiserum, and sera of TG nude mice, normal BALB/c mice, and normal BALB/c nu/nu mice.

Enzyme-linked immunosorbent assay. Microplates coated with purified bovine retinal S antigen or IRBP were incubated with serum from TG nude, normal BALB/c mice, or normal BALB/c nu/nu mice. These sera were tested in the range of 200 to 12,800-fold dilution. The microplates were stained with horse-radish peroxidase-labeled anti-mouse IgG, and read by a 2-wave microplate photometer (Corona, Japan) at 492 nm.

RESULT AND DISCUSSION

Grafted embryonic rat thymuses generally developed well macroscopically, and histologically formed a proper thymus architecture with cortex and medulla zones. In the eyes of TG nude mice, uveo-retinitis developed as early ocular lesions, i.e., as illustrated in Fig. 1, irregular or partial destruction of retinal layers with mild mononuclear cell infiltration around basement membrane and in ciliary body was noticed. Eventually, atrophic retinae with complete loss of photoreceptor layers from layer of rods and cones to outer nuclear layer was observed. Such lesions were found in 40 % (14/35) of 7-month-old TG nude mice, and the lesions developed always bilaterally. In the TG nude mice, a high incidence of severe inflammatory lesions was also found in several other organs, such as thyroid and stomach, as reported previously (5). These lesions were never found in euthymic BALB/c and normal BALB/c nu/nu mice.

As shown in Fig. 2, a circulating IgG antibody reacting with the pigment epithelium and the layer of rods and cones was detected in TG nude mice with uveo-retinitis. The antibody was also reacted with the same retinal layers of bovines. Identification of target antigen of the antibody was analyzed by

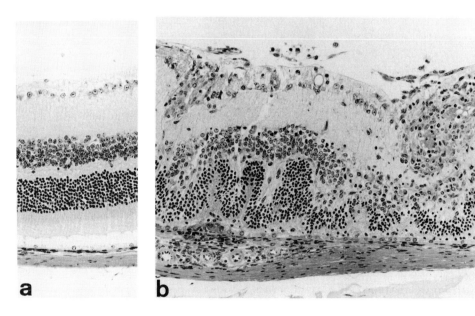

Fig. 1. (a) Normal retina of a normal BALB/c nu/nu mouse. (b) An early ocular lesion of a TG nude mouse.

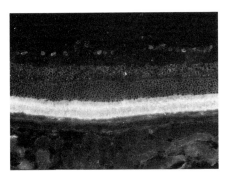

Fig. 2. A circulating IgG antibody reacting with the pigment epithelium and the layer of rods and cones.

immunoblotting assay using crude retinal antigens (Fig. 3) and also by enzyme-linked immunosorbent assay using retinal S antigen and IRBP. Both assays showed strong reactions with IRBP, but not S antigen, indicating that endogenous IRBP antigen is the target of autoimmunity in the TG nude mice.

The most important function of the thymus is to educate T cells to properly recognize self and nonself. The basis of this function is dependent upon the interactions between T cell precursors and non-lymphoid components such as the thymic epithelial cells. In the grafted thymuses of TG nude mice, the epithelial cells were of donor origin, but other tissues such as dendritic cells

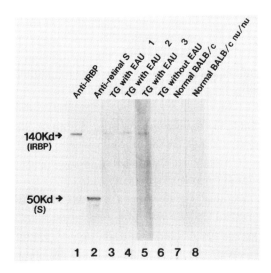

Fig. 3. Western immunoblot analysis of the antigen detected by an autoantibody against the photoreceptor layer in TG nude mice. Crude antigen preparation from bovine retinae fractionated with ammonium sulfate solution is used. Lanes 1 and 2 indicate IRBP and S protein that are detected by antiIRBP and anti-retinal S antiserum, respectively. Lanes 3-5, the band which shows the similar size of IRBP is stained with serum from TG nude mice with uveo-retinitis. Lanes 6-8, no blot is stained, when serum from TG nude mouse with normal retinae, from normal BALB/c mouse, and from BALB/c nu/nu mouse, is used.

186

and macrophages were of host origin (unpublished data). In our previous study (5), we demonstrated that T cell-mediated immune function in TG nude mice was recovered by the education in the grafted rat thymic environment. Severe organ-localized autoimmune lesions were, however, recognized in several organs including eyes. These lesions could be transferred to syngeneic BALB/c nu/nu mice by splenic L3T4 positive cells (6). These results altogether suggested that rat/mouse chimeric thymus micro-environment is able to reconstitute effector T cell function, but may not properly recover proper regulatory T cell function, probably because maturation or education of such T cells requires a more refined interaction in the thymus, as we proposed with the autoimmune disease model after newborn thymectomy (7, 8). Another possibility is that xenogeneic thymus may provide conditions to induce abnormal effector T cells, which can not be controlled by endogenous regulatory T cells. Pathogenesis of autoimmune diseases has long been associated with disorder of education cell-to-cell interactions in the thymus and our TG nude mouse model may be the case. Our model may provide a new useful tool for analysis of pathogenesis of uveo-retinitis.

ACKNOWLEDGMENTS   We thank Dr. H. Hiai for his encouragement and advice throughout this study. We also thank M. Izawa for technical assistance. This study was supported by a Special Coordination Fund from the Science and Technology Agency, Japan.

REFERENCES

1. Wacker WB, Lipton MM (1868) J Immunol 101:157-165

2. Donoso LA, Merryman CF, Sery TW, Shinohara T, Dietzschold B, Wistow G, Graft C, Morley W, Henry TT (1986) Curr Eye Res 6:1151-1159

3. Faure JP (1980) In: Zadunaisky JA, Davson H (eds) Curr Topics in Eye Research, Vol. 2. Academic Press, New York, 215-302

4. Sanui H, Redmont TM, Hu L-H, Kuwabara T, Margalit H, Cornette JL, Wiggert B, Chader GJ, Gery I (1988) Curr Eye Res 7:727-735

5. Taguchi O, Takahashi T, Seto M, Namikawa R, Matsuyama M, Nishizuka Y (1986) J Exp Med 164:60-71

6. Ikeda H, Taguchi O, Takahashi T, Itoh G, Nishizuka Y (1988) J Exp Med 168:2397-2402

7. Taguchi O, Nishizuka Y (1987) J Exp Med 165:146-156

8. Taguchi O, Takahashi T, Nishizuka Y (1990) Current Opinion Immunol 2: in press

© 1990 Elsevier Science Publishers (Biomedical Division)
Ocular Immunology Today. M. Usui, S. Ohno and K. Aoki, editors.

POLYMORPHONUCLEAR LEUKOCYTE-INDUCED RETINAL DAMAGE IN EXPERIMENTAL AUTOIMMUNE UVEITIS (EAU)

HIROSHI GOTO, GUEY-SHUANG WU, FEN CHEN, LILY ATALLA, NARSING A RAO

Doheny Eye Institute, 1355 San Pablo Street
Los Angeles, California, USA

INTRODUCTION

In inflammation, tissue damage is caused by various chemical mediators derived from either plasma proteins or inflammatory phagocytic cells, i.e., polymorphonuclear leukocytes (PMNs) and macrophages. It has been shown that these phagocytes undergo "respiratory burst" and release reactive oxygen metabolites, including superoxide and hydrogen peroxide. These metabolites and their secondary oxygen radicals cause tissue damage by various mechanisms, one of the prominent process being peroxidation of cell membrane lipids. As retina contains abundant polyunsaturated fatty acids that are susceptible to in vivo peroxidation, it is plausible that those activated phagocytes cause retinal damage via lipid peroxidation. In experimental uveitis induced by retinal S-antigen, Lewis rats develop acute retinitis and pan uveitis. The infiltrating inflammatory cells consist of mononuclear cells admixed with polymorphonuclear leukocytes. Histopathologically, it appears that degree of PMN infiltration depends on the severity of uveo-retinitis.

In recent studies, the myeloperoxidase (MPO), which is present in large amounts in the azurophil granules of PMN, has often been applied as a marker for PMN infiltration in tissues.

In this study, we investigated the damaging effects of free radicals generated by phagocytes in experimental autoimmune uveoretinitis (EAU) by correlating the levels of MPO with various products of retinal lipid peroxidation.

MATERIAL AND METHODS

Lewis rats weighing approximately 175 g were given a single hind foot-pad injection of 50 μg of purified bovine retinal S-antigen (1) in complete Freund's adjuvant and an intravenous injection of 1 μg of pertussis toxin. Animals were sacrificed 7, 9, 12, 15 and 18 days after immunization. The eyes were enucleated at these time points, fixed in 10% formalin and stained with hematoxylin and eosin to evaluate histopathologic changes.

Superoxide production in the inflammatory infiltrate was measured by the reduction of nitroblue tetrazolium (NBT) (2). Retinas and choroids were dissected from rats with EAU, and the tissue fragments placed on a glass slide were exposed to 0.1% NBT. The slide was covered and incubated at 37° C in 5% CO_2 for 1 hour.

Myeloperoxidase assay

To determine the level of MPO activity in the retinas and choroids, the method described by Bradley was used (3). One unit of MPO activity was defined as that degrading 1.0 μ mole of peroxide per minute at 25°C. The degradation of 1.0 μl mole of peroxide gives a change in extinction per minute of 1.13 x 10^{-2}(4).

Measurement of lipid peroxidation products

Three distinct products of lipid peroxidation were measured using the retinas and choroids on various time points after immunization. These consisted of conjugated dienes, malondialdehyde (MDA) and fluorescent chromolipids. The details of the method were described before (5,6).

RESULTS

Histopathologic Examination

Retina showed no inflammatory damage 7 days postimmunization of S-antigen. On day 9, focal degeneration of outer retina along with edema and a few acute inflammatory cells were noted in the retina. However, the photoreceptor layers were relatively well-preserved. At the peak of the inflammation, on day 12, the infiltrate was markedly increased in the retina, which showed degeneration and necrosis of the outer retina. The cellular infiltrate consisted mostly of PMNs. On day 15, severe retinal destruction was noted. However, the number of inflammatory cells was less than that on day 12. The inflammation was considerably reduced by day 18 and the retina was atrophic and gliotic. The infiltrate was mostly made up of mononuclear cells at this stage.

The retinas and choroids obtained from rats with EAU revealed a positive reaction consisting of intracellular blue staining granules when exposed to NBT. Most of these positive cells apear to be PMNs. Several mononuclear cells with abundant cytoplasm were also positive.

Measurement of PMN infiltration using myeloperoxidase assay
Retinas and choroids obtained from normal control rats showed no MPO activity. No significant elevation of MPO activity was detected on day 7. Begining with the onset of the disease on day 9, there was a sharp increase in MPO level, to a maximum on day 12, and then the activity decreased relatively slowly to day 18.

Measurement of lipid peroxidation products

Elevated levels of conjugated dienes, MDA and fluorescent chromolipid were noted in the inflamed eyes, however the levels of these peroxidation products varied at different time periods. The amounts of conjugated dienes increased from day 9 to 12, peaked on day 12 to 2.7 fold that of the control level decreased slowly thereafter. The levels of MDA increased rapidly to a maximum on day 12, then fell rather rapidly on day 18 to a level even lower than that of the control. At the maximum, on day 12, the increase of conjugated dienes above the control level (13 nmole/eye) was much higher than that resulting from MDA (1 nmole/eye). The production of fluorescent chromolipids was slightly delayed compared with the other two parameters. On day 9, control level was observed which increased sharply to the maximum recorded on day 12, followed by decrease.

DISCUSSION

Histopathologic examination of the development of EAU revealed sequential retinal damage with inflammatory infiltrate increasing during the initial phase. The MPO activity was detected on day 9, following which the enzyme levels correlated with histopathologic findings. This enzyme is found in large amounts in PMN, comprising up to 5% of the dry weight of the cell, while other inflammatory cells possess little or no MPO (7). Although this enzyme level does not directly indicate the number of PMN infiltrate in the tissue, this method appear to be useful to estimate the extent or severity of acute uveoretinitis.

Inflammatory phagocytes such as PMNs and macrophages are known to liberate oxygen free radicals (8). We demonstrated the production of superoxide in the PMNs and presumably macrophages in the retina and choroid of experimental animals. The granular staining detected intracellularly is considered to be the superoxide dependent reduction of NBT to an insoluble formazan (2). The retina, in particular, the outer segment of the photoreceptors contain abundant amounts of polyunsaturated fatty acids, which are susceptible to peroxidation. Although mechanisms that initiate the peroxidation of cell membrane lipids in vivo are unknown, free radicals liberated from phagocytes or hydroxy radicals generated by the reaction of superoxide and hydrogen peroxide are known to cause chain reactions of lipid peroxidation (6,9).

Our results show various products of lipid peroxidation in the retina during development of EAU. It has been suggested that no one method by itself can be considered an accurate measure of lipid peroxidation due to the nonspecificity of some methods. In addition, due to the labile nature of some products of lipid peroxidation, it is necessary to utilize more than one parameter for their detection. Hence, it has been suggested that an attempt should be made to measure several products of lipid peroxidation in order to confirm its occurence in a given tissue (2,10). All products of lipid peroxidation determined in this study followed a similar pattern of time-dependent kinetics during the course of EAU. In addition, these changes generally appeared to parallel PMN infiltration, as estimated by MPO assay. Peroxidation of the polyunsaturated fatty acid of cell membrane lipids can lead to breakdown of the membrane secretory function and transmembrane ionic gradients (11). Such alteration can result in cellular edema, degeneration and necrosis. Even though the precise mechanism of initiation of lipid peroxidation is not clear in this experimental model, our present study suggests that the retinal damage caused by the infiltrating leukocytes is from free radicals mediated lipid peroxidation. Presence of high levels of lipid peroxidation products in the initial stages of uveitis and low levels during the late stage indicates that the lipid peroxidation is the cause of retinal damage rather than the consequence of retinal necrosis. These studies provide basis for developing drugs with antioxidant properties to prevent retinal damage in uveitis.

ACKNOWLEDGEMENTS

Supported in part by NIH Grant Nos. EY 06953 and EY 05662

REFERENCES

1. Dorey C, Cozette J, Faure JP (1982) Ophthalmic Res 14:249-255

2. Ryer-Powder JE, Forman HJ (1989) Free Radical Biol Med 6:513-518

3. Bradley P, Priebat DA, Christensen RD, Rothstein G (1982) Invest Dermatology 78:206-209

4. Worthington Enzyme Manual (1972) Worthington Biochemical, Freehold, NJ, pp 43-45

5. Buege JA, Aust SD (1978) Methods Enzymol 52:302-310

6. Ward PA, Till GO, Hatherill JR, Annesley, Kunkel RG (1985) J Clinical Invest 76:517-527

7. Schultz J, Kaminker K (1962) Arch Biochem Biophys 96:465-467

8. Weiss SJ, LoBuglio AF (1982) Lab Invest 47:5-18

9. Rao NA, Fernandez MA, Cid LL, Romero JL, Sevanian A (1987) Arch Ophthalmol 105:1712-1716

10. Tribble DL, AW TY, Jones DP (1987) Hepatology 7:377-387

11. Halliwell B, Guteridge JMC (1985) In: Halliwell B, Gutteridge JMC (eds) Free Radicals in Biology and Medicine. Clarendon, Oxford, pp 139-170

© 1990 Elsevier Science Publishers (Biomedical Division)
Ocular Immunology Today. M. Usui, S. Ohno and K. Aoki, editors.

EXPERIMENTAL   PROLIFERATIVE   VITREORETINOPATHY   EVOKES   AUTOIMMUNE
RESPONSIVENESS TO RETINAL PHOTORECEPTOR ANTIGENS

AJJM RADEMAKERS, AHM VAN VUGT, HJ WINKENS, RM BROEKHUYSE.
Institute of Ophthalmology, University of Nijmegen, The Netherlands

INTRODUCTION

Proliferative vitreoretinopathy (PVR) remains the most significant
cause of surgical failure in the management of retinal detachment. It
is characterized by the proliferation of macrophages, fibroblasts,
glial cells and pigment epithelial cells as cellular elements (1).
Inflammatory cells have been seen in the initial stage of experimental
traction retinal detachment (2; present results). The possibility of
intraocular inflammatory and macrophage responses in direct relation
to wound healing and so to the pathogenesis of PVR has been argued
(3).

We investigated the immune responsiveness to S-antigen, opsin and
interphotoreceptor retinoid binding protein (IRBP) in animals with
experimental PVR.

MATERIALS AND METHODS

PVR was induced in New Zealand rabbits by intravitreal injection of
homologous fibroblasts. After dilation of the pupils the animals were
anesthetized by Hypnorm, and 500,000 fibroblasts were injected in the
vitreous cavity of both eyes. Animals injected similarly with buffer
alone or with fixed fibroblasts served as controls. Under indirect
binocular ophthalmoscopic control, the cells were carefully deposited
in the vitreous in front of and close to the optic nerve head. For a
period of eight weeks the development of PVR was studied by slit-lamp
and indirect ophthalmoscopy. Staging of the PVR was recorded according
to Fastenberg et al. (4). Inflammatory cell reaction in the anterior
chamber and in the vitreous was scored as well.

Bovine S-antigen, opsin (extensive washed rod outer segments), IRBP
and rabbit antisera to these test antigens were prepared as described
previously (5,6). Humoral immune responses to the three antigens were
essayed by ELISA (7). Cellular immune responses were determined by
lymphocyte transformation in vitro and were expressed as stimulation
indices (8).

RESULTS

PVR developed in the first 2 to 3 weeks after cell injection. Moderate inflammatory cell infiltration in the vitreous was observed predominantly in the posterior segment and the score peaked at day 5 after injection.

We subdivided the animals in a group with maximum PVR score 3 and a group with severe PVR, score 4-5. It was striking that the difference in the inflammation scores of these two groups occurred already in the earliest stages. These were highest in the group exhibiting severe PVR later on.

Rabbits with PVR score 4-5 exhibited variable and yet consistently elevated stimulation indices (Table 1). Most animals with elevated cellular immune responses were found in the period from 3-6 weeks after fibroblast injection, i.e. 1-2 weeks after severe PVR had developed. Remarkable was the more frequently found reactivity against the soluble retinal photoreceptor cell layer proteins (S-antigen, IRBP) than against the rod visual pigment protein (opsin), which is insoluble. No elevated humoral immune responses were found.

TABLE 1

INFLUENCE OF PVR STAGE AND CELLULAR AUTOIMMUNE RESPONSES TO PHOTORECEPTOR ANTIGENS

Test antigen	Percentages of animals with elevated SI[a]		Significance[b]
	PVR scores 0-3 (n = 5)	PVR scores 4-5 (n = 17)	
S-antigen	13 (2-40)%	82 (52-94)%	< 0.01
IRBP	0 (0-18)%	76 (47-94)%	< 0.01
Opsin	20 (4-48)%	65 (36-83)%	< 0.01

a Mean values (with 95% confidence intervals) of the percentages of rabbits with an elevated stimulation index (SI). SI was elevated if it was higher than all SI values in the controls during 8 weeks after injection of fibroblasts. These levels were 2.1, 2.5 and 3.3 for the three antigens, respectively.

b Level of significance for the difference in SI according to Fisher's exact test.

COMMENTS

Retina S-antigen, IRBP and opsin are now accepted as potent uveitogenic agents in animals. The fact that epiretinal membrane formation can be evoked by intraocular inflammation (9), and the possibility to reduce PVR by corticosteroids (10) point to an interaction between PVR and inflammation. We suggest that in the early stage of retinal detachment small amounts of soluble autoantigens are released. In advanced stages in which the blood retina-barrier is damaged, further autosensitization may be stimulated. Surgical treatment may enhance this effect and even can result in boosting. If the immune response exceeds a critical level marked inflammatory responses as observed in human PVR may arise. These phenomena may be taken into consideration in the treatment and further study of human PVR.

REFERENCES

1. Newsome DA, Rodrigues MM and Machemer R (1981) Arch Ophthalmol 99: 873-880

2. Usman JH, Lazarides E and Ryan SJ (1981) Arch Ophthalmol 99: 869-872

3. Miller B, Miller H, Patterson R and Ryan SJ (1986) Arch Ophthalmol 104: 281-285

4. Fastenberg DM, Diddie KR, Sorgente N and Ryan SJ (1982) Am J Ophthalmol 93: 559-564

5. Broekhuyse RM, Winkens HJ and Kuhlmann ED (1986) Curr Eye Res 5: 231-240

6. Broekhuyse RM, Rademakers AJJM, Van Vugt AHM and Winkens HJ (1990) Exp Eye Res 50: 197-202

7. Schalken JJ, Winkens HJ, Van Vugt AHM, Bovée-Geurts PHM, De Grip WJ and Broekhuyse RM (1988) Exp Eye Res 47: 135-145

8. Broekhuyse RM and Van Vugt AHM (1990) Ophthalmic Res 21: 436-439

9. Hiscott PS, Unger WG, Grierson I and McLeod D (1988) Curr Eye Res 7: 877-890

10. Chandler DB, Hida T, Sheta S, Proia AD and Machemer R (1987) Graefe's Arch Clin Exp Ophthalmol 225: 259-265

© 1990 Elsevier Science Publishers (Biomedical Division)
Ocular Immunology Today. M. Usui, S. Ohno and K. Aoki, editors.

GENETIC SUSCEPTIBILITY OF RAT STRAINS TO INDUCTION OF EAU IN RELATION WITH THE IMMUNE RESPONSE TO A PARTICULAR EPITOPE OF S-ANTIGEN

M. MIRSHAHI[1], Y. DE KOZAK[1], D.S. GREGERSON[2], R. STIEMER[3], C. BOUCHEIX[4] and J.P. FAURE[1]

[1]INSERM U 86, Centre de Recherche des Cordeliers, 15 rue de l'Ecole de Médecine, 75270 Paris 06, France; [2]University of Minnesota, Minneapolis, USA; [3]EMBL, Heidelberg, FRG; [4]INSERM U 268, Villejuif, France

INTRODUCTION

Different rat strains display different susceptibilities to induction of experimental autoimmune uveoretinitis (EAU) with S-antigen (1): Lewis rats are highly susceptible whereas Brown Norway are refractory. However, all strains develop a humoral response against S-antigen.

Immunization of Lewis rats against some murine monoclonal antibodies (mAbs) to S-antigen inhibits EAU induction by subsequent challenge with S-antigen (2) (see De Kozak et al., this symposium). These mAbs, S2D2 (the most effective for EAU suppression), S6H8 and S7D6, recognize an epitope ("S2 epitope") highly conserved during evolution (3) and located in the N-terminal region of the amino acid (aa) sequence of S-antigen: they react with the N-terminal 12 kDa fragment from chymotrypsin digest (fragment 99) and with N-terminal fragments CB 74 (74 aa) and CB 47 (47 aa) from cyanogen bromide digest of S-antigen. Precise localization of the S2 epitope was determined using Pepscan method (4) in the sequence of aa 40 to 50 (peptide S2) (R. Stiemer et al., article in preparation). It is distant from the uveitopathogenic region (fragment CB 123, aa 198-320) which contains the antigenic sites involved in EAU production (5). Another mAb, S9E2, without protective activity against EAU, recognizes an epitope near the C-terminus (CNBr fragment CB 46, aa 361-369).

The suppressive activity of mAb S2D2 suggests that the S2 epitope plays a special role in susceptibility to EAU. In this study, we compared the humoral response to this epitope in rats of the susceptible Lewis and the refractory BN strains immunized with S-antigen.

METHODS

Lewis and BN rats were immunized with 50 μg of S-antigen with complete Freund's adjuvant and H. pertussis vaccine (6).Two methods were used to analyse epitopic specificity of antibodies in their serum.

Reactivity of rat sera with peptide fragments of S-antigen

Digestion of S-antigen (2 mg) by chymotrypsin (20 μg in 1 ml of PBS with 0.1% polyethylene glycol 4000) for 48 h at 4°C led to several peptide fragments which were separated by reverse phase HPLC. A 12 kDa fragment (fragment 99) reacted in ELISA with S2D2, S6H8 and other mAbs. Sequencing its 10 N-terminal amino acids showed that this fragment represents the N-terminal region of S-antigen. Another fragment, 79, was recognized by S9E2. The reactivity of rat sera was tested by ELISA on plates coated with purified fragments 79 or 99.

Peptide fragments were produced by a limited CNBr digestion of S-antigen. These fragments (CB peptides) have been located in the aa sequence of the protein. They are identified on Western blots by their reactivity with polyclonal antibodies to each CB peptide (7). Such blots were used for assaying the reactivity of sera from S-antigen-immunized Lewis and BN rats with CB peptides.

Antibodies were also determined on ELISA plates coated with two synthetic peptides: the immunopathogenic peptide M (aa 303-320) and the peptide S2 bearing the epitope recognized by mAbs S2D2 and S6H8.

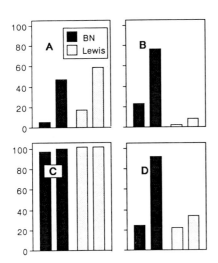

Fig. 1. Reactivity of antibodies in sera of S-antigen-immunized BN and Lewis rats with peptide fragments of S-antigen: chymotrypsin fragments 79 (A) and 99 (B), synthetic peptides M (C) and S2 (D). Antibody levels are expressed as the ratio of ELISA reading on peptide-coated plate over ELISA reading on S-antigen-coated plate, at two different times after immunization, 10 and 18 days in A and B and 11 and 32 days in C and D (mean of 5 rats in each group). EAU-susceptible Lewis rats have a low response to peptides of the N-terminal region of S-antigen containing the S2 epitope (B, D), compared to EAU-refractory BN rats.

Competition assay for the presence of "S2D2 blocking antibodies" in rat sera

S-antigen-coated plates (1 µg/ml) were incubated with serial dilutions of rat serum, then with mAb S2D2 at subsaturating concentration (0.5 µg/ml). The binding of S2D2 was detected using a biotinylated rat mAb specific for mouse kappa chain and not cross reacting with rat immunoglobulins (RAMK, Immunotech, Marseille-Luminy, France) followed by streptavidin-peroxidase complex (Amersham, UK) revealed by orthophenylene diamine-hydrogene peroxide.

RESULTS

Humoral response of rats to selected peptides of S-antigen

After S-antigen immunization, the serum content (ELISA) of antibodies to the whole S-antigen molecule and to chymotrypsin fragment 79 was similar in Lewis and BN rat strains. The amount of antibodies reacting with chymotrypsin fragment 99, containing the S2 epitope, and with the synthetic peptide S2 was much lower in Lewis than in BN rats (Fig. 1). Likewise, on immunoblots of CB peptides, Lewis sera presented a low reactivity to the N-terminal fragments CB 74 and CB 47 (Fig. 2).

Days after S-antigen immunization:
30 14 10   30 14 10

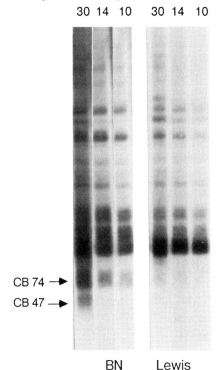

CB 74 →
CB 47 →

BN   Lewis

Fig. 2. Immunoblot of CNBr peptide fragments of S-antigen. Immunoreaction of sera from a Brown Norway rat (BN) and a Lewis rat at days 10, 14 and 30 after immunization with S-antigen. BN sera recognize the CB peptide 74 and, after 30 days, the CB peptide 47. Lewis sera have a very low reactivity with these N-terminal fragments.

Inhibition of the binding of mAb S2D2 to S-antigen by anti-S-antigen rat sera

Sera from BN rats impeded S2D2 binding to S-antigen-coated plates, while sera from Lewis rats did not inhibit significantly the binding of S2D2 to the protein (Fig. 3).

CONCLUSIONS

Two genetically distinct rat strains, Lewis and BN, differ in their antibody response to a particular epitope of S-antigen. After S-antigen immunization, the S2 epitope is well recognized by BN rats, which produce "S2D2-like" antibodies. Lewis rats had a low response to this epitope, as shown by the low reactivity of their serum with the synthetic peptide reproducing this epitope, and its failure to compete with S2D2. We suggest that the susceptibility of Lewis rats to develop EAU in response to S-antigen immunization could be related to a genetically determined relative incapacity to develop an immune response against this epitope. This observation is another indication of the role of this region of S-antigen in immunoregulation of EAU.

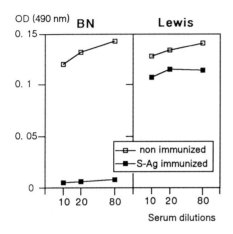

Fig. 3. Competition between rat sera and mAb S2D2. The binding of S2D2 to S-antigen-coated plates is inhibited by BN serum but not by Lewis serum (mean of ELISA values for 5 BN and 5 Lewis sera taken 21 days after S-antigen immunization).

REFERENCES

1. Gery I, Mochizuki M, Nussenblatt RB (1986) In: Osborne N, Chader J (eds) Progress in Retinal Research. Pergamon Press, Oxford, pp 75-109
2. De Kozak Y, Mirshahi M, Boucheix C, Faure JP (1987) Eur J Immunol 17:541-547
3. Mirshahi M, Boucheix C, Collenot G, Thillaye B, Faure JP (1985) Invest Ophthalmol Vis Sci 26:1016-1021
4. Geysen HM, Rodda SJ, Mason TJ, Tribbick G, Schoofs PG (1987) J Immunol Methods 102:259-274
5. Donoso LA, Merryman CF, Sery TW, Shinohara T, Dietschold B, Smith A, Kalsow CM (1987) Curr Eye Res 6:1151-1159
6. De Kozak Y, Sakai J, Thillaye B, Faure JP (1981) Curr Eye Res 1:327-337
7. Knospe V, Fling SP, Gregerson DS (1988) Curr Eye Res 7:181-189

MOLECULAR BIOLOGY

© 1990 Elsevier Science Publishers (Biomedical Division)
Ocular Immunology Today. M. Usui, S. Ohno and K. Aoki, editors.

IMMUNOPATHOGENICITY OF A BACTERIALLY EXPRESSED IRBP FUSION PROTEIN

TM REDMOND, S KOTAKE, B WIGGERT, I GERY, GJ CHADER AND JM NICKERSON

Laboratories of Retinal Cell and Molecular Biology and Immunology,

National Eye Institute, National Institutes of Health, Bethesda, MD

20892, USA.

INTRODUCTION

Experimental Autoimmune Uveoretinitis (EAU) is an animal model for the assemblage of human ocular autoimmune and inflammatory diseases termed "uveitis". EAU may be induced in a variety of animal species by immunization with several ocular-specific antigens (1), including bovine interphoto-receptor retinoid-binding protein (IRBP), a 140-kDa glycolipoprotein of the interphotoreceptor matrix (2). EAU and its collateral, Experimental Autoimmune Pinealitis (EAP) may be induced in the Lewis rat by immunization with the intact IRBP protein (3,4), by proteolytic fragments thereof (5) and by synthetic peptides derived from the sequence of IRBP (6).

Because of a need for larger amounts of specific large fragments of IRBP than can be conveniently prepared by proteolysis of purified protein or by peptide synthesis, we have turned to the use of bacterial expression vectors to overproduce specific IRBP fragments in Escherichia coli. In this communication, we describe the production and immunological testing of one such bacterially synthesized IRBP fusion protein. For a more complete treatment of the findings outlined here, see ref. 7.

MATERIAL AND METHODS

A 2-kb EcoR I insert from a 3' IRBP cDNA clone was subcloned into the three expression plasmids pWR590-0, 1 and 2 (8) by standard methods (9). Recombinant plasmid-transformed cells expressing a β-galactosidase-IRBP (βGal-IRBP) fusion protein were identified by antibody screening. LE392 E. coli cells containing plasmid were grown in 2xYT medium + 100 μg ampicillin/ml to stationary phase (18-20 hr) and harvested by centrifugation. The cells were fractionated (10), and the expressed fusion protein was further purified by reversed-phase HPLC.

SDS-PAGE was undertaken using 12% gels and western blotting was carried out using E.coli-absorbed anti-bovine IRBP antiserum as the primary antibody.

202

Lewis rats (male, 8-10 wk) were immunized via the hind foot pad with 10 µg samples of the HPLC-purified fusion protein dissolved in 8 M urea emulsified in complete Freund's adjuvant (CFA) using the procedure described in detail elsewhere (5).

RESULTS AND DISCUSSION

Construction of the expression plasmid

The 2-kb EcoR I insert of pIRBP2-2000, which expresses the C-terminal 136 aa of IRBP, was subcloned into the three pWR590 vectors. The recombinant plasmids were transformed into competent LE392 cells and screened for the expression of a βGal-IRBP fusion protein. As expected, pWR590-1, the version predicted to express an in-frame IRBP fusion protein, was the only one to do so. EcoR I digestion of pXS590-IRBP, the resultant recombinant plasmid, shows the presence of the 2-kb EcoR I insert (Fig. 1).

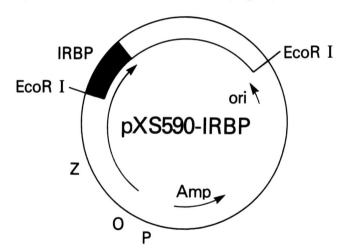

Fig. 1 Recombinant expression plasmid, pXS590-IRBP. The black segment indicates the cDNA encoding the C-terminal 136 aa of IRBP.

Expression and isolation of the fusion protein

Cells expressing the βGal-IRBP fusion protein were grown to stationary phase. The harvested cell pellet was subjected to successive detergent and chaotrope extractions to enrich for the fusion protein. SDS-PAGE analysis showed it was most abundantly present as putative inclusion bodies in the final 2 M KSCN-insoluble pellet. SDS-PAGE and immunoblotting of the final pellet fraction of expressing and non-expressing LE392 cells demonstrated that the former synthesized an 86 kDa fusion protein containing the 583 N-terminal aa of βGal fused to the 136 C-terminal aa of IRBP, and that had IRBP immunoreactivity. The encoded C-terminal 136 residues contains the entire CNBr fragment CB-71, previously shown to be immunopathogenic (4).

A 7 M guanidine HCl extract of the final 2 M KSCN-insoluble was subjected to reversed-phase HPLC to further purify the fusion protein. Although the fusion protein was not completely homogeneous, all of the previous major contaminants were removed (not shown).

Induction of EAU/EAP by the βGal fusion protein

EAU and EAP were induced in rats immunized with 10 μg of the HPLC-purified protein. The disease induced was identical (not shown) to that induced by authentic bovine IRBP (3). Briefly, there was extensive infiltration of both the anterior and posterior segments of the eye by inflammatory cells, resulting in severe edema of the retina, photoreceptor cell destruction and retinal detachment. Pineal gland changes included focal infiltration of inflammatory cells. No disease was induced by either the BSA or β-galactosidase controls.

To our knowledge, this is the first study to employ a recombinant autoantigen for the successful induction of an autoimmune pathology. As such, it serves as a baseline for further experiments to study the role of different epitopes of IRBP in the induction of EAU/EAP or perhaps modulation of the course of the disease. The biochemistry of IRBP may also be studied using plasmid-coded fragments. Such studies are currently underway.

SUMMARY

1) We have constructed a plasmid, pXS590-IRBP, which expresses an 86 kDa fusion protein containing the 136 C-terminal aa of IRBP and that has IRBP immunoreactivity.

2) The fusion protein was isolated by fractionation of the expressing cells followed by reversed-phase HPLC.

3) The partially purified IRBP fusion protein induced an EAU/EAP in immunized Lewis rats indistinguishable from that induced by authentic bovine IRBP, showing that a biological property of the C-terminal 136 aa of IRBP is retained by the fusion protein.

REFERENCES

1. Gery I, Mochizuki M, Nussenblatt RB (1986) Prog Retinal Res 5:75-109

2. Chader GJ, Wiggert B, Lai Y-L, Lee L, Fletcher RT (1983) Prog Retinal Res 2:163-189

3. Gery I, Wiggert B, Redmond TM, Kuwabara T, Crawford MA, Vistica BP, Chader GJ (1986) Invest Ophthalmol Vis Sci 27:1296-1300

4. Broekhuyse RM, Winkens HJ, Kuhlmann ED (1986) Curr Eye Res 5:231-240

5. Redmond TM, Sanui H, Nickerson JM, Borst DE, Wiggert B, Kuwabara T, Chader GJ, Gery I (1988) Curr Eye Res 7:375-385

6. Sanui H, Redmond TM, Kotake S, Wiggert B, Hu L-H, Margalit H, Berzofsky JA, Chader GJ, Gery I (1989) J Exp Med 169:1947-1960

7. Redmond TM, Si J-S, Barrett DJ, Borst DE, Rainier S, Kotake S, Gery I, Nickerson JM (1989) Gene 80:109-118

8. Guo L-H, Stepien PP, Tso JY, Brousseau R, Narang S, Thomas DY, Wu R (1984) Gene 29:251-254

9. Maniatis T, Fritsch EF, Sambrook J (1982) Molecular cloning: a laboratory manual. Cold Spring Harbor Laboratory, Cold Spring Harbor, New York

10. Krippl B, Ferguson B, Rosenberg M, Westphal H (1984) Proc Natl Acad Sci USA 81:6988-6992

© 1990 Elsevier Science Publishers (Biomedical Division)
Ocular Immunology Today. M. Usui, S. Ohno and K. Aoki, editors.

MOLECULAR MIMICRY PLAY A ROLE IN UVEITIS

KUNIHIKO YAMAKI* , V.K. SINGH, TOHRU ABE, SHOZO SAKURAGI* AND
TOSHIMICHI SHINOHARA.

*Department of Ophthalmology, Akita University School of
Medicine, Akita, Japan
Laboratory of Retinal Cell and Molecular Biology, National Eye
Institute, NIH, Bethesda, USA

ABSTRACT
    Experimental autoimmune uveitis(EAU) serves as an animal
model of ocular inflammation. The disease is caused by
immunization with microgram amounts of a soluble retinal
protein, designated S-Ag, in susceptible animal strains,
including primates. One of the uveitopathogenic peptide
(peptide M) has sequence homology with some bacterial, fungal,
viral, and food proteins. Lymphocytes from animals immunized
with peptide M show significant proliferation when incubated
with synthetic peptides corresponding to the amino acid
sequence of the above mentinoned foreign proteins. In
addition, these peptides and native baker's yeast histon
induce EAU and experimental antoimmune pinealitis(EAP) in
Lewis rats. These findings provide a basis for studying
autoimmune inflammatory disease of the eye.

INTRODUCTION
    Autoimmunity to ocular antigen is thought to play a role in
the pathogenesis of uveitis, comprising a diverse group of
numerous intraocular inflammations. Retinal S-antigen(S-Ag)
is a soluble photoreceptor protein, when injected with
complete Freund's adjuvant(CFA) into susceptible animal
species, EAU and EAP develop[1]. EAU may serve as an animal
model for human ocular inflammations[2].
    Recently amino acid sequences of retinal and pineal S-Ag
from different species were determined[3-7]. Four uveito
pathogenic sites in bovine and human S-Ag were identified
using synthetic peptides[8,9].
    Many theories have been proposed to account for induction of
autoimmune disease. One plausible mechanism which accounts
for the development of autoimmune disease involes molecular
mimicry, whereby selected microbial pathogens may trigger an
autoimmune response. In this process immunogenic determinants
of a nonself protein can elicit the formation of antibodies or
effector lymphocytes, which in turn may react with homologous
epitopes in a host protein[10-12]. Depending on the biologic
function of the host protein which is recognized and the
magnitude of immune response elicited, the outcome of the
interaction may be disease. Thus we were interested in
searching for proteins from microbial sources which have
sequence homology with S-Ag and can induce EAU in susceptible
animal strains under our experimental conditions.
    Here we report that one of the uveito pathogenic peptide
(peptide M) has sequence homology with proteins from
bacterial, viral, fungal and food proteins (table I). These

Souce	Sequence	Position	Abbreviation
S—Antigen	DTNLASSTIIKEGIDKTV	(303-320)	Peptide M
Berker's yeast	DTNLAAIHAKRVTIQK	(106-121)	BYHH3
E. coli	LANLASSTQLCKKN	(11-24)	ECHP11
E. coli	DWLANLASSTQLCK	(9-22)	ECHP9
Hepatitis B Virus	LTNLLSSNLSWL	(404-415)	HBVDP
Baboon Virus	PTNLAKVRTITQ	(354-365)	BEVGP
AKV Mur. Leu. V.	PTNLAKVKGITQ	(347-358)	AKVMLVGP
Murine Leu. Virus	PTNLAKVKGITQ	(348-359)	MMLVGP
Murine Sar Virus	PTNLAKVKGITQ	(348-359)	MMSVGP
Patato Proteinase	DTNIASYKSVCE	(25-36)	PPIIIa

Table I
Amino acid sequence homology with peptideM and other proteins

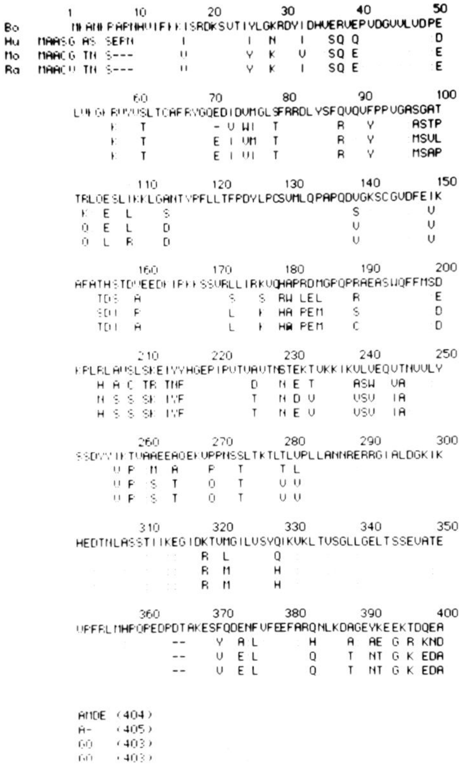

Fig.1
Amino acid sequcences of S-Ag
Bo:Bovine, Hu:Human, Mo:Mouse
Ra:Rat

above mentioned peptides induced EAU in Lewis rats. In addition, lymphnode cells from animals immunized with either peptide M or above mentioned peptides showed significant cross reaction when tested in vitro for mitogenesis in the presence of peptide M or above mentioned peptides.

RESULTS AND DISCUSSION

Amino acid sequence of S-antigen and uveitopathogenic site
We determined amino acid sequcences of Bovine, Human, Mouse and Rat retina and Rat pineal, deduced from cDNA sequencing (Fig.1). The cDNAs and deduced amino acid sequences for the S-Ag from retina and pineal are identical in rat[7]. Four uveitopathogenic site in bovine S-Ag was determined as 3, K, M and N[8]. Fig.2 shows sequence comparison of corresponding amino acid sequences from Bovine, Human, Mouse and Rat. Peptide N and M has virtually identical sequences among these species, wheras 3 and K have some differences among these species.

Lymphocyte in vitro proliferation assays
Proliferative response was determined by the lymphocyte mitogenesis assay using popliteal and inguinal lymphnode cells by [³H] thymidine uptake. The results of proliferation assay of lymphnode cells from rats immunized with peptide M, fungal, bacterial, viral and food peptids are summarized in table Ⅰ. Lymphnode cells of rats immunized with peptide M proliferated significantly in the presence of peptide M as well as other peptides derived from fungus, bacteria, virus and food. Similary lymphnode cells of rat immunized with above mentioned peptides proliferated well when stimulated with either immunizing peptide or peptide M. All of the above mentioned cultures proliferated against PPD, a component of CFA and ConA, a mitogen[13-16].

Uveitopathogenecity of different synthetic peptides and native protein
The Lewis rats were immunized with various doses of different peptides and native protein emulsified in CFA. The development of EAU was evaluated by the observation of slit lamp microscope between 12 to 28 days. The development of EAU was summerized in tableⅡ. The clinical signs of an inflammatory responses were induced between 14 to 28 days and was same as induced by peptide M or Bovine S-Ag. The histopathological changes in the eyes were also same as induced by peptide M or Bovine S-Ag(Photography was not shown)[13-16]. These results provide important clues to understanding autoimmune disease of the eye. It is thought that autoimmune responses provoked by molecular mimicry occur when the nonself and host determinants are similar enough to cross-react, yet different enough to break immunologic tolerance[10-12]. An immune response against a determinant shared by host and nonself proteins can elicit tissue-specific responses that are presumably capable of eliciting cell and tissue destruction. The mechanism by which this occurs probably involves cytotoxic cross-reactive effector lymphocytes that recognize specific determinants on target cells.

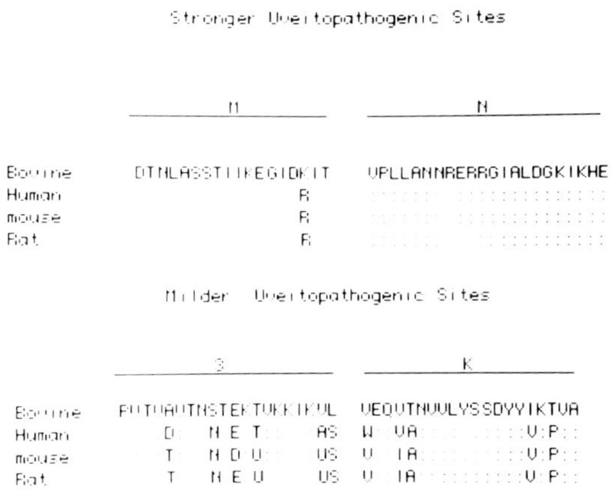

Stronger Uveitopathogenic Sites

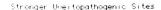

	M	N
Bovine	DTNLASSTIIEGIDKIT	UPLLANNRERRGIALDGKIKHE
Human	R	
mouse	R	
Rat	R	

Milder Uveitopathogenic Sites

	3	K
Bovine	FUTUAUTNSTEKTUKKIKUL	UEQUTNUULYSSDYYIKTUA
Human	D N E T AS U UA U P
mouse	T N D U US U IA U P
Rat	T N E U US U IA U P

Fig.2
Amino acid sequences of uveitopathogenic sites

Proliferative response of primed lymph node cells from rats immunized with different Antigen

Immunizing Antigen	Stimulant					
	Peptide M	Histome H3 peptide	Native histone	Thymus Histone	PPD	Con A
Peptide M	17.3	9.6	4.1	1.1	19.6	28.8
Histome H3 peptide	5.2	24.5	3.9	1.3	14.3	19.9
Native histone	3.7	4.3	11.2	1.0	16.4	33.5

	Peptide M	ECHP 11	ECPH 9	PPD	Con A
Peptide M	8.9	6.5	3.5	18.0	30.0
ECHP 11	3.2	5.9	4.0	22.7	9.6
ECPH 9	2.5	3.7	5.1	7.2	24.3

	Peptide M	HBVDP	BEVGP	AKVMLVGP	Con A	PPD
Peptide M	7.8	2.9	3.2	3.9	7.7	6.5
HBVDP	2.4	4.6	2.8	3.2	7.9	5.9
BEVGP	2.9	2.5	5.9	2.5	8.3	4.9
AKVMLVGP	3.2	2.1	2.9	4.0	4.6	5.1
PBS	0.9	0.9	1.0	1.0	7.9	5.3

Table II

In our study, we examined the ability of various synthetic peptides or native proteins that have sequence homology to the amino acid sequence of the uveitopathogenic site (peptide M) of S-Ag to induce EAU in Lewis rats.

Using high doses of synthetic peptides (400 to 2000µg/rat) or native protein we have induced an EAU in Lewis rats, which is dose dependent. In those experiments we found that sharing of three or more amino acids were sufficient to produce immunologic crossreactivity. Only three or four subsequent amino acids of the viral peptides and peptide M are identical, although these identical fragments are part of larger peptides, 12-18 mer amino acid long. The approach described here provides another useful investigative tool to understand molecular mimicry.

Uveitopathogenicity of different doses of various peptides
in Lewis rats

Immunizing Agent	Immunizing Dose, µg	No. with EAU/ No. Immunized
Baker's yeast		
BYHH3	100	2/4
BYHH3	200	3/4
BYHH3	400	5/15
E. coli		
ECHP11	400	2/5
ECHP11	500	3/5
ECHP11	2000	5/5
ECHP9	400	2/5
ECHP9	500	2/5
ECHP9	2000	5/5
HBV		
HBVDP	500	2/4
HBVDP	2000	3/4
BEV		
BEVGP	500	1/4
BEVGP	2000	3/4
AKVMLV		
AKVMLVGP	500	2/4
AKVMLVGP	2000	2/4
Potato		
ppIIIa	500	1/4
ppIIIa	1000	1/4
ppIIIa	2000	2/4
Native Histone H3	500	5/5

Table III

ACKNOWLEDGMENTS

We appreciate the secretarial assistance of Miss Yumiko Fukuda in the preparation of this manuscript.

REFERENCES

1. Wacker,W.B.,L.A.Doso,C.M.Kaslow,J.A.Yankeelov and D.T. Organisciak.1977.J.Immunol.119:1494.
2. Nussenblatt,R.B.,I.Gery.E.J.Ballinitine,and W.B Wacker. 1980.Am.J.Ophthalmol.89:173.
3. Yamaki,K.,Y.Takahashi,S.Sakuragi and K.Matsubara.1987. Biochem.Biophys.Res.Commun.142:904.
4. Shinohara,T.,B.Dietzschold,C.M.Craft,G.Wistow,J.J.Early, L.A.Donoso,J.Horwitz and R.Tao.1987.Proc.Natl.Acad.Sci.USA 84:6975.
5. Yamaki,K.,M.Tsuda,and T.Shinohara.1988.FEBS Lett.243:39.
6. M.Tsuda,M.Syed,K.Bugra,J.P.Whelan,J.F.Meginnis and T.Shinohara.1988.Gene 73:11
7. T.Abe,K.Yamaki,M.Tsuda,V.K.,Singh,S.Suzuki,R.Mckinnon,D.C. Klein,L.A.donoso and T.Shinohara.1989.FEBS Lett.247:307.
8. Singh,V.K.,R.B.Nussenblatt,L.A.Donoso,K.Yamaki,C.Chan, and T.Shinohara.1988.Cell.Immunol.115:413.
9. Donoso L.A.,K.Yamaki,C.F.Merryman,T.Shinohara,S.Yue and T.W.Sery.1988.current Eye Research.1077:7.
10. Oldstone,M.B.A.,and A.L.Norkins.1986. Molecular mimicry.In Concepts in Viral Pathogenesis.A.L.Notkins and M.B.A. Oldstone,eds.Springer Verlag,New York,p.195.
11. Cohen,I.R.1988. The self,the world and autoimmunity.Sc.Am. April:52.

12. Oldstone,M.B.A.1987.Cell 50:819.
13. Singh,V.K.,K.Yamaki,L.A.Donoso,and T.Shinohara.1989.
    J.Immunol.142:1512.
14. Singh,V.K.,K.Yamaki,L.A.Donoso,and T.Shinohara.1989.Cell.
    Immunol.119:211.
15. Singh,V.K.,K.Yamaki,T.Abe and T.Shinohara.1989. Cell.
    Immunol.122;262.
16. Singh.V.K.,H.K.Kalra,K.Yamaki,T.Abe,L.A.Donoso and
    T.Shinohara.1990.J.Immunol.in press.

© 1990 Elsevier Science Publishers (Biomedical Division)
Ocular Immunology Today. M. Usui, S. Ohno and K. Aoki, editors.

CHARACTERIZATION OF 33-KDa PROTEIN OF RETINA AND PINEAL GLAND

TOHRU ABE‡°, HIROFUMI TAMADA°, TAKESHI TAKAGI°, SHOZO SAKURAGI°, HIROKI NAKABAYASHI※, KUNIHIKO YAMAKI° AND TOSHIMICHI SHINOHARA‡

‡Laboratory of Retinal Cells and Molecular Biology, National Eye Institute, ※Endocrinology and Reproduction Research Branch, NICHD, NIH, Bethesda, MD 20892 (USA). °Department of Ophthalmology, Akita University School of Medicine, Akita-shi, Akita, 010 (Japan)

INTRODUCTION

The photoreceptor cells of retina have a phosphoprotein called "33-KDa protein" that may participate in the regulation of visual phototransduction (1-3). This protein is phosphorylated by cAMP-dependent protein kinase, mostly in dark-adapted retina (4).

Although the pineal gland in mammalian species has lost its photoreceptor function, retina and pineal gland share some proteins in common such as interphotoreceptor retinoid-binding protein and S-antigen. We and the other group found that 33-KDa protein was also present in pineal gland (5,6).

In order to characterize 33-KDa protein, a monoclonal antibody against 33-KDa protein was raised. Using this antibody, cDNAs of 33-KDa protein of rat retina and pineal gland was analyzed.

MATERIALS AND METHODS

Establishment of anti-33-KDa protein monoclonal antibody (MAb-TS-SC-6). Rats were hyperimmunized with crude bovine retinal homogenates. Hybridomas between spleen cells of the rats and myeloma cells were made by conventional methods. Monoclanal antibodies were analyzed by Western blotting and immunohistochemistry.

Phosphorylation and immunoprecipitation of retinal proteins. The retinal homogenates from dark-adapted rats were phosporylated with γ -^{32}P-ATP, in the presence or absence of cAMP (4). Phosphorylated 33-KDa protein was immunoprecipitated with MAb-TS-SC-6 and immobilized-anti-rat IgG. The resulting immune complexes were analyzed by 12% gel SDS-PAGE, and visualized by autoradiography.

cDNA screening, characterization and DNA sequence determination. The rat pineal λ gt11 cDNA library (gift from Drs. McKinnon and Klein) were used for screening of cDNAs with MAb-TS-SC-6. The obtained pineal cDNA was used as a probe of cDNA hybridization method to isolate rat retinal 33-KDa protein cDNA clones from the λ gt10 cDNA library (gift from Drs. Liou and Gonzalez-Fernandez).

212

The sequence determination of the DNAs was performed by the
dideoxy chain termination method.

RESULTS

Anti-33-KDa protein monoclonal antibody (MAb-TS-SC-6) bound to
the protein present in retina and pineal gland, but did not bind
to proteins from other tissues by Western blotting. The
immunohistochemical study of rat retina and pineal gland indicated
that 33-KDa protein was present in photoreceptor cells and in
pinealocytes. The study of immunoprecipitation showed that 33-KDa
protein was phosphorylated by cAMP-dependent manner (Fig.1).

The entire cDNA sequences and predicted amino acid sequences of
rat retinal and pineal 33-KDa protein were determined, and the
retinal sequence is summarized in Fig.2. The sequences of cDNAs
derived from retina and pineal gland were almost identical except
four nucleotides. The pineal nucleotides were "A" at the position
of 483, "G" at the position of 571, "A" at the position of 990 and
"T" at the position of 1033, in the Fig.2. The size of these cDNAs
was almost full, since the Northern blot analysis indicated that
the mRNAs from both rat retina and pineal gland were approximately

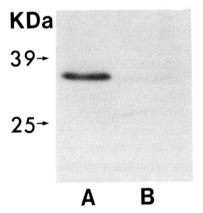

Fig.1. cAMP-dependent phosporylation of 33-KDa protein. The level
of the phosphorylation of 33-KDa protein in the presence of cAMP
(lane A) is higher than that in the absence of cAMP (lane B). The
numbers in the left margin indicate the molecular weight.

```
        -70         -60         -50         -40         -30         -20         -10
CAGAGATTCTCACCCACTGGACATAATCTAGGACTCCAGGAACAGAGACCCCAAACTACTACACCGAACACAACC
    1          10          20          30          40          50          60
CATAAAATGGAAGAAGCCGCAAGCCAAAGCTTAGAGGAAGATTTTGAAGGACAGGCCACACACACAGGACCCAAA
       M   E   E   A   A   S   Q   S   L   E   E   D   F   E   G   Q   A   T   H   T   G   P   K   23
         80          90         100         110         120         130         140
GGAGTAATAAATGACTGGAGAAAGTTTAAATTAGAAAGTGAAGATGGTGATTCAATTCCACCCAGCAAGAAGGAG
  G   V   I   N   D   W   R   K   F   K   L   E   S   E   D   G   D   S   I   P   P   S   K   K   E   48
    150         160         170         180         190         200         210
ATCCTCAGACAAATGTCCTCTCCTCAGAGCAGAGATGACAAAGACTCGAAAGAAAGAATGAGCAGAAAGATGAGC
  I   L   R   Q   M   S   S   P   Q   S   R   D   D   K   D   S   K   E   R   M   S   R   K   M   S   73
    230         240         250         260         270         280         290
ATTCAAGAATATGAACTAATTCATCAGGACAAAGAAGATGAAGGTTGCCTTCGCAAATACCGCAGACAGTGCATG
  I   Q   E   Y   E   L   I   H   Q   D   K   E   D   E   G   C   L   R   K   Y   R   R   Q   C   M   98
    300         310         320         330         340         350         360
CAGGATATGCATCAGAAGCTGAGCTTTGGGCCTAGGTATGGGTTTGTGTATGAGCTGGAAACAGGGGAGCAATTC
  Q   D   M   H   Q   K   L   S   F   G   P   R   Y   G   F   V   Y   E   L   E   T   G   E   Q   F   123
    380         390         400         410         420         430         440
CTGGAAACCATCGAAAAGGAGCAGAAGGTCACCACCATCGTGGTTAACATTTACGAGGATGGTGTCAGGGGCTGT
  L   E   T   I   E   K   E   Q   K   V   T   T   I   V   V   N   I   Y   E   D   G   V   R   G   C   148
    450         460         470         480 ⇩   490         500         510
GACGCACTCAACAGCAGTTTAGAATGCCTTGCAGCAGAGTACCCAATGGTCAAGTTCTGTAAAATAAGAGCTTCG
  D   A   L   N   S   S   L   E   C   L   A   A   E   Y   P   M   V   K   F   C   K   I   R   A   S   173
    530         540         550         560         570 ⇩   580         590
AATACTGGAGCTGGGGACCGCTTTTCCTCAGACGTACTCCCGACATTGCTCATATACAAAGGTGGGGAGCTCATA
  N   T   G   A   G   D   R   F   S   S   D   V   L   P   T   L   L   I   Y   K   G   G   E   L   I   198
    600         610         620         630         640 ⇩   660
AGCAATTTTATTAGTGTCGCTGAACAATTTGCCGAAGATTTTTTCGCTGCGGATGTGGAGTCTTTCCTAAATGAA
  S   N   F   I   S   V   A   E   Q   F   A   E   D   F   F   A   A   D   V   E   S   F   L   N   E   223
    680         690         700         710         720         730         740
TATGGCTTACTACCAGAAAGAGAGATACATGACCTAGGGCAGACCAACACGGAAGATGAAGATATCGAGTAAGCA
  Y   G   L   L   P   E   R   E   I   H   D   L   G   Q   T   N   T   E   D   E   D   I   E   *   246
    750         760         770         780         790         800         810
CGCACGGTGCAGTATCTCGTGACTATCCTTTGCACAGTGAACATCGATGGTTTTTTTGGTAGTATCTATATTCCT
    830         840         850         860         870         880         890
TTAGCAAACACTAAATACAGTCAGGCCAACTCAAATTGGGGAGGGGACACTAAAATTATGTAAATAGCATTTTTA
    900         910         920         930         940         950         960
GTACTAATTATTCAAATTGAGATAATATTTTACTGCAAAAAATATTGTGGTTCTGAGCAAATAACTACTGAACAG
    980          ⇩    1000        1010        1020        1030  ⇩   1040
AGGAGGTGGGTGATGTCAACGTTAGGTCATTGTAAAAATCCCTTTCCAGTTCCGTGTTAGCTTATTACTCCTCCT
    1050        1060        1070        1080        1090        1100        1110
TTTCCCCTTGGCATTTATTTTTGGGCTTTTGAGGCTGAATGCTACTTATAAATTGGTTTGTATGATAAGAATAAA
    1130
GTCCTATGAAG
```

Fig.2. The nucleotide and deduced amino acid sequence of 33-KDa protein from rat retina. The underlined "ATG", "TAA" and "AATAAA" indicate the initiation codon, termination codon and putative polyadenylation signals, respectively. The numbers above nucleotide sequence indicate the position of bases, starting with the first base of the initiation "ATG". The amino acid sequence is indicated by one letter code, below the nucleotide sequence. The numbers in the right margin indicate the numbers of the amino acid residues from the amino terminal (methionine). A putative phosphorylation site (RKMS) and a putative carbohydrate attaching site (NSS) are underlined. The arrowed nucleotides and amino acid are different from those of pineal gland (see text).

1300 nucleotides long. The open reading frame of 738 nucleotides encodes 246 amino acid residues in retina and pineal gland. The predicted amino acid sequences were virtually identical between retina and pineal gland. The difference of the amino acid residue in pineal gland was only one. The pineal amino acid was "Val" at the position of 191. The predicted molecular weight of 33-KDa protein is 28143 in rat retina and 28129 in rat pineal gland. Thus, 33-KDa protein present in retina and pineal gland probably derives from the same gene and difference in the sequences are perhaps due to the polymorphism. The predicted amino acid sequence has a putative phosphorylation site, by cAMP-dependent protein kinase, at the position of 73 serine (RKMS) residue (7).

These results may provide a step to initiate a molecular study of 33-KDa protein in retina as well as in pineal gland.

ACKNOWLEDGEMENTS

We wish to thank Ms. Hisae Kayama and Ms. Takumi Satoh for their great technical assistance.

REFERENCES

1. Lolley RN, Brown BM, Farber DB (1977) Biochem Biophy Res Comm 78:572-578

2. Lee RH, Lieberman BS, Lolley RN (1987) Biochemistry 26:3983-3990

3. Lee RH, Brown BM, Lolley RN (1982) Biochemistry 21:3303-3307

4. Lee RH, Brown BM, Lolley RN (1984) Biochemistry 23:1972-1977

5 Tamada H, Takagi T, Abe T, Yamaki K, Sakuragi S (1990) Folia Ophthalmol Jpn, in press

6. Reig RH, Yu L, Klein DC (1990) J Biol Chem, in press

7. Engstrom L, Ekman P, Humble E, Ragnarsson U, Zetterqvist O (1984) In: Wold F, Moldave K (eds) Methods in Enzymology (vol 107). Academic Press, New York, 130-154

© 1990 Elsevier Science Publishers (Biomedical Division)
Ocular Immunology Today. M. Usui, S. Ohno and K. Aoki, editors.

THE EXPRESSION OF αB-CRYSTALLIN IN RETINOBLASTOMA: EVIDENCE FOR TRANSDIFFERENTIATION

R. PINEDA II, CHI-CHAO CHAN, NI MING, G.J. CHADER
National Eye Institute, National Institutes of Health, Bethesda, Maryland 20892, U.S.A.
Howard Hughes Medical Institute, Bethesda, Maryland, U.S.A.

INTRODUCTION

Retinoblastoma (Rb) is the most commonly occurring intraocular malignancy in childhood[1]. Cells from this tumor were first isolated and cultured in suspension by Reid et al. in 1974[2]. Current evidence indicates that retinoblastoma tumor cells are multipotential in origin and are capable of terminal differentiation (i.e. into glial, neuronal or pigmented epithelial cells)[3].

Recently, αB-crystallin, the basic subunit of α-crystallin and major class of soluble lens protein, has been observed in normal non-lenticular tissues[5-7] (heart, lung, skeletal muscle, kidneys and brain). This lends support to the concept of a "dual role" for crystallins as performing both structural and other functions in lens and non-lenticular tissues[9]. Pathologically, αB-crystallin accumulates in scrapie-infected brain tissue[8]. It is also highly expressed in "Rosenthal fibers" within enlarged astrocytes in Alexander's disease[7], a degenerative neurological disorder of childhood. αB-crystallin thus may be involved in disease processes in a primary or secondary manner.

Although the presence of αB-crystallin in the retina has been previously described[6], it has not been examined in Rb tissue or cell culture lines. Okada et al.[10,11] first reported the appearance of lens crystallins in primary cultures of human fetal retinal cells demonstrating the potential of these cells to *"transdifferentiate"*. We now report that αB-crystallin is observed in Rb tissue and Rb cultured lines(Y-79, WERI Rb-1 and GM01232C) as assessed by the avidin-biotin-peroxidase complex method[4] and Northern blot technique. Thus, not only do our positive findings in Rb tissue and cells support the potential for transdifferentiation *in vitro* but also *in vivo*. Moreover, the expression of a major vertebrate crystallin in Rb supports the view that these tumor cells are pleuripotential in origin. Alternatively, it may indicate an important role of these proteins as "stress" proteins in normal and diseased tissue.

MATERIALS & METHODS

Materials

Antibodies generated to a 13 amino acid synthetic peptide of the carboxy terminus of αB-crystallin were kindly donated by Joseph Horwitz (Jules Stein Eye Institute, UCLA). Robert Dubin (National Eye Institute) donated the partial human genomic fragment to αB-crystallin (250bp of the

3' half of exon 3 of the human αB-crystallin gene). The Rb tissue was procured from the enucleated eyes of a 3 year old girl and a 2 month old girl. There was a no family history of Rb in both cases.

Retinoblastoma Tissue and Cell Cultures

Y-79, WERI-Rb1(American Type Culture Collection Rockville, MD) and GM01232C(Human Genetic Mutant Cell Repository Institute, Camden, NJ) were grown in Dulbecco's modified Eagle's medium (DMEM), penicillin-streptomycin, 10% fetal bovine serum (Flow Laboratories), and L-glutamine at 37° C/ 5% CO_2. Rb cultured cells were plated on poly-D-lysine[13](Sigma, St. Louis, MO) coated glass slide chambers(Lab-Tek, Nunc, Inc., Naperville, IL) for 2 days prior to drying and immunostaining. Cells used for Northern blotting were plated on PDL-coated 250 ml flasks (Costar, Cambridge, MA) for 3 days, harvested, and stored at -80° C .

Immunohistochemistry

Both the Rb tissue (frozen, unfixed) and cell lines were stained using the avidin-biotin-peroxidase complex (ABC) technique as previously described[15]. Polyclonal antibodies raised against the following antigens were used: a 13 amino acid synthetic peptide to the carboxy terminus of αB-crystallin (1:200); neuron-specific enolase (NSE, 1:100, Accurate Chemical & Scientific Corp.); glial fibrillary acidic protein (GFAP, 1:500 ,Dakopatts); interphotoreceptor retinoid-binding protein (IRBP, 1:200; courtesy of B.J.Hayden); S-58 (1:200); γ-crystallin (1:1000; courtesy of L. Takamoto).

Northern Blot

Total RNA was extracted from the Rb cells by acid guanidinium thiocyanate-phenol-chloroform extraction method as described by Chomczynski and Sacchi[16]. Briefly, total RNA was fractionated on 1.5% formaldehyde-agarose gel and transferred to nitrocellulose in 20x SSC. Prehybridization and hybridization conditions included 40% formamide at 42° C. 2X SSC-0.1 % SDS at room temperature and 0.1X SSC-0.1% SDS at 59°C were used in the final washes for the nitrocellulose blot[4]. RNA integrity was confirmed with a human β-actin cDNA.

RESULTS

The results of immunostaining for the two cases of Rb are summarized below in Table I. Both tumors stained nearly identically for the various neuronal, glial and lens markers, although morphologically they appeared very different. Case 1 was from a 3 year old girl with a poorly differentiated tumor which contained no identifiable Flexner-Wintersteiner rosettes or other evidence of differentiation. Case 2 was from a 2 month old girl with a well-differentiated tumor. This tumor contained numerous Flexner-Wintersteiner rosettes but no fleurettes were noted. A Muller cell marker, S-58, was observed to a greater degree in case 1 than case 2. Case 1 also expressed γ-crystallin which was not found in case 2 but both cases were positive for αB-crystallin. These differences may reflect the stage of differentiation of these tumors and their ability to express specific gene products.

TABLE I

The Comparison of Antibody Markers for Rb Case 1 and Case 2

ANTIBODY			CASE 1	CASE 2
Neuronal Marker				
	1.	NSE	+	+
	2.	IRBP	+	+
Glial Marker				
	1.	GFAP	+	+
	2.	S-58 (Muller)	+	+/-
Lens Marker				
	1.	αB-cyrstallin	+	+
	2.	γ-crystallin	+	-

All the Rb cell culture lines (Y-79, WERI Rb-1 and GM01232C) were shown to express αB-crystallin as demonstrated by either immunohistochemistry or Northern blot (not shown). These cells have also been shown to express neuronal and glial marker which can be modulated when the cells are treated with agents like butyrate or dibutyryl cyclic-AMP[12].

DISCUSSION

Our results demonstrate that αB-crystallin is expressed in Rb both *in vivo* and *in vitro* as shown by either immunohistochemistry or Northern blot analysis. In addition, the expression of lens crystallins in Rb may support the concept of transdifferentiation in these tumor cells and the embryonic retina. The expression of αB-crystallin in Rb is consistent with Kyritsis's [3] speculation of the pleuripotential nature of this tumor and its ability to differentiate along widely divergent lines. With the finding of αB-crystallin expression in non-lenticular tissues and disease states, it is interesting to speculate on the function of this protein. It may represent a response to cellular stress in normal and diseased non-lenticular tissue as αB-crystallin has been shown to have homology to the small heat shock proteins[9] or it may perform a yet unknown function in the normal or tumorigenic retina.

Further research is needed to elucidate the function of αB-crystallin and other crystallin proteins in non-lenticular tissues. Our results indicate that the Rb cell lines may serve as an *in vitro* model for crystallin gene expression in non-lenticular tissues. Future work on lens crystallin gene expression in treated Rb cells (i.e., butyrate, cAMP) may help to clarify a role for these proteins outside of the lens. Alternatively, correlating the expression of lens crystallins to the state of differentiation of Rb might result in predictive therapeutic management of patients with this tumor.

REFERENCE

1. Pendergrass, TW and Davis, S. Arch Ophthalmol. 98:1204-1210, 1980.

2. Reid, TW, Albert, DM, Rabson, AS, Russell, RP, Craft, J, Chu, EW, Tralka, TS and Wilcox, JC. J. Natl. Cancer Inst. 53:347-360, 1974.

3. Kyritsis, A, Tsokos, M, Triche, T and Chader, GJ. Nature. 307:471-473, 1984.

4. Dubin, RA, Wawrousek, EF and Piatigorsky, Mol. Cell. Biol. 9:1083-1091, 1989.

5. Bhat ,SP and Nagineni, CN. Biochem. Biophys. Res. Commun. 158:319-325, 1989.

6. Iwaki, T, Kume-Iwaki, A and Goldman, JE. J. Histochem. Cytochem. 37:000-000, 1989.

7. Iwaki, T, Kume-Iwaki, A, Liem, RKH and Goldman, JE. Cell. 57:71-78, 1989.

8. Duguid, JR, Rohwer, RG, Seed, B. Proc. Natl. Acad. Sci. 85:5738-5742, 1988.

9. Piatigorsky, J and Wistow, GJ. Cell 57:197-199, 1989.

10. Okada, TS, Itoh, Y, Watanabe, Y and Eguchi, G. Dev. Biol. 45:318-329, 1975.

11. Okada, TS. Develop. Growth and Differ. 28(3):213-221, 1986.

12. Rodrigues, MM, Wiggert, B, Shields, J, Donoso, L, Bartenstein, D, Katz, N, Friendly, D and Chader, GJ. Ophthalmology. 94:378-387, 1987.

13. Campbell, M and Chader, GJ. Ophthalmic Paediatr. and Genet.. 9(3):171-199, 1988.

14. De Pomerai, DI. Zoological Science. 5:1-19, 1988.

15. Hsu, SM, Raine, L and Frangeor, H. J. Histochem. Cytochem. 29:577-580, 1981.

16. Chomczynski, P and Sacchi, N. Anal. Biochem. 162:156-159, 1987.

© 1990 Elsevier Science Publishers (Biomedical Division)
Ocular Immunology Today. M. Usui, S. Ohno and K. Aoki, editors.

USE OF THE POLYMERASE CHAIN REACTION TO AMPLIFY PUTATIVE UVEITOGENIC DNA FRAGMENTS OF RAT IRBP

A. ARTHUR, D. SAPERSTEIN, I. GERY, G. CHADER, AND J. M. NICKERSON. Laboratory of Retinal Cell and Molecular Biology, National Eye Institute, National Institutes of Health. Bethesda, MD 20892 U.S.A.

INTRODUCTION

"Uveitis" is a generic term used to describe the myriad intraocular inflammatory conditions known to lead to visual impairment in man. Animal disease models for uveitic conditions hold promise for further elucidating the factors responsible for immune mediated disease processes.

IRBP (interphotoreceptor retinoid-binding protein), originally identified as "7S Protein" of the retina, is a 140 kDa glycoprotein found in the extracellular interphotoreceptor matrix; between the neural retina and retinal pigment epithelium layers. IRBP is also present in the pineal gland and is thought to function as a mediator of retinoid and fatty acid transport in the visual cycle. For example, IRBP promotes the incorporation of all-trans retinol from the photoreceptors to the retinal pigment epithelium. (1)

The IRBP cDNA and gene has been cloned. The gene is 11.6 kb in size and contains four exons and three introns. All three introns fall into the region encoding the fourth protein repeat. Dot matrix analysis demonstrates a four-fold repeat in both the nucleic acid and the protein sequence. (2)

IRBP has been shown to cause Experimental Autoimmune Uveitis (EAU) and Experimental Autoimmune Pinealitis (EAP) when injected into the footpads of Lewis rats. (3) IRBP was also found to induce EAU in other species and is suspected to play a role in the etiology of human uveitis. (4)

The immunopathogenic epitopes of bovine IRBP have been identified by examining the capacity of several CNBr cleavage products of IRBP and synthetic peptides to induce EAU and EAP in Lewis rats. The epitope with residues 1169-1191 in bovine IRBP has been found to be immunodominant and highly immunogenic and immunopathogenic in Lewis rats. This immunodominant area of rat IRBP is contained entirely within the the fourth repeat. (5,6)

Human, bovine and mouse IRBPs have been shown to exhibit significant homology. Our studies have been aimed at amplifying DNA sequences which potentially code for the immunopathogenic and/or immunodominant sequences of Lewis rat IRBP. Enzymatic amplification of these regions using the polymerase chain reaction (PCR), followed by DNA sequencing and synthesis of corresponding peptides, may prove to be a method of generating autologous antigen to produce a more informative model of EAU in Lewis rats. In this study we have applied PCR to amplify the DNA sequence which codes for the fragment of rat IRBP that corresponds to the highly immunopathogenic site of bovine IRBP (sequence 1169-1191).

MATERIALS AND METHODS

DNA was extracted from Lewis rat livers obtained from fresh cadavers using Applied Biosystems 340A DNA extractor. This DNA served as a template for the polymerase chain reaction.

The polymerase chain reaction protocol by Perkin Elmer Cetus (Norwalk, CT) was utilized with the following modifications: 1.0 ug of rat genomic DNA was used and mixed with 1 uM of each primer. The dNTPs used had a total concentration of 200 uM. To each tube 1x PCR Reaction Buffer was added along with 2.5 Units/assay of Taq polymerase. The final volume was adjusted to 100 ul with distilled water. Each tube was overlaid with 100 ul of mineral oil to prevent evaporation during the thermal cycling. The reaction was subjected to 31 cycles of amplification. In each cycle DNA was denatured at 94^0 C for 2 minutes, annealed at 37^0C to 70^0 C for 1 minute, elongated at 72^0 C for 1 minute and the amplified product was denatured for 9.8 minutes at 72^0 C. Annealing temperatures and $MgCl_2$ concentrations were adjusted to determine optimum conditions for amplifications. After amplification, samples were electrophoresed on 8% polyacrylamide gels. In samples with identifiable bands at the 250 b.p. region, the bands were excised and the DNA extracted using the "Crush and Soak" method of Maxam and Gilbert.(7) The purified aliquot was dried on a speed vac apparatus and resuspended in 10 ul of TE buffer (10mM Tris and 0.1 mM EDTA). 0.7% Agarose gels were used for blotting and hybridization by standard techniques.

RESULTS

Enzymatic amplification of a potentially uveitogenic region of rat IRBP using a variety of annealing temperatures revealed the following:

1.   Oligonucleotides based on the bovine IRBP sequence can be used as primers to generate short fragments of rat and mouse IRBP from a suitable DNA template. This suggests that there is a significant amount of cross-species homology between human, rat, bovine, and mouse in the area flanking the highly uveitogenic region.

2.   The optimum temperature for PCR amplification appeared to be 62^{0}C.

3.   The optimum $MgCl_2$ concentration for PCR amplification was 3.5 mM.

4.   PCR can be used to amplify fragments of IRBP, from cloned or genomic DNA. However, our experiments demonstrated a high level of extraneous sequence amplification when genomic DNA was used as a template. Isolation and extraction of the DNA after one complete round of PCR, and subsequent use of this product as a template for a second round of PCR produced a more enhanced signal with less background.

5.   Southern blot analysis of the PCR product with a labelled human cDNA oligonucleotide yielded a positive signal. The signal increased in intensity for each round of PCR performed, correlating with the geometric expansion of the desired short products with each amplification.

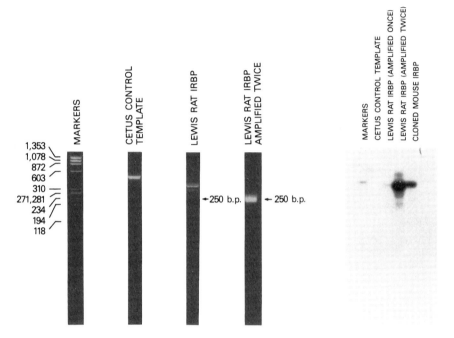

Figure 1. PCR amplification of 250 b.p. fragment of Lewis rat IRBP at annealing temperature of 62 °C.

Figure 2.   Southern blot of Lewis rat 250 b.p. fragment probed with labelled human cDNA oligonucleotide.

DISCUSSION

The exciting new technology - the polymerase chain reaction - has been used successfully to amplify fragments of rat IRBP genomic DNA.   Further studies designed to optimize the reaction are currently being undertaken. Subsequent subcloning of PCR derived DNA fragments which code for immunopathogenic sites may provide a system for large scale expression of antigen. Utilization of new protocols to perform direct sequencing from the PCR product may obviate the need for subcloning this fragment into an appropriate vector system. Determination of the degree of cross-species sequence homology in the uveitogenic regions of IRBP will help to clarify the relationship between the conservation of particular sequences and disease producing capability. This series of investigations will allow us to determine if short, overlapping or contiguous amino acid sequences of rat IRBP induce EAU and whether such sequences are homologous to immunopathogenic sequences found in bovine IRBP.

REFERENCES

1. Okajima T, Pepperberg D, Ripps H, Wiggert B, and Chader G   (1989) Exp. Eye Research 49: 629-644

2. Borst D, Redmond TM, Elser J, Gonda M, Wiggert B, Chader G   and Nickerson JM (1987) J. of Bio. Chem. 264: 1115-1123

3. Gery I, Wiggert B, Redmond TM, Kuwabara T, Crawford MA, Vistica BP and   Chader G (1986) Invest. Ophthalmol. Vis. Sci. 27:1296-1300

4. Hirose S, Kuwabara T, Nussenblatt RB, Wiggert B, Redmond TM and Gery I (1986) Arch. Ophthalmol. 104: 1698-1702

5. Sanui H, Redmond TM, Kotake S, Wiggert B, Hu L, Margalit H, Berzofsky J, Chader G and Gery I (1989) J. of Exp. Med. 169:1947-1960

6. Sanui H, Redmond TM, Hu L, Kuwabara T, Margalit H, Cornette J, Wiggert B, Chader G, and Gery I (1988) Current Eye Research 7: 727-735

7. Sambrook J, Fritsch EF T. Maniatis (1989) Molecular Cloning - A Laboratory Manual Cold Spring Harbor Laboratory Press

© 1990 Elsevier Science Publishers (Biomedical Division)
Ocular Immunology Today. M. Usui, S. Ohno and K. Aoki, editors.   223

ANALYSIS OF T-CELL RECEPTOR VARIABLE REGION GENES IN UVEITOGENIC T-CELL LINES

CHARLES. E. EGWUAGU, CHRISTOPHER Y. C. CHOW, EVELYNE P. BERAUD, RACHEL. R. CASPI, RASHID M. MAHDI, ROBERT. B. NUSSENBLATT, IGAL GERY. LABORATORY OF IMMUNOLOGY, NEI/NIH, BETHESDA MARYLAND, U.S.A.

INTRODUCTION:

Experimental autoimmune uveoretinitis (EAU) is an intraocular inflammatory disease which is induced in various animals by immunization with ocular-specific antigens, mainly S-Antigen or the interphotoreceptor retinoid binding protein (IRBP) (1,2). EAU is considered a model for certain uveitic conditions in man, such as sympathetic ophthalmia, birdshot retinochoroidopathy, Behçet's disease and Vogt-Koyanagi-Harada's (VKH) syndrome. Transfer studies have established that EAU is mediated by helper (CD4+) T-lymphocytes with MHC class II restriction (3,4).

Specificity of T-lymphocytes for antigens in the context of MHC molecules resides with the dimeric complex of α and β-chains of the T-cell receptor (TCR). In the mouse the enormous diversity of TCR-β specificities is generated during ontogeny by the rearrangement of more than 50 germline variable (V), 2 diversity (D), 13 junction (J) and 2 constant (C) region gene segments to give rise to the functional V-D-J-C receptor (5). In experimental allergic encephalomyelitis (EAE), another animal model of autoimmune diseases, it has been shown that the T-lymphocytes predominantly express the Vβ8.2 gene element (6).

In the present study we have investigated V-region gene usage in several uveitogenic T-cell lines and clones. The major goal of these analyses was to evaluate whether EAU, like EAE, is mediated by T-cells which predominantly rearrange and express the Vβ8.2 gene element.

MATERIALS AND METHODS

T-Cell Lines and Clones:

All T-cell lines were derived from lymph nodes of Lewis rats immunized in complete Freund's adjuvant with S-Antigen (3) or peptides corresponding to uveitogenic determinants of IRBP (7). All T-cell lines and clones expressed the CD4+,CD8- membrane phenotype and recognized antigen in the context of MHC Class II. T-cell lines

ThS8 and LR16 are highly pathogenic, requiring 5x10^6 and 2x10^6 cells respectively to adoptively transfer EAU to naive syngeneic recipients. ThS4 T-cell line is considered non-uveitogenic; even 2x10^7 cells are insufficient for induction of disease. Clones C3 and C4 derived from LR16 T-cell line are non-pathogenic although they share the same fine specificity with the parental line. A pathogenic cell line specific to myelin basic protein (MBP) that expresses Vβ8.2 message was used as a positive control for Vβ8.2 expression.

Probes:

The murine TCR Vβ8 cDNA probe is a 0.3 kb EcoRI/HindIII fragment that is homologous (87% on the DNA and 83% on the protein level) to the rat Vβ8.2 segment (9). The probe was labeled with deoxycytidine 5'-[α-^{32}P]triphosphate (>3000 Ci/mmol) by the random priming method to high specific activity (>10^9 cpm/μg) and purified by passage over a sephadex G-25 quick spin column (Boehringer Mannheim Biochemicals).

The Vβ8.2 specific oligonucleotide probe is complementary to nucleotides coding for amino acids 53-59 of rat TCR Vβ8.2. The oligomer was synthesized on an applied Biosystem 380B DNA synthesizer, gel-purified, end-labeled with adenosine 5'-[γ-^{32}P]triphosphate (>5000 Ci/mmol) and T4 polynucleotide kinase to high specific activity (>10^8 cpm/μg) and purified as described above.

Northern blot analyses:

Total RNA for northern blot analysis was prepared from T-cells purified by passage through ficoll gradients. Fifty million cells were suspended in guanidinium isothiocynate and centrifuged through 5.7M CsCl cushion at 22,000 rpm, 20°C for 24 hours in SW41 rotor. Twenty micrograms RNA were electrophoresed onto a 1.2% agarose-formaldehyde gel, transferred to nylon membrane and prehybridized in 5xSSPE, 5xDenhardt's, 0.1% SDS, 100μg/ml salmon sperm DNA for 2 hours at 65°C (10). Murine Vβ8.2 cDNA was then added at 2x10^6 cpm/ml and hybridized overnight in the same solution. Filters were washed twice in 2xSSPE, 0.1% SDS for 20 minutes at room temperature followed by two 15-minutes high stringency washes in 0.1xSSPE, 0.1% SDS at 65 °C. The filter was autoradiographed at -70°C with Kodak X-Omat AR film and Cronex intensifying screen. In northern analysis using the synthetic oligonucleotide probe, the filter was prehybridized in 6xSSPE, 5xDenhardt's, 0.1% SDS, 100μg/ml salmon sperm DNA. Hybridization was performed in the same solution containing 5x10⁶ cpm/ml of end-labeled Vβ8.2 oligonucleotide probe for 20 hours at 65°C. The filter was washed three times at room temperature in 6xSSPE, 0.1%SDS followed by a 1 minute wash at 50°C. Autoradiography was as described above.

RESULTS AND DISCUSSION

Northern analysis using the 0.3 kb murine Vβ8 cDNA probe shows that uveitogenic T-cell lines (ThS8 and LR16) express Vβ8 genes (Fig.1a). It is noteworthy that the intensity of the hybridization signals of these two T-cell lines were three times less than that of the MBP-specific T-cell line. In contrast, no hybridization signals are detectable in lanes corresponding to the non-pathogenic T-cell line and clones (ThS4, C3 and C4). These results indicate that Vβ8 expressing T-cell clones are enriched in pathogenic, but not in non-pathogenic T-cell lines.

In order to determine whether our T-cell lines also express the Vβ8.2 subfamily gene as is the case in EAE (6), northern analysis was performed using the 21-mer oligonucleotide probe that is specific to the hypervariable CDR2 (complementarity-determining region 2) of rat Vβ8.2. In the mouse this region shows the highest sequence diversity between the three members of the murine Vβ8 gene family (5). This analysis is shown in Fig.1b and indicates that the pathogenic T-cells that induce EAU do not express the Vβ8.2 gene; only the MBP-specific positive control T-cell line gave a positive hybridization signal.

Taken together, these results suggest that other members of the Vβ8 family are being used by T-lymphocytes which induce EAU. Thus, in different autoimmune diseases, pathogenic T-cells may preferentially express one or more members of the three-member Vβ8 gene family. We hope that the information derived from our analyses would provide the experimental basis for development of immunotherapeutic strategies aimed at the control of ocular autoimmunity.

226

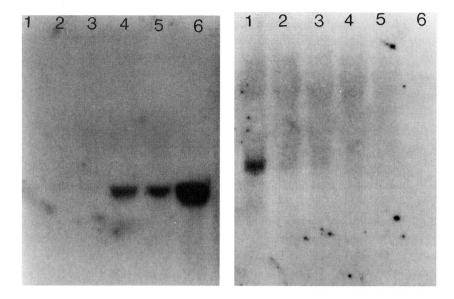

Figure 1. Expression of Vβ8 and Vβ8.2 mRNA in rat S-Antigen and IRBP-specific T-cell lines and clones. Total RNA (20 µg/lane) was fractionated on 1.2% agarose-formaldehyde gels, transfered onto nylon membranes and hybridized as described in materials and methods. (a): Hybridization is with the hexamer-primed 0.3 kb murine cDNA probe. Lanes 1 through 6 are T-cell lines and clones C4, C3, ThS4, LR16, ThS8, and MBP respectively. (b): The end-labeled synthetic oligonucleotide was used as hybridization probe. Lane 1 is total RNA from the MBP-specific line that serves as a positive control for Vβ8.2 gene expression. Lanes 2,3,4 and 5 are RNAs from T-cell lines ThS8, LR16, ThS4 and T-cell clone C3 respectively. Lane 6 is molecular weight standard. For more details see Materials and methods.

REFERENCES

1. Wacker, W.B. (1981) In: Proceceeding 'Immunology of the Eye; Workshop II' (R.J. Helmsen, A. Suran, I. Gery and R.B. Nussenblatt, eds) pp11-32 Information Retrieval, Washington,DC
2. Gery, I., Mochizuki, M. and Nussenblatt, R. B. (1986) In: Progress in Retinal Research (Osborne, N. and Chader, J., eds) 5:75-109
3. Caspi, R.R. et al. (1986), J. Immunol. 136(3):928-933
4. Hu, L., et al. (1989), Cell. Immunol. 122:251-261
5. Kronenberg, M. et al. (1986), Ann. Rev. Immunol. 4:529-591
6. Zamvil, S.S., et al. (1988), J. Exp. Med. 167: 1586-1596
8. Sanui, H. et al. (1989), J. Exp. Med. 169:1947-1960
9. Chluba, J. et al. (1989), Eur. J. Immunol. 19:279-284
10. Maniatis, T., Fritsch, E.F. and Sambrook, J., (1989), Molecular cloning: a laboratory manual, Cold Spring Harbor Laboratory Press, Cold Spring Harbor, New York.

INFECTION

© 1990 Elsevier Science Publishers (Biomedical Division)
Ocular Immunology Today. M. Usui, S. Ohno and K. Aoki, editors.

LANGERHANS CELLS IN THE CORNEA PROMOTE IMMUNOPATHOGENIC HSV-1 RELATED KERATITIS, IRITIS, AND ENCEPHALITIS

MARTINE J. JAGER, DEBRA BRADLEY, SALLY S. ATHERTON, J. WAYNE STREILEIN

Department of Microbiology and Immunology, University of Miami Medical School, P.O. Box 016960 (R138), Miami, Florida 33101, USA.

INTRODUCTION

Herpetic stromal keratitis occurs primarily in immunocompetent individuals infected with HSV-1. It is believed that recurrent stromal keratitis is initiated by reactivation of latent HSV-1 infection in the trigeminal ganglion. Damage to the cornea after reactivation of the virus is probably due to T cells (Russell 1984). Since T cells require that antigen is first processed by antigen-presenting cells like Langerhans cells (LCs), the presence of such cells may influence the development of stromal keratitis. Since the central cornea is usually devoid of LCs, we sought to determine whether the induced presence of LCs influences the severity of ocular disease due to HSV-1.

For this purpose we used an animal model for zosteriform spread of HSV-1 that partly resembles Herpes Simplex secondary infection, and more closely corresponds to Herpes Zoster infection in man (Tullo 1982, Hill 1987). Infection with HSV-1 (strain sc16) on the snout of a BALB/c mouse leads to a skin lesion around the eye on the infected side four days after snout infection, and to mydriasis, iris hyperemia and in some cases to clouding of the cornea. Sporadically, an infected mouse may die, showing signs of paralysis on the side where snout infection took place. This unusual outcome may indicate that the viral infection and the local T cell response against the Herpes virus are not localised to the eye but also involve the brain stem. We therefore included observations concerning the possible neurological symptoms during the development of ocular disease, in our analysis.

Previous studies from this laboratory (McLeish 1989) showed that cautery of the superficial cornea induces the migration of Langerhans cells into the central cornea. Such corneas are highly susceptible to the development of stromal keratitis if the anterior segment of these eyes becomes infected with HSV-1 delivered to that site via zosteriform spread. To investigate further the possible relationship between corneal LC, ocular, and CNS disease, we determined the number of LC in the central cornea and performed unilateral snout infections in four groups of mice: (a) lightly cauterized corneas, (b) corneas scratched mechanically with a 25 gauge needle, (c) corneas with a naturally occurring dystrophy, (4) normal corneas.

MATERIALS AND METHODS

Experimental animals.

Seven to twelve week old female BALB/c mice (Taconic Farms, Germantown, NY) were infected on the lateral side of the snout with HSV-1 virus (strain sc16, 1.5 x 105 PFU in 5 microl) and examined daily with a slitlamp for the development of skin or eye involvement. Snout inoculation, cauterization, and scratching were carried out using pentobarbital (0.30 mg/gm body weight) as the anesthetic agent.

Treatment of the cornea.

Cautery of the corneal surface took place with a hand-held Accu-Temp thermal cauter (Concept, Inc.). Eight to ten light burns were applied to the center of the cornea (McLeish 1989). Scratching of the cornea took place with a 25 gauge needle, which was moved over the corneal surface ten times in two perpendicular directions.

Virus.

Virus stocks were maintained in Vero cells grown in Dulbecco's minimal essential medium containing 5% bovine calf serum and antibiotics. Virus stocks were titrered on Vero cells using a standard plaque assay and stored at -70 C.

Langerhans cell assay. Corneas were obtained from mice treated according to the different protocols mentioned above and epithelial sheets were prepared by soaking the eye in EDTA (Gillette 1981). The epithelial sheets were stained with an immunofluorescence assay employing a monoclonal antibody directed against I-Ad. The sheets were mounted on slides and the number of LC was counted in the central third of the cornea.

RESULTS

During the study, mice would die sporadically during the development of the full-blown herpetic disease. It was noted that such animals showed signs of paralysis in the front and hind limbs ipsilateral to snout infection. The relationship between the development of early pupil dilatation, early corneal involvement and death due to herpetic involvement was studied in mice with normal corneas before snout infection. Iris-hyperemia (before or on the ninth day after infection, $P = 0.037$), and corneal disease (before or on day eight, $P = 0.0016$) were correlated with death due to herpetic nervous system disease.

The number of Ia positive cells in corneal sheets was determined ten days after cauterization or scratching. The number of LC after scratching was slightly higher than than that observed in control corneas (Fig. 1), whereas the number of LC was much higher after cauterization. Mice with the naturally occurring corneal dystrophy showed intermediate and varying numbers of LC.

Snout infection led to different incidences of corneal involvement in the four groups (Fig. 2), with the lowest frequency in control eyes and eyes after scratching, and higher rates in eyes after cauterization and in eyes with a dystrophy.

DISCUSSION

Herpes infection on the snout of immunocompetent mice leads to severe disease in immunocompetent mice, not only involving the eye, but also extending to the central nervous system, even culminating in

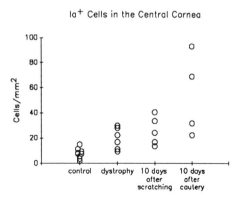

Figure 1. Number of Ia^+ cells in the central cornea in various situations.

death. Our findings show that early expression of iris hyperemia (as an indicator of uveitis), and an early involvement of the cornea are prognostic factors for death due to Herpes Simplex infection. This suggests that the severity of the disease is not limited to the eye, and that the immune response in the eye is part of a more general process. Whether this generalized process involves the brain stem and/or other structures of the brain remains to be studied.

Our data suggest that an increased number of antigen presenting cells in the central cornea at the time of viral infection leads to an early and more vigorous local and systemic immune response. We suspect that subsequent infiltration with immunologically active virus-specific T cells may result in deleterious reaction against virally infected corneal cells. It may be that the virtual absence of LC in the central cornea (which is the case in normal eyes) delays local presentation of viral antigen and therefore (sometimes temporarily) prevents a locally harmful immune response. This ultimately leads to opacification of the cornea and the loss of visual function. It is possible that the absence of LC from the normal central

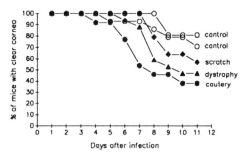

Figure 2. Development of herpetic corneal disease depends on local corneal condition.

cornea is not associated with local resistance to viral infections, but instead helps to preserve the integrity of the cornea, supporting the hypothesis that stromal keratitis has an immunogenic basis in which antigen presenting cells play an important intermediary role.

REFERENCES

1. Easty DL, Shimeld C, Claoue CMP, Menage M (1979). Herpes simplex virus isolation in chronic stromal keratitis: human and laboratory studies. Curr Eye Res. 6:69-74.

2. Gillette TH, Chandler JW (1981). Immunofluorescence and histochemistry of corneal epithelial flat mounts: use of EDTA. Curr Eye Res. 1:249-253.

3. Hill TJ (1987). Ocular pathogenicity of herpes simplex virus. Curr Eye Res 6:1-7.

4. McLeish W, Rubsamen P, Atherton SS, Streilein JW (1989). Immunobiology of Langerhans cells on the ocular surface. II. Role of central corneal Langerhans cells in stromal keratitis following experimental HSV-1 infection in mice. Reg. Immnunol. 2:236-243.

5. Russell RG, Nasisse MP, Larsen HS, Rouse BT (1984). Role of T-lymphocytes in the pathogenesis of herpetic stromal keratitis. Invest. Ophthalmol. Vis Sci 25:938-944.

6. Tullo AB, Shimeld C, Blyth WA, Hill TJ, Easty DL. Spread of virus and distribution of latent infection following ocular herpes simplex in the non-immune and immune mouse. J. Gen Virol 63, 95-101, 1982.

© 1990 Elsevier Science Publishers (Biomedical Division)
Ocular Immunology Today. M. Usui, S. Ohno and K. Aoki, editors.

REACTIVATION OF LATENT MURINE CYTOMEGALOVIRUS IN THE EYE BY IMMUNOSUPPRESSIVE TREATMENT

THEODORE RABINOVITCH, JANG O. OH, PETROS MINASI.
F.I. Proctor Foundation, University of California, San Francisco. CA, USA

INTRODUCTION

Ocular involvements of cytomegalovirus (CMV) such as uveitis and retinochoroiditis have been reported in the literature as a manifestation of systemic CMV infection (1-4). Furthermore, recent studies indicate that CMV retinopathy is the most common ocular infection in AIDS patients (5). Whether these ocular infections are due to reactivation of latent virus within the eye or are from dissemination from peripheral organs to the eye is unknown. Although Hayashi et al. (6) and Bale et al. (7) reported the existence of latent murine CMV (MCMV) in murine ocular tissues, there is still no convincing evidence that indicates the presence of latent CMV in the human eye. It is also unknown whether defects in the host's immunity can lead to the reactivation of latent virus in the eye. Our results indicate that the eye is a site of latency of MCMV and that latent virus in the eye can indeed be reactivated *in vivo* by immunosuppression.

MATERIALS AND METHODS

Three week-old BALB/c male mice obtained from a local vendor were used throughout the experiments. They were free from MCMV infection as shown by negative antibody against the virus. Smith strain of salivary gland-passed MCMV (SG-MCMV) was obtained from the American Type Culture Collection and maintained in BALB/c mice. A working stock of MCMV was prepared by passing the SG-MCMV once in primary BALB/c mouse embryo fibroblast cells and had a titer of 10^5 plaque-forming units (pfu)/ml. Monolayer cultures of secondary BALB/c embryo fibroblast cells grown in wells of 24-well plastic cell culture plates (Costar, Cambridge, MA) were used for virus isolation from specimens. The blood was separated into mononuclear cells and plasma by Ficoll-Hypaque gradation. Mononuclear cells (10^4 cells) or 0.1 ml of plasma were inoculated onto each of the duplicate wells of mouse embryo fibroblast cells. Ten percent tissue homogenate of each organ was prepared and 1.0 ml of the supernatant was then inoculated into each of the duplicate wells of mouse embryo cells in a 24-well culture plate. Co-culture of tissue was carried out by placing a 1-2 mm^3 fragment of tissue in each of two wells containing monolayer culture of mouse embryo fibroblast cells. The culture plates were then incubated at 37°C in a humid atmosphere of 5% CO_2 and 95% air, and the cell culture medium was completely replaced with fresh medium twice a week during the experimental period. The plates were examined for cytopathic effect (CPE) twice a week for 8 weeks, and any virus isolate from culture with positive CPE was confirmed as MCMV by immunofluorescence assay with fluorescein-conjugated specific anti-MCMV serum.

EXPERIMENTAL DESIGNS AND RESULTS

Latency of MCMV in the Eye Following Primary Eye Infection

Mice received bilateral intravitreal injections of MCMV (10^3 pfu/eye). At weekly intervals, 2 to 3 mice were sacrificed, and organs including the eyes were collected for MCMV isolation from homogenate cultures and co-cultures of each organ. Both eyes were cut into two equal portions, and one portion of each eye was used for the homogenate culture and the other for the co-culture. Infectious virus could be recovered from three of four eye homogenates in week 1, from one of four in week 2, but from none thereafter. In co-cultures, virus could be recovered from two of four eyes on week 4 and one of the four eyes on week 5, but no virus was detected thereafter suggesting that virus in the eye becomes latent after week 4. No virus was recovered from trigeminal ganglia homogenates, but one of four co-cultures at week 2 and week 4 were positive for MCMV. Salivary gland samples were most consistently positive for virus isolation with almost 100% of both homogenates and co-cultures positive up to week 5, and with 25% of co-cultures on week 6. Other than isolation of virus from mononuclear cells in one of four mice on week 6, no virus was recovered from any blood specimen at any other time.

In Vivo Reactivation of Latent MCMV in Eyes by Cyclosporine and Cortisone

Two groups of mice received bilateral intravitreal injections of MCMV (10^3pfu/eye). Mice in the third group served as a control and received bilateral intravitreal injections of saline instead of the virus. Nine weeks later, well after latency of the virus was established in eyes of mice in virus-injected groups, mice in one of the virus-injected groups and mice in the saline injected group were subjected to an immunosuppressive treatment with daily injections of CsA (40 ug/g IM) and cortisone (125 ug/g IP) while mice in the remaining virus-injected group received sham immunosuppressive treatment with daily saline injections. At three weekly intervals, two to three mice from each group were sacrificed, and eyes and other organs were obtained for MCMV isolation from tissue homogenates. This experiment was repeated three times.

In the virus-injected mice with immunosuppression, ocular homogenates were positive for virus isolation in ten of forty-four eyes in ten of twenty-two mice. Most of the virus isolates (9/10) were obtained during the first two weeks of immunosuppression. Virus was also recovered from 4 of 22 salivary gland homogenates. Virus isolation was positive in two of twenty-two mononuclear cell cultures from immunosuppressed mice but homogenates of trigeminal ganglia and blood plasma remained negative. In the virus-injected mice with sham immunosuppression (saline injection), no virus could be isolated from homogenates of any tissue except mononuclear cells; mononuclear cells from one of eighteen previously infected mice yielded virus without immunosuppressive treatment. The saline-injected mice with immunosuppression failed to yield virus from homogenates of any organs. All the virus isolates were confirmed as MCMV by immunofluorescence assay with fluorescein-conjugated specific anti-MCMV serum.

DISCUSSION

In the past, the murine model of MCMV infection has been widely used to study *in vivo* reactivation of latent MCMV. Cytotoxic agents such as cyclophosphamide (8-11), or antithymocyte serum with or without corticosteroids (8) have been used to reactivate latent MCMV from various organs. Also immunologic stimulation by whole blood (12) or spleen cell transfer (9) also led to reactivation of latent virus. However, as far as we know, no such *in vivo* reactivation of latent CMV in the eye has been previously reported. In our attempts to reactivate latent MCMV in the eye, we recovered virus from eye homogenates in ten of twenty-two animals following the immunosuppressive treatment with CsA and cortisone, while no virus was recovered from animals receiving saline (p<0.001). The virus recovered from the eye homogenates could not be of extraocular origin, such as from the trigeminal ganglia, since no virus could be recovered from homogenates of this tissue. Similarly, it was unlikely that the salivary gland was disseminating the virus to the eye because the recovery rate of the virus from homogenates of the gland (18.2%) was far lower than that from the eye (45.5%). Furthermore, the possibility of hematogenous spread of the virus to the eye from other organs, such as salivary glands, is remote because the virus was infrequently present in the blood (9.0%) at anytime. Therefore, the immunosuppression by daily injection of CsA and cortisone must have induced reactivation of latent MCMV within the eye *in vivo*. Our present study is the first to our knowledge to report such *in vivo* reactivation of latent MCMV in the eye.

SUMMARY

The eye can serve as a site of latent infection of MCMV which can be reactivated *in vivo* by immunosuppressive means.

ACKNOWLEDGMENT

This work was supported in part by EY 01578 and EY 08037.

REFERENCES

1. Burns RP (1959) Arch Ophthalmol 61:376

2. Aaberg TM, Cesarz TJ, and Rytel MW (1972) Am J Ophthalmol 74:407

3. England AC, Miller SA, and Maki DG (1982) New Engl J Med 307:94

4. Meredith TA, Aaberg TM, and Reeser FH (1979) Am J Ophthalmol 87:793

5. Holland GN, Pepose JS, Pettit TH, Gottlieb MS, Yee RD, and Foos RY (1983) Ophthalmology 90:859

6. Hayashi K, Kurihara I, and Uchida Y (1985) Invest Ophthalmol Vis Sci 26:486

7. Bale JF, O'Neill ME, Hogan N, and Kern ER (1987) Arch Ophthalmol 102:1214

8. Jordan ML, Shanley JD, and Stevens JG (1977) J Gen Virol 37:419

9. Mayo D, Armstrong JA, and Ho M (1978) J Infect Dis 138:890

10. Mayo D, Armstrong JA, and Ho M (1977) Nature 267:721

11. Dowling JN, Saslow AR, Armstrong JA, and Ho M (1976) J Infect Dis 133:399

12. Cheung KS, and Lang DJ (1977) J Infect Dis 135:841

© 1990 Elsevier Science Publishers (Biomedical Division)
Ocular Immunology Today. M. Usui, S. Ohno and K. Aoki, editors.

CO-FACTORS ASSOCIATED WITH CYTOMEGALOVIRUS INFECTION OF THE RETINA

JAY S. PEPOSE,[*][+] KEITH A. LAYCOCK,[*] MAX Q. ARENS[#] and GREGORY A. STORCH[#]

Departments of Ophthalmology,[*] Pathology[+] and Pediatrics,[#] Washington University School of Medicine, St. Louis, Missouri, USA, 63110.

INTRODUCTION

Cytomegalovirus (CMV) infection of the retina is the most common blinding ocular manifestation of AIDS, resulting in total retinal necrosis if left untreated.[1] It is estimated that 35,000 AIDS patients will develop CMV retinitis in 1991 in the United States alone, and that this also represents the leading cause of suicide amongst AIDS victims.

The reported incidence of CMV retinitis is 0% among healthy homosexual males,[2] 4% in ambulatory AIDS patients,[3] 15% in hospitalized AIDS victims,[4] and 34% in an autopsy series of AIDS patients. Whereas CMV retinitis had been previously reported in patients with other forms of immunosuppression such as leukemia, lymphoma, solid tumors, Hodgkin's disease, and organ transplant recipients,[6,7] the incidence of CMV retinitis in these groups does not approach that seen in AIDS.[6,7] This could reflect different rates of viremia, more virulent, retinotropic or multiple strains of CMV, differences in the nature of the immunosuppression in these different disorders, or immunogenetic factors. We studied the role of the AIDS virus--HIV type 1--in retinal tissue as an agent that could interact at the cellular level with hematogenously spread CMV and potentiate productive CMV replication and subsequent retinal necrosis.

MATERIALS AND METHODS

HIV and CMV Antigen Staining and Culture Techniques: The methods utilized for viral culture, immunohistochemistry and sequential antigen staining were as described by Skolnik et. al.[8]
Polymerase Chain Reaction: The HIV primers and reaction conditions were as described by Ou et al.[9] The primer pair SK 68/69 was used.
CD4 Antigen and Macrophage Detection: CD4 antigen staining was performed using Leu3a (Becton-Dickinson, Mountain View, CA) and OKT4a (Ortho Diagnostic, Raritan, NJ) monoclonal antibodies and an enhanced 4-step avidin biotin technique.[10] Macrophages were detected using the Leu-M3 antibody (Becton-Dickinson). Co-staining for HIV and macrophage markers was performed using the avidin-biotin immunoperoxidase method followed by glucose oxidase staining[8] (Vector Laboratories, Burlingame, CA).

RESULTS

Demonstration of HIV in CMV-Infected Retinas from AIDS Cadavers

Of 10 retinas that were culture positive and/or antigen positive for cytomegalovirus, HIV co-infection was demonstrated in 6 by polymerase chain reaction (Figure 1).

238

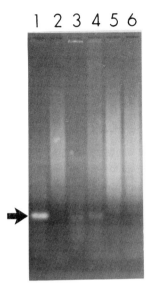

Figure 1. PCR analysis of DNA from HIV-infected H9 cells using HIV-specific primers (lane 1) amplified a 142 bp sequence (arrow). With the same primers, this HIV sequence was detected in 2 of 5 CMV-infected retinas (lane 3 and 4) tested in this run.

Detection of HIV Antigens in CMV-Infected Retinas

HIV antigens (Figure 2) were demonstrated on vascular endothelial cells and macrophages in 4 of the 10 CMV-infected retinas. In addition, HIV-antigen positive cells were demonstrated on

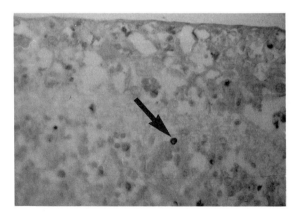

Figure 2. HIV antigens are demonstrated on scattered cells (arrow) in a necrotic CMV-infected retina.

macrophage-like cells in the conjunctiva, ciliary body, iris, choroid, optic nerve and nervehead. Many of these cells co-stained with the Leu-M3 macrophage marker in sequential labeling studies. Occasional retinal cells with glial morphology were also HIV-antigen positive. Many megalic retinal cells were co-stained with antibodies against HIV and CMV, and were presumably co-infected. Cotton-wool spots did not react with HIV or CMV antibodies using the avidin-biotin immunoperoxidase technique.

Retinal Tissue is CD4 Antigen Negative

Retinas from AIDS patients and controls were processed for the presence of the CD4 antigen using the OKT4a and Leu3a monoclonal antibody and an enhanced avidin-biotin technique. No positive cells were identified in retinal tissue from either AIDS or controls, although occasional CD4-positive cells were seen scattered in the choroid in control tissues.

DISCUSSION

The reason for the tenfold higher incidence of CMV retinitis in AIDS patients as compared to renal transplant recipients[6] is unclear. Several groups of investigators have recently documented HIV-type 1 infection of human retina.[8,12-14] In this study, we focus on the frequency of dual infection of the retina of AIDS patients with HIV and CMV. The polymerase chain reaction was in our hands, more sensitive than HIV recovery in tissue culture, showing amplification of a specific HIV sequence with DNA extracted from 3 CMV-infected retinas that were HIV-culture negative. CMV and HIV-type 1 co-infections have been similarly demonstrated in human brain tissue of AIDS victims.[15]

In vitro studies have demonstrated reciprocal enhancement of gene expression and viral replication between HIV-type 1 and human CMV[8,16-21] The mechanisms underlying bi-directional enhancement may include transactivation of the CMV or HIV enhancer/promoters by cellular or viral transcription factors,[16-21] alterations in binding affinity or phenotypic mixing.[8]

The majority of retinal cells bearing HIV antigens had macrophage-like morphology and many co-stained with macrophage markers. These cells may represent the primary vehicle initiating HIV-retinal infection. The vascular endothelium was also focally involved with HIV, although no CMV antigens were demonstrated on these cells. Occasional cells with glial characteristics bore HIV antigens, as did cytomegalic retinal cells. It is presumed that these later cells, which we have shown to be negative for CD4 antigen, were infected by HIV via an alternative CD4-independent mechanism. Whereas it is well documented that the CD4 antigen serves as a receptor for HIV-1,[22] there is increasing evidence for an alternative pathway(s) by which HIV can enter and replicate in CD4-negative cells of diverse origin.[23]

In summary, CMV co-infection of human retinal tissue along with HIV may allow biological interactions that enhance productive infection and retinal necrosis, and may account for the high incidence of CMV retinitis in AIDS patients as compared with other immunocompromised hosts. These bi-directional interactions may, in part, account for documented regression of CMV retinitis in patients treated with zidovudine alone,[27-29] an anti-HIV drug with no reported effect on CMV replication in vitro.

ACKNOWLEDGEMENTS

Supported in part by Public Health Service Grant EY08143-01 from the National Eye Institute (JSP) and a grant from Research to Prevent Blindness, Inc. Dr. Pepose is the recipient of the American College of Surgeons Faculty Fellowship. Dr. Laycock is the recipient of an ARVO-ALCON Postdoctoral Fellowship.

REFERENCES

1.   Palestine AG, Rodrigues MM, Macher MM, et al (1984) Ophthalmology 91:1092-1099

2.   Khadem M, Kalish SB, Goldsmith J, et al (1984) Arch Ophthalmol 102:201-206

3.   Rosenberg PR, Uliss AE, Friedland GH, et al (1983) Ophthalmology 90:874-884

4.   Freeman WR, Lerner CW, Mines JA, et al (1984) Am J Ophthalmol 97:133-142

5.   Pepose JS, Holland GN, Nestor MS, et al (1985) Ophthalmology 92:472-484

6.   Porter R, Crombie AL, Gardner PS, Vidall RP (1972) Br M J 3:133-136

7.   Murray HW, Knox DL, Green WR, Susel RM (1977) Am J Med 63:574-

8.   Skolnik PR, Pomerantz RJ, de la Monte SM, et al (1989) Am J Ophthalmol 107:361-372

9.   Ou CY, Kwok S, Mitchell SW, et al (1988) Science 239:295-297

10.   Gupta PK, Myers JD, Baylin SB, et al (1985) Diagnostic Cytopathol 2:133-6

11.   Holland GN, Pepose JS, Pettit TH, et al (1983) Ophthalmology 90:859-873

12.   Pomerantz RJ, Kuritzkes DR, de la Monte SM, et al (1987) N Engl J Med 317:1643-1647

13.   Cantrill HL, Henry K, Brooks J, et al (1988) Ophthalmology 95:1458-1463

14.   Qavi HB, Green MT, SeGall GK, Font RL (1987) Curr Eye Res 8:379-387

15.   Nelson JA, Reynolds-Kohler C, Oldstone MBA, Wiley CA (1988) Virology 165-286-295

16.   Davis MG, Kenney SC, Kamine J, et al (1987) Proc Natl Acad Sci, USA 84:8642-8646

17.   Elfassi E, Michelon S, Bachelevis F, et al (1987) Virology 138:461-470

18.   Rando RF, Pellett PE, Luciw PA, et al (1987) Oncogene 1:13-18

19.   Gendelman HE, Phelps W, Feigenbaum L, et al (1986) Proc Natl Acad Sci, USA 83:9759-9763

20.   Skolnik PR, Kosloff BR, Hirsch MS (1988) J Infect Dis 157:508-514

21.   Ho WZ, Harouse JM, Rando RF, et al (1990) J Gen Virol 71:97-103

22.   Maddon PJ, Dagleish AG, McDougal JS, et al (1986) Cell 47:333-348

23.   Li XL, Moudgil T, Vinters HV, Ho DD (1990) J Virol 64:1383-1387

24.   Clapham P, Weber JN, Whitby D, et al (1989) Nature 337:368-370

25.   Harouse JM, Kunsch C, Hartle HT, et al (1989) J Virol 63:2527-2533

26.   Tateno M, Gonzalez-Scarano F, Levy JA (1989) Proc Natl Acad Sci, USA 86:4287-4290

27.   D'Amico DJ, Skolnik PR, Kosloff BR, et al (1988) Arch Ophthalmol 106:1168-1169

28.   Guyer DR, Jabs DA, Brant AM, et al (1989) Arch Ophthalmol 107:868-874

29.   Fay MT, Freeman WR, Wiley CA, et al (1988) Am J Ophthalmol 105:483-490.

© 1990 Elsevier Science Publishers (Biomedical Division)
Ocular Immunology Today. M. Usui, S. Ohno and K. Aoki, editors.

ATYPICAL INTERMEDIATE UVEITIS (PARS PLANITIS) ASSOCIATED WITH LYME BORRELIOSIS

WILLIAM W. CULBERTSON, M.D., KIRK E. WINWARD, M.D., J. LAWTON SMITH, M.D.
Bascom Palmer Eye Institute, Miami, Florida, U.S.A.

Lyme borreliosis is a recently described multisystem disorder caused by the spirochete Borrelia burgdorferi. The infection is transmitted from animals, particularly deer, to humans by the bite of various species of the Ixodes deer tick.(1). The disease appears to be worldwide in distribution although infection is usually acquired during exposure in specific endemic areas such as the Northeastern and Great Lakes regions of the United States. Similar to syphilis, there are three overlapping clinical stages of Lyme disease. Stage one is characterized by the erythema chronicum migrans (ECM) skin lesion and flu-like constitutional symptoms. In the secondary stage, meningitis, cranial nerve palsies and myocarditis may occur. The tertiary stage is manifested by arthritis, demyelinating-like syndromes, and chronic fatigue. Previous reports of ocular manifestations have described cranial nerve palsies, interstitial keratitis, optic neuropathy, pseudotumor cerebri, panuveitis, choroiditis and orbital myositis, usually occuring in the secondary or tertiary stage of Lyme disease. We recently diagnosed tertiary Lyme disease in a 26 year old woman (Index case-LC) with pars planitis. This prompted a search for evidence of Lyme disease in 21 additional randomly selected patients with pars planitis, yielding six additional patients with both pars planitis and Lyme disease.

The index case is a 26 year old woman (LC) who developed a typical ECM lesion on her right ankle in 1975 followed by a flu-like illness and temporary bilateral facial palsy. In 1981 she had a recurrent right facial palsy. In 1984 she was diagnosed as having bilateral pars planitis with vitritis, cystoid macular edema and snowbanked exudates over the pars plana. Small granulomatous keratic precipitates and iris nodules with posterior synechia were present in both eyes. She was treated with oral and periocular corticosteroids with gradually deteriorating vision. A right facial palsy recurred in 1988, and she noted fatigue, arthralgias and myalgias. Serologic testing for Lyme disease was positive with a Lyme IFA IgG of 1:128 and a Lyme ELISA of 1.7 (normal less than 1.0). All other evaluations were negative including FTA-ABS, VDRL, antinuclear antibody, rheumatoid factor, angiotensin converting enzyme, chest x-ray, and tuberculin skin testing. She initially responded to a ten day course of intravenous ceftriaxone with a decrease in intra-ocular inflammation. After several months, the inflammation recurred and she again responded to a month course of intravenous ceftriaxone, 2.0g./day. Her fatigue resolved, but she continues to experience myalgias and arthralgias. However, after four months the inflammation increased again, but not as severely as previously, and her inflammation has been managed on modest doses of topical corticosteroids. A lumbar puncture performed after treatment was normal but magnetic resonance imaging of the brain demonstrated large areas of possible demyelination.

This case prompted serologic testing of an additional 21 randomly selected patients diagnosed as having pars planitis. Six of these patients had positive serologic (either positive IFA-IgG, ELISA and/or Western blot) and clinical evidence of previous Lyme infection. Six had lived in endemic areas for Lyme disease and three reported a definite history of a tick bite. Two patients recalled an ECM-like lesion, two had recurrent facial palsies, and two had a pauciarticular arthritis consistent with Lyme disease and only one, an 11 year old girl, had had no systemic manifestations of Lyme disease.

All patients had been diagnosed as having pars planitis with predominantly vitreous inflammation, inferior snowbanking and snowballs, and an otherwise negative evaluation. The anterior segment inflammation however was somewhat atypical for pars planitis with small granulomatous keratic precipitates, iris nodules and posterior synechia associated with episcleral injection and photophobia.

The intraocular inflammation initially responded to anti-borrelia antibiotic therapy in all seven patients. Four patients were initially treated with oral antibiotics and two responded. The two failures were then treated with intravenous antibiotics with response. The other three patients were treated with intravenous antibiotics alone with a prompt decrease in intraocular inflammation two to nine months following initial treatment and five required additional oral maintenance treatment with oral doxycycline.

In a previously conducted survey of 75 randomly selected Bascom Palmer Eye Institute patients, two patients (3%) were found to be seropositive for Lyme antibodies (2). Comparing our percentage of seven of 22 (32%) seropositive pars planitis patients with this 3% incidence in the local population gives a significant difference statistically (P less than .001).

DISCUSSION

Approximately one-third of our pars planitis patients appear to also have Lyme disease. This is similar to the 32% found by Scholes et al in a study of fifteen pars planitis patients in Utah (3). Ongoing chronic borrelia infection probably plays a role in the ocular inflammation in these patients since all responded to anti-borrelia antibiotic therapy. It is uncertain whether this represents the effects of living borrelia within the eye or whether the extraocular organisms are causing a remote secondary ocular inflammatory effect. In some late manifestations of Lyme disease such as interstitial keratitis (4) and arthritis, antibiotic therapy has not been helpful (1), whereas in others, such as myocarditis, antibiotics have been curative and borrelia have been demonstrated in the affected tissue (5). Further investigation employing immunocytologic techniques, polymerase chain reaction and borrelia culture performed on intraocular samples will be necessary to determine whether intraocular borrelia infection is responsible for some cases of pars planitis.

The serologic diagnosis of Lyme disease is inexact with diversity in testing technique, antigen and limits for positivity creating inconsistent results between laboratories and within the same laboratory (1). "Seronegative" (6) and false positive Lyme disease compounds the difficulty in diagnosis and it is possible that our percentage of Lyme disease and pars planitis (32%) is inaccurately low or high. The possibility of "seronegative" borrelia infection in a patient with atypical pars planitis could be considered an indication for antibiotic therapy if the history or other findings suggest Lyme disease.

REFERENCES

1. Steere AC. Lyme disease. N Engl J Med 1989; 321:586-96.

2. Smith JL, Parsons TM, Paris-Hamelin AJ, Porschen RK. The prevalence of Lyme disease in a non-endemic area. J Clin Neuro-ophthalmol 1989; 9:148-55.

3. Scholes GN, Teske MP, Zimmerman PL. Lyme disease and pars planitis. Poster. American Academy of Ophthalmology Annual Meeting, 1989, New Orleans, LA.

4. Baum J, Barza M, Weinstein et al. Bilateral keratitis as a manifestation of Lyme disease. Am.J Ophthalmol 1988; 105:75-6.

5. Stanek G, Klein J, Bittner R, Glogar D. Isolation of Borrelia burgdorferi from the myocardium of a patient with longstanding cardiomyopathy. N Engl J Med 1990; 322:249-52.

6. Schutzer SE, Coyle PK, Belman AL, Golightly MG, Drulle J. Sequestration of antibody to Borrelia burgdorferi in immune complexes in seronegative Lyme disease. Lancet 1990; 335:312-5.

© 1990 Elsevier Science Publishers (Biomedical Division)
Ocular Immunology Today. M. Usui, S. Ohno and K. Aoki, editors.

IMMUNOHISTOCHEMICAL STUDY OF CYTOMEGALOVIRUS RETINOUVEITIS :
IMMUNODIAGNOSIS WITH ANTI-CYTOMEGALOVIRUS MONOCLONAL ANTIBODY

Y MASUYAMA, A SAWADA, Y EIZURU*, Y MINAMISHIMA*, A SUMIYOSHI**
Department of Ophthalmology, *Department of Microbiology,
**Department of Pathology, Miyazaki Medical College, Kiyotake,
Miyazaki (Japan)

INTRODUCTION

Cytomegalovirus(CMV) retinitis is one of the most common cause of
blindness in patients with organ transplantation or patients with
acquired immunodeficiency syndrome. Pathologically, CMV retinitis
is usually diagnosed by detecting cytomegalic cells with inclusions
and CMV particles. However, each virus of the herpesvirus family
shares a common morphological appearance. Therefore, the histopathological findings alone are unsatisfactory for a definitive diagnosis of this disease.

To make a definitive diagnosis of CMV retinitis, we employed a
direct immunoperoxidase technique with a CMV-specific monoclonal
antibody(MAb). The MAb was valuable in detecting CMV antigens in
paraffin-embedded sections of the ocular tissues.

MATERIALS AND METHODS

Case history: The patient was a 29-year-old male with longstanding
so-called Banti's syndrome and he complained of visual impairment in
both eyes as previously described (1). In the fundus examination,
the optic disc was pale and the retinal arteries and veins were nar-
rowed with perivascular sheathing. The striking findings were multiple large patches of granular yellow-white retinal necrosis associated with flame-shaped hemorrhages. Four months after the initial
visit, he died of pneumonia. The ocular specimens of suspected CMV
retinouveitis were obtained at autopy and fixed in 5% formaldehyde
fixative for light microscopy and in 3% glutaraldehyde fixative for
electron microscopy.

Pathological and immunohistochemical examination: The specimens
were examined by light and electron microscopy. The paraffin-
embedded specimens were further examined by direct immunoperoxidase
technique using horseradish peroxidase(HRP)-labeled anti-CMV MAb.
The MAb used is the Fab'fragment of human IgG1 against an immediate-
early antigen.

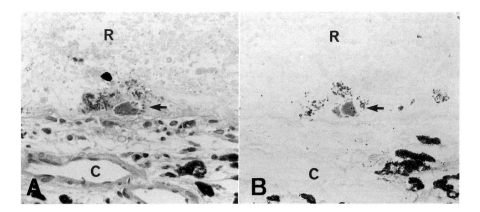

Figure 1. A. Photomicrograph of the retina. The retina is extensively necrotic. A cytomegalic cell with intranuclear inclusion
is present. HE.x400   B. Direct immunoperoxidase staining of the
serial section. Inclusion body is stained with HRP-labeled MAb
against CMV (arrow).   x400   C: choroid, R: retina

RESULTS

   Histopathologic examinations revealed extensive loss of cellular
architecture and severe, massive necrosis of the retina. A large
number of cytomegalic cells with intranuclear and intracytoplasmic
inclusion bodies were seen throughout the retina. Although the
origin of the majority of these affected cells was uncertain, some
of them were apparently vascular endothelial cells or pigment epithelial cells of the retina (Fig. 1A). In contrast, a small number
of cytomegalic cells were scattered throughout the uveal tissues
(Fig. 2A). Within the intranuclear and intracytoplasmic inclusion
bodies, particles of the herpesvirus type and dense bodies, respectively were found by electron microscopy (Fig. 3).

   Immunohistologically, the inclusion bodies of cytomegalic cells
were stained specifically with HRP-labeled anti-CMV MAb (Fig. 1B &
2B).

DISCUSSION

   Each herpesvirus infection causes virtually the same severe necrotizing retinitis. An enlarged cell with the intranuclear inclusion is thought to be characteristic of CMV infection in the paraffin
-embedded sections. However, the mere presence of cytomegalic cells
with inclusions is not pathognomonic for CMV infection. Occasionally CMV affected cells may remain normal in size and similar inclusions may be produced herpes simplex(HSV)- and varicella-zoster

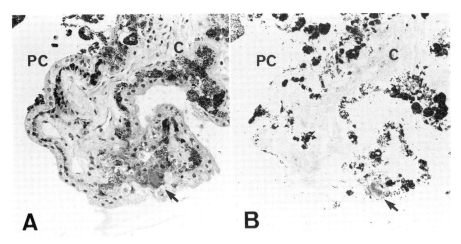

Figure 2. A. Photomicrograph of the ciliary body. A cytomegalic
cell is seen in the ciliary pigment epithelium. HE.x400 B. Direct
immunoperoxidase staining of the serial section. The intranuclear
inclusion body specifically stained by the MAb. x400 C: ciliary
body, PC: posterior chamber

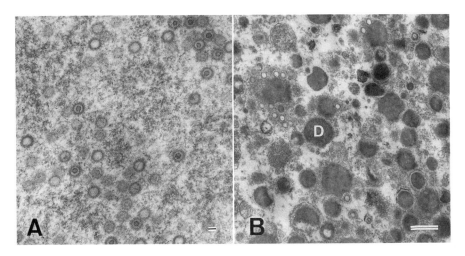

Figure 3. A. Electron micrograph of an intranuclear inclusion body.
CMV particles display three different types; empty capsids, capsids
with electron-lucent cores and with electron-dense cores. Bar=100nm
B. A number of dense bodies with limiting membrane are observed in
the cytoplasmic inclusion body. Bar=1µm

virus(VZV). Although the presence of dense bodies is unique for CMV infection (2), all herpesviruses generally share a common morphologic appearance, which makes it difficult to identify the causative virus by a conventional pathologic method.

The MAb used in this study is human IgG1 against an immediate-early antigen of CMV(3). This MAb reacted neither with other human herpesviruses including HSV-1, HSV-2, VZV, or Epstein-Barr virus, nor with CMVs of primate or rodent origin (4). The antigen reactive with this MAb appears in the cells immediately after virus inoculation, which affords rapid diagnosis of CMV infection by virus isolation. It also enables us to detect an early CMV lesion in paraffin-embedded sections. Some MAbs against early protein were not applicable to detect CMV antigen in paraffin-embedded tissue sections, though they were useful in cell culture system (5). However, the MAb used in this study is readily applicable to paraffin-embedded tissue sections. The direct immunoperoxidase technique was superior to any other methods and it will facilitate rapid diagnosis of CMV infection.

CONCLUSION

CMV retinitis was virologically diagnosed by a direct immunoperoxidase technique with paraffin-embedded materials. A HRP-labeled MAb against an immediate-early antigen of CMV is valuable for definitive diagnosis of CMV retinitis.

REFERENCES

1. Masuyama Y, Baba Y, Sawada A, Sumiyoshi A (1981) In: Sundmacher R (eds) Herpetische Augenkrankungen. J.F. Bergmann, Munchen, pp495-500.

2. Smith JD, de Harven E (1973) J Virol 12:919-930

3. Masuho Y, Matsumoto Y, Sugano T, Fujinaga S, Minamishima Y (1987) J gen Virol 68:1457-1461.

4. Y. Eizuru, Y Minamishima et al. in preparation.

5. Goldstein LG, McDougall J, Hackman R, Meyers JD, Thomas ED, Nowinski R (1982) 38:273-281.

© 1990 Elsevier Science Publishers (Biomedical Division)
Ocular Immunology Today. M. Usui, S. Ohno and K. Aoki, editors.

CORRELATION BETWEEN HIV-INDUCED SEROLOGIC FINDINGS AND RETINAL LESIONS IN PATIENTS WITH AIDS

PIVETTI-PEZZI P.,TAMBURI S.,MEZZAROMA I.*, PINTER E.*, ACCORINTI M. Istituto di Oftalmologia. *Cattedra di Allergologia e Immunologia Università degli Studi di Roma "La Sapienza" - Rome. Italy.

INTRODUCTION

The more frequent retinal lesions in patients with AIDS are opportunistic infections (mainly cytomegalovirus retinitis) and microangiopathy; this consists of retinal cotton-wool spots, haemorrages, microaneurysms, ischemic maculopathy.(Holland, 1983; Freeman,1989; Jabs, 1989).

The retinal microangiopathy observed in AIDS could be related to an endothelial damage induced by HIV. However not all the patients with AIDS develop microangiopathy and the determinant factors are unknown. The HIV might induce an endothelial damage directly and/or indirectly (Pepose,1985). Indeed the virus was isolated by Pomerantz (1987) in neuronal and endothelial cells of the retina but in the pathogenesis of ocular lesions immunomediated mechanisms cannot be disregarded. We carry out a study on the correlations between serologic markers of HIV infection and retinal changes.

PATIENTS AND METHODS

Forty-eight patients with full-blown AIDS were submitted to ophthalmic evaluations and serologic studies for HIV-specific antibodies (Western blot) and antigenemia (ELISA). They were divided into two groups: the first grouped 16 patients with retinal cotton-wool spots (CWS); the second 32 patients with no opportunistic ophthalmic lesions or without ocular involvement.

Both these groups were divided again regarding the absence of antibodies against p 24 and antigenemia in the serum. The antibodies directed against other viral proteins were also evaluated.

The statistic analysis of the results was performed by Chi-square test.

RESULTS

In the group with CWS 56.25% of patients was negative for antibodies against p 24 and positive for antigenemia, 25% was positive for antibodies against p 24 and positive for antigenemia, 6.25% was positive for antibodies against p 24 and negative for antigenemia and 12.5% was negative for antibodies against p 24 and for antigenemia.

On the contrary in the group with other ocular lesions or without ocular involvement 15.6% was negative for antibodies against p 24 and positive for antigenemia; 40.6% was positive for antibodies against p 24 and for antigenemia; 34.4% was positive for antibodies against p 24 and negative for antigenemia and 9.4% was negative for antibodies against p 24 and for antigenemia.

The statistic analysis demonstrated a significative difference (X^2=6.6681; p < 0.01) between the group with CWS versus the other group regarding the negative reaction for the presence of antibodies against p 24 and positive antigenemia.

A lesser statistic significance between the two groups, probably due to few observations, was found considering patients with positive antibodies to p 24 and negative antigenemia (6% vs 34.4%; X^2=3.125; p < 0.1) (Tab.1).

No significative differences were found between the two groups considering the other viral proteins (i.e. gp 160, gp 120, gp 41, p 64, p 55, p 53, p 31, p 18, p 15), however in the first group the humoral reaction frequently was impaired and directed against a lesser number of proteins. Particularly antibodies against p 41 were more persistent.

Tab. 1 - SEROLOGIC FINDINGS IN AIDS PATIENTS WITH AND WITHOUT CWS.

ANTI p 24	ANTIGENEMIA	PATIENTS WITH CWS %	PATIENTS WITHOUT CWS %
+	—	6.25 *	34.4 *
—	—	12.5	9.4
+	+	25	40.6
—	+	56.25 **	15.6 **

* POSITIVE p 24 REACTIVITY WITH NEGATIVE ANTIGENEMIA $\chi^2 = 3.125$ $p < 0.1$
** NEGATIVE p 24 REACTIVITY WITH POSITIVE ANTIGENEMIA $\chi^2 = 6.6681$ $p < 0.01$

CONCLUSIONS

We think that CWS in HIV infected patients without other causes of microangiopathy (i.e. mellitus diabetes, hypertension, etc.) are a marker for AIDS with negative prognostic value. Infact we demonstrated, in a previous study (Pivetti-Pezzi, 1989), that they are well related to the decrease of the number of CD4+ cells, and in this study we have found their correlation with some markers of HIV infection predictive for a bad prognosis as the decrease of antibodies against p 24 and the positive antigenemia.

The antibodies to p 24 (an HIV-core protein) in fact decrease in the later phases of the infection and may go with a repositivization of antigenemia as result of an increase in viral replication and/or immunological failure.

Therefore considering the serologic findings we think that CWS are related to a more severe state of immunodeficiency when compared with patients without these retinal lesions. According to this opinion we could explain how only some ocular manifestations are characteristic of full-blown AIDS and have a negative prognostic value.

In fact other retinal lesions as isolated haemorrhages are

present also in earlier stages of the disease and seem not to have a similar negative prognostic value; they could be explained by piastrinopenia. The pathogenesis of CWS remain to be cleared but we underline the possibility that they could be related to the impairment of humoral response against viral proteins.

Indeed we were not able to demonstrate some significative differences regarding the pattern of antibodies directed against other HIV proteins (i.e. gp 160, gp 120, gp 41, p 64, etc.) between the two groups of patients considered, but the more frequently reduction in the types expressed in the first group may be of interest and require further studies.

ACKNOWLEDGEMENTS

This study was supported in part by grants from Ministero della Sanità Istituto Superiore di Sanità-Progetto AIDS 1989 - Roma-Italy

REFERENCES

1. Holland G.N., Pepose J.S., Pettit T.H. et. al.: Acquired immune deficiency syndrome. Ocular manifestations. Ophthalmol 90:858-873, 1983.

2. Freeman W.R., Chen A., Henderly D.E. et al.: Prevalence and significance of acquired immunodeficiency syndrome-related retinal microvasculopathy. Am. J. Ophthalmol 107:229-235, 1989.

3. Jabs D.A., Green R.W., Fox R.et al.: Ocular manifestations of acquired immune deficiency syndrome. Ophthalmol 96:1092-1099, 1989.

4. Pepose J.S., Holland G.N., Nestor M.S., et al.: Acquired immune deficency syndrome. Pathogenic mechanisms of ocular disease. Ophthalmol 92:472-484, 1985.

5. Pomerantz R.J., Kurit D.R., Delamonte S.R. et al.: Infection of the retina by human immunodeficiency virus type I. N. Eng. J. Med. 317:1643-1647, 1987.

6. Pivetti-Pezzi P., Tamburi S., D'Offizi G.P., et al.: Cotton-wool like spots: a marker for AIDS? Ann. Ophthalmol. 21:31-33, 1989.

GENERAL OCULAR IMMUNOLOGY

© 1990 Elsevier Science Publishers (Biomedical Division)
Ocular Immunology Today. M. Usui, S. Ohno and K. Aoki, editors.

EVIDENCE THAT ANTERIOR CHAMBER AND INTRAVENOUS ANTIGEN INJECTIONS HAVE DISTINCTLY DIFFERENT SYSTEMIC IMMUNE CONSEQUENCES

J. WAYNE STREILEIN and GARTH A. WILBANKS

Departments of Microbiology and Immunology and of Ophthalmology University of Miami School of Medicine, P.O. Box 016960 (R-138), Miami, Florida 33101, USA

INTRODUCTION

Immune deviation is a term first used in the 1960's by investigators who discovered that intravenous inoculation of soluble antigens elicited specific antibodies, but impaired delayed hypersensitivity in guinea pigs (1). Although the physiologic basis for immune deviation has not been fully explained, it is known that the intravenous (IV) route of antigen administration is crucial, and that soluble, rather than particulate, antigens are usually required. In 1975, Kaplan and Streilein (2) first reported that rats, which received anterior chamber (AC) injections of semi-allogeneic lymphoid cells, produced circulating alloantibodies, but were impaired in their capacity to reject orthotopic skin grafts genetically identical with the intracamerally injected cells. More recently, Niederkorn et al (3), Wetzig et al (4), and Waldrep et al (5) have independently demonstrated in mice that intracameral injections of hapten-modified syngeneic spleen cells or tumor cells bearing minor transplantation alloantigens elicit systemic immune responses selectively deficient in delayed hypersensitivity. In the intracameral allogeneic tumor model system, tumor antigen-specific serum antibodies were detected, and as a consequence, the phrase, Anterior Chamber Associated Immune Deviation (ACAID), was coined to identify this phenomenon, and to link it with immune deviation described earlier. Based on our own experimental findings of the past 15 years, we have proposed that ACAID is a physiologic mechanism that is uniquely designed to modify the nature of immune effector responses in the eye (6).

Since the great bulk of aqueous humor normally flows directly through the trabecular meshwork into the venous outflow of the anterior intraocular segment, it has been assumed that antigen injected intracamerally escapes intravascularly (7). Moreover, since the internal eye lacks an effective lymphatic drainage pathway, it is likely that virtually all antigen that escapes the AC leaves by the venous outflow. Because of these anatomical considerations, it has been argued that injections of antigens into the AC are merely the equivalent of IV injections, and it has been concluded/conjectured by some (sic) that there is nothing interesting or unique about the way antigens from the AC impact the immune system.

The literature of ACAID provides ample evidence to support the contention that immune responses to anterior chamber antigens are unique, i.e. different from the response to IV antigens. Although P815 mastocytoma cells (DBA/2 origin) elicit ACAID when injected into the AC of BALB/c mice, IV injections of P815 cells induce vigorous delayed hypersensitivity (DH) (8). Enucleation of eyes into which P815 cells (8) or TNP-derivatized syngeneic spleen cells (5) have been injected prevents ACAID induction, and promotes DH. Finally, AC-induced, but not IV-induced, splenic T cells are able to suppress the efferent limb of the cell-mediated immune response (4,5,9). Despite this published evidence, there are still investigators who refuse to believe that ACAID exists as a unique phenomenon, and who argue that experiments of this type are superfluous.

In this report we have re-explored the basis of ACAID induction in mice using a soluble antigen (bovine serum albumin - BSA). By comparing the immune consequences of AC, IV, and subconjunctival (SC) routes of antigen administration, we confirm that the systemic immune response to AC antigens is unique, and thereby we hope to lay to rest the unjustified criticism of this important area of investigation

MATERIALS AND METHODS

Mice. 6-12 week old BALB/c mice were obtained from our domestic mouse colony.

Inoculations into the anterior chamber (AC), subconjunctiva (SC), and intravenously (IV) have been described elsewhere (3).

Antigen. Bovine serum albumin (BSA) was dissolved in PBS as appropriate. Radioiodination with ^{125}I was conducted as described elsewhere (10).

Delayed hypersensitivity induction and expression has been described previously (9).

Suppressor cell studies employed assays for efferent suppression as described previously (11), and for afferent suppression by a modification of a method described by Moorhead (12). Where appropriate, surface markers on suppressor cells were assessed by negative selection with specific monoclonal antibodies (anti Thy 1, anti CD4, anti CD8) plus complement.

TABLE 1

CHARACTERIZATION OF SUPPRESSOR CELLS INDUCED BY AC AND IV INJECTED BSA

TYPE OF SUPPRESSORS	AMOUNT OF SUPPRESSION OBSERVED (%)				
	AC	IV	SC	POS CONTROL	NEG CONTROL
EFFERENT (Ear Swelling Responses)	68	1	5	0	75
AFFERENT (^{125}IUDR Incorporation)	61	72	13	0	76

TABLE 2

SURFACE MARKERS ON DIFFERENT SUPPRESSOR CELLS

ROUTE	SUPPRESSOR	Thy 1	CD4	CD8
IV	Afferent	+	−	+
AC	Afferent	+	+	−
AC	Efferent	+	−	+

RESULTS

AC and IV routes of BSA injection induce immune deviation. Panels of BALB/c mice (5 each) received 50 ug BSA into the AC, IV, or SC. One week later, each received 50 ug BSA in CFA injected subcutaneously. When their ears were challenged with BSA 7 days later, mice pretreated with BSA by AC and IV routes failed to mount DH responses, whereas recipients of antigen SC displayed vigorous DH (13). Thus, both AC and IV routes elicit deviant systemic immune responses.

AC and IV routes of BSA injection induce different types of suppressor T cells. Spleen cells were harvested from mice that received soluble BSA by AC or IV routes 7 days previously. These cells were then subjected to negative selection with appropriate antibodies plus complement (in order to determine expression of Thy 1, CD4, CD8), and assayed for afferent or efferent suppression. To assay efferent suppression, unfractionated or negatively-selected regulatory spleen cells (10^6) were mixed with soluble BSA (200 ug) plus BSA-primed spleen cells (10^6) (from mice sensitized with BSA in CFA 7 days previously) and injected into the ears of naive, adult mice. The data, presented in Table 1, reveal that only spleen cells from AC-injected donors were capable of suppressing the expression of DH; the relevant cells proved to be Thy 1+, CD8+. (See Table 2). To assay afferent suppression, negatively selected spleen cells (2×10^6) were mixed with 50 ug BSA incorporated into Incomplete Freund's

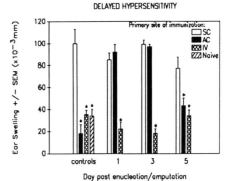

Figure 1. Effect of enucleation on induction of BSA-ACAID. * = mean value significantly differs from SC group (p<0.05).

Adjuvant and injected into the footpads of naive BALB/c mice. After four days, the mice received ^{125}IUDR (2 uCi) intraperitoneally, and five hours later their popliteal lymph nodes were assessed for radioactive content (reflecting incorporation into newly synthesized DNA, i.e. proliferation). The results, displayed in Table 1, indicate that afferent suppressor T cells are elicited by both AC and IV injections of BSA. However, AC suppressor cells are CD4+, whereas IV suppressor cells are CD8+. Thus, the suppressor T cells elicited by AC and IV injections of BSA are distinct, different and non-overlapping.

Excision of antigen injection site prevents AC-, but not IV-, induced immune deviation. Panels of BALB/c mice received AC or IV injections of 50 ug BSA. At periodic intervals thereafter (a) injected eyes were enucleated or (b) tail injection sites were amputated. The animals were then tested for deviant immunity. The results, presented in Figure 1, indicate that ACAID requires that antigen-bearing eyes remain anatomically intact for at least 5 days post-inoculation; no such requirement exists for tail inoculation sites.

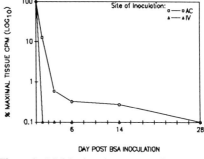

Figure 2. AC injection sites act as antigen depots. Mean cpm for AC and IV groups significantly differ at all time points (p<0.001).

Anterior chamber, but not intravenous, injection sites act as antigen depots. BSA was radiolabelled with ^{125}I and injected (50 ug) into the AC or IV. In one set of experiments, injection sites were enucleated/amputated at periodic intervals and assayed for radioactive content. In complementary experiments, blood samples were harvested at periodic intervals post-antigen injection and similarly assayed. As the results summarized in Figure 2 indicate, AC injection sites function as antigen "depots", retaining significant amounts of antigen for at least 14 days post-injection. Moreover, BSA-associated radiolabel persisted in the blood in excess of three weeks after AC injection, whereas all label was cleared from the blood within 2 weeks of IV injection (See Figure 3). The slope of the curve that depicts clearance of BSA following AC injection suggests that new radiolabel was being added to the blood between days 5 and 21, as though antigen was being released from the eye during this interval.

Blood after AC, but not IV, antigen injection contains immune deviation-inducing signals. Blood was harvested from splenectomized mice that received BSA by AC, IV or SC routes 48 hours previously. 0.5 cc was then injected IV into naive BALB/c mice. Five days later, the mice received 50 ug BSA in CFA subcutaneously. When their ears were challenged with BSA 7 days later (see Figure 4), recipients of blood from IV- and SC-injected donors displayed vigorous DH, whereas recipients of blood from AC-injected donors mounted feeble DH responses. Thus, only blood from mice that received BSA intracamerally contained immune deviation-inducing activity, implying that an antigenic signal is created uniquely by the eye, and that this signal is the agent of ACAID.

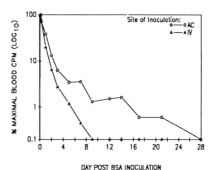

Figure 3. Blood clearance of ^{125}I-BSA following AC and IV inoculations. Mean cpm for AC and IV groups differ significantly after day 4 (p<0.05).

DISCUSSION

The results forming the basis of this report confirm and extend the findings reported from our laboratory and from other laboratories concerning the differing immune consequences of AC and IV routes of antigen administration. The most compelling new observations are that (a) distinctly different T suppressor cells are generated by the two injection routes, (b) the eye functions as an antigen depot, and (c) the eye creates an antigen-specific ACAID-inducing signal that can be detected in the blood. Since CD4 and CD8-bearing T cells use different MHC restricting elements (class II and class I, respectively), our results indicate that AC-induced afferent suppressors down-regulate different target cells from those acted upon by IV-induced suppressors. Moreover, the absence of efferent suppression following IV injection of soluble antigen, which has been reported several times (3,4,5), further emphasizes the importance of efferent suppression in the expression of ACAID.

258

Discovering that the eye serves both as an antigen depot and as the generator of the so-called ACAID-inducing signal is particularly exciting. Not only does this offer an explanation why immune regulation is different after IV injection of antigen (where no comparable depot or circulating immune deviation-inducing signal was detected), but it serves to focus our attention on the eye as playing an active role in modifying systemic immune responses to ocular antigens. This finding is reminiscent of that of Ferguson and Kaplan (14) who identified suppressor factors in the blood of mice that received AC injections of hapten-derivatized spleen cells 24 hours previously. At present, the molecular identity of the ACAID-inducing signal in the blood of recipients of AC BSA is unknown, although we do know that the ACAID induced is antigen-specific and exerts its effect through efferent suppression.

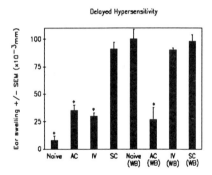

Figure 4. ACAID inducing capacity of whole blood (WB) 2 days after AC, IV and SC injections. * = significantly differs from SC group (p<0.05).

In light of these newer findings, and in recognition of similar results that already exist in the literature of ACAID, we conclude that antigen injected into the AC of the eye impacts the immune system in a manner very different from antigen delivered IV. Although the immune outcomes are superficially similar, the regulatory mechanisms initiated by these routes are fundamentally different. We believe that it is time to put this "controversy" behind us and to move forward to elucidate the complex immunoregulation that is initiated by ocular antigens. We are convinced that further analysis of ACAID - its manifestations and physiologic basis - will eventually lead to a better understanding of the pathogenesis of ocular inflammatory diseases, and offer hope for prevention and therapy of these diseases.

REFERENCES

1. Asherson GL & Stone SH (1965) Immunology 9:205

2. Kaplan HJ & Streilein JW (1977) J Immunol 118:809

3. Niederkorn J, Streilein JW & Shadduck JA (1980) Ophthal & Vis Sci 20:355

4. Wetzig RP, Foster CS & Greene MI (1982) J Immunol 128:1753

5. Waldrep JC & Kaplan HJ (1983) Invest Ophthal & Vis Sci 24:1986

6. Streilein JW (1987) FASEB J 1:199

7. Bill A (1975) Physiol Rev 55:383

8. Niederkorn JY & Streilein JW (1982) J Immunol 128:2470

9. Streilein JW & Niederkorn JY (1985) J Immunol 134:1381

10. Wilbanks GA & Streilein JW (1990) Regional Immunology (IN PRESS)

11. Williamson JSP & Streilein JW (1988) Regional Immunology 1:15

12. Moorhead JW (1976) J Immunol 117:802

13. Mizuno K, Clark AJ & Streilein JW (1989) Invest Ophthal Vis Sci 30:1112

14. Ferguson TA, Hayashi JD & Kaplan HJ (1989) J Immunol 143:821

© 1990 Elsevier Science Publishers (Biomedical Division)
Ocular Immunology Today. M. Usui, S. Ohno and K. Aoki, editors.

CHARACTERIZATION OF HUMORAL IMMUNE RESPONSES FOLLOWING ANTERIOR CHAMBER AND INTRAVENOUS ADMINISTRATION OF SOLUBLE ANTIGEN. B-CELL SECRETION OF COMPLEMENT-FIXING ANTIBODY IS SELECTIVELY AND ACTIVELY SUPPRESSED

GARTH A. WILBANKS and J. WAYNE STREILEIN
The Department of Microbiology and Immunology, and The Department of Ophthalmology, University of Miami School of Medicine and Bascom Palmer Eye Institute, P.O. Box 016960 (R-138), Miami, FL 33101.

INTRODUCTION

Inoculation of soluble antigen into the Anterior Chamber (AC) of the eyes of mice and rats induces a distinctive form of immune deviation known as Anterior Chamber Associated Immune Deviation (ACAID). ACAID to soluble antigens is characterized by (a) impaired cell mediated immunity [of the delayed hypersensitivity (DH) type], and (b) preservation of humoral immunity (1). With regard to this latter characteristic, we recently noted that radiolabeled bovine serum albumin (BSA) was not eliminated in an immune fashion from the blood of animals primed with antigen via AC and IV routes. The apparent failure to immune eliminate an antigen from blood that contains specific antibodies may be due to: (1) a quantitative difference in the total amount of anti-BSA antibody produced, or (2) a qualitative difference in the isotype of anti-BSA antibody produced. For example, isotypes of antibodies which fix complement (such as murine IgG_2) are involved in immune elimination; these antibody isotypes may not be elicited by antigen placed in the anterior chamber (2). To gain insight into the cellular basis of ACAID, we have studied in detail the isotypic nature of the humoral immune response which normal mice generate following AC injections of BSA. Results confirm that antigen is not eliminated from the blood after AC injection and reveal the probable cause to be active suppression of IgG_2 (complement-fixing) antibody production.

MATERIALS AND METHODS

Animals. Six to 12 week old BALB/c mice were obtained from the University of Miami mouse colony.

Iodination of bovine serum albumin (BSA) was accomplished with 5 mCi of [125]Iodine (^{125}I) using lactoperoxidase by a standard technique.

Antigen inoculations. Anterior chamber (AC), subconjunctival (SC) and intravenous (IV) inoculations of BSA were carried out as described elsewhere (1, 3).

Assessment of gamma emissions. Blood samples (20 μl/sample) were counted using a 4 channel γ-counter.

Assessment of ^{125}I-BSA present in the blood following inoculation. 1 μCi of ^{125}I-BSA (50μl) was administered IV. Blood samples were collected for the ensuing 28 days and assessed for γ-emissions.

Determination of serum anti-BSA antibody. Serum samples were obtained on various days and assayed for the presence of anti-BSA IgA, IgM, IgG_1, IgG_2, and IgG_3 using an enzyme-linked immunosorbant assay. Results were expressed as titer[1].

Adoptive Transfer of Splenocytes was carried out as previously described (3).

Statistical Analysis was accomplished using a two-tailed Student's t-test. All p-values less than 0.05 were deemed significant. All experiments were repeated at least twice.

RESULTS and DISCUSSION

Our experimental goal was to assess quantitatively and qualitatively systemic humoral immune responses to BSA injected into the AC of eyes of adult BALB/c mice. We examined the effect of pretreatment with soluble BSA inoculated via AC, IV or SC routes on the character of a subsequent humoral immune response to BSA in adjuvant. We determined (a) whether mice that received intracameral injections of antigen were capable of immune eliminating radiolabeled antigen from the blood, (b) the total serum titers of specific anti-BSA antibody produced through time, and (c) the titers of specific anti-BSA antibody of each isotype (except IgE) produced.

Effect of pretreatment with soluble BSA on the ability of BSA-CFA immunized mice to immune eliminate ^{125}I-BSA from the blood. Panels of adult BALB/c mice received 50 μg BSA either AC, IV or SC. This last route

260

was chosen as a positive control because previous work has demonstrated that SC inoculations prime for DH responses. Six days later, all groups received a subcutaneous inoculum containing BSA-CFA, a process known to induce a vigorous humoral immune response. A naive group of mice served as a negative control. Ten days later (experimental day 16), all groups received intravenous challenges with 50 μg of radiolabeled BSA. Serum was collected periodically to measure antibody levels (by isotype) and to assess BSA clearance from the blood. Mice that initially received BSA via the SC route cleared the

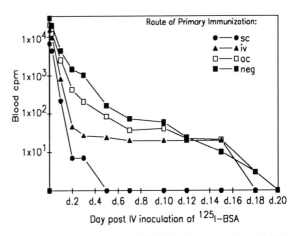

Figure 1. Immune elimination of ^{125}I-BSA. Mean cpm for AC, IV and Neg. control groups differ significantly from SC group after day 2 (p<0.05).

radiolabel from the blood very rapidly, reaching baseline values within 5 days (Figure 1). In contrast, mice first exposed to soluble BSA via IV and AC routes and then immunized with BSA-CFA cleared radiolabel from the blood very slowly; their blood still contained significant amounts of radioactivity 15 days following IV injection of ^{125}I-BSA and finally reached baseline values between 18 and 20 days, respectively. Thus AC and IV inoculations of BSA impair the capacity of recipients to clear antigen from their blood in an immune fashion, even when these mice subsequently receive BSA in a highly immunogenic form (emulsified in CFA).

Effect of AC, SC and IV BSA inoculations on the quantity of BSA-specific antibody produced following conventional immunization with

BSA in adjuvant. To test the possibility that pretreatment with AC or IV inoculations of BSA down-regulates the total amount of anti-BSA antibody produced, serum titers of anti-BSA antibody produced by the mice discussed in Figure 1 were determined. All groups of mice, regardless of the route of primary inoculation produced comparable anti-BSA titers by days 6 and 16 of the experiment (1:800 and 1:3000 respectively) (Figure 2). Thus, the failure of AC- or IV-pretreated mice to immune eliminate BSA is not due to a global deficiency in antigen-specific immunoglobulin production.

Effect of AC, SC and IV BSA injections on the isotypic profile of

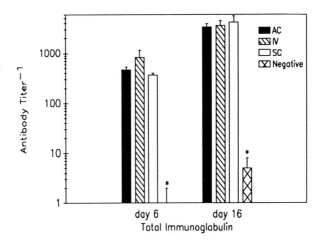

Figure 2. Humoral immune response to BSA inoculated AC, SC or IV. Days 6 and 16. * = differs significantly from SC group (p<0.05).

the humoral response to a subsequent immunization with BSA in adjuvant. We next examined the individual isotypic anti-BSA profiles of the serum of these same mice, with a special interest in IgG_2 titers. That is, the capacity of IgG_2 to fix mouse complement (mouse IgG_1, IgG_3, IgM, and IgA do not fix mouse complement) (2) and to bind with high affinity to the macrophage Fc-receptor (4) renders this isotype a prime candidate for immune elimination capabilities during memory humoral immune responses. Sera from the previously described panels of adult BALB/c mice were assayed for BSA-specific IgM, IgG_1, IgG_2, IgG_3 and IgA.

Results indicate that titers of BSA-specific IgG_1 were significantly elevated 10 days after the SQ injection of BSA-CFA (experimental day 16), indicating that B cells making this isotype had been primed by soluble BSA (Figure 3). However, significant differences among groups were seen for the IgG_2 isotype. The titers of anti-BSA IgG_2 found in mice pretreated with soluble BSA by the SC route were significantly greater than titers of this isotype found in the sera of mice that initially received BSA by either AC or IV routes. Thus, mice pretreated AC and IV with soluble BSA are impaired selectively in the ability to mount IgG_2 responses, when immunized subsequently with BSA in CFA. Serum IgA and IgM titers were moderately elevated to an equivalent extent in all groups (IgA ≈ 1:100, IgM ≈ 1:200).

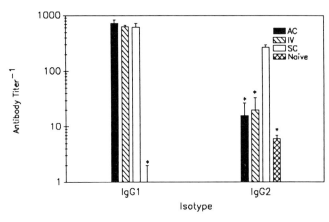

Figure 3. Effect of AC, SC and IV BSA injections on the humoral response to BSA in adjuvant. Day 16. * = differs significantly from SC group (p<0.05).

Adoptive transfer of impaired IgG_2 production with splenocytes from AC or IV inoculated mice. To explore the possibility that AC and IV injections of soluble BSA induce active suppression of complement-fixing antibody formation, we attempted to transfer adoptively the deficient IgG_2 response with splenocytes from AC and IV recipients of BSA. Groups of mice received 50 μg BSA either AC, SC or IV. Seven days later, 5×10^7 splenocytes from each animal were inoculated into naive syngeneic recipients. One hour later, all recipients received a subcutaneous BSA-CFA inoculum. Serum was collected from all groups 10 days later and assayed for BSA-specific IgG_1 and IgG_2. As expected, all groups, regardless of

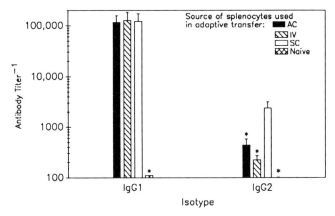

Figure 4. Adoptive transfer of impaired IgG_2 production post AC and IV BSA inoculation. Day 17. * = differs significantly from SC group (p<0.05).

the source of splenocytes used in the adoptive transfer, mounted vigorous IgG_1 responses. Interestingly, recipients of splenocytes from AC or from IV primed donors were significantly impaired in their ability to mount BSA-specific IgG_2 responses. This provides direct evidence for the presence of a cell population present in the spleens of AC or IV recipients that can actively suppress BSA-specific IgG_2 production.

Taken together, these results indicate that AC and IV inoculations of soluble BSA have vastly different effects on the B-cell compartment than do SC inoculations. Even when challenged with a sensitizing regimen of BSA-CFA, AC and IV groups still failed to mount effective IgG_2 antibody responses (Figure 3), probably accounting for the fact that they never acquired the ability to eliminate BSA in an immune fashion from the blood (Figure 1). The same sensitizing regimen produced vigorous IgG_2 responses in SC groups, and these mice were also able to immune eliminate BSA. The failure to develop either the capacity to immune eliminate antigen or to mount an effective anti-BSA IgG_2 response, even after exposure to a sensitizing regimen, combined with our ability to adoptively transfer this effect (Figure 4), suggests that T cell help required for activation and differentiation of IgG_2-secreting B cells is actively suppressed as a consequence of AC and IV pretreatment with antigen.

It has recently been proposed, on the basis of the analysis of *in vitro*-generated T helper cell clones, that there are two categories of T_H cells, based on different lymphokines secreted in response to antigen stimulation (5). T_{H1} cells secrete uniquely IL-2, IFN-γ, and lymphotoxin, whereas T_{H2} cells secrete uniquely IL-4 and IL-5. In providing help to B cells *in vitro*, IL-4 and IL-5 (secreted only by T_{H2} cells) promote the secretion of IgM, IgG_1, IgA and IgE (not IgG_2), whereas IFN-γ/IL-2 (secreted only by T_{H1} cells) promote the secretion of IgM, IgG_1 and IgG_2 (5). If, as recent evidence suggests (6), the *in vitro*-described dichotomy of T helper cells accurately reflects T-helper cell function *in vivo*, we infer that only IL-4-secreting T_H cells (T_{H2}) are activated in ACAID, whereas IFN-γ/IL-2-secreting T_H cells (T_{H1}) are actively suppressed. Experiments to test this possibility are currently underway.

REFERENCES

1. MIZUNO K, CLARK AF & STREILEIN JW (1989) *Invest Ophthalmol Vis Sci 30:1112*

2. KLAUS GGB, PEPYS MB, KITAJIMA K & ASKONAS BA (1979) *Immunology 38:687*

3. STREILEIN JW & NIEDERKORN JY (1985) *J Immunol 134:1381*

4. HEUSSER CH, ANDERSON CL & GREY HM (1977) *J Exp Med 145:1316*

5. COFFMAN RL, SEYMOUR BWP, LEBMAN DA, HIRAKI DD, CHRISTIANSEN JA, SHRADER B, CHERWINSKI HM, SAVELKOUL HFJ, FINKELMAN FD, BOND MW & MOSMANN TR (1988) *Immunol Rev 102:5*

6. BASS H, MOSSMANN T & STROBER S (1989) *J Exp Med 170:1495*

© 1990 Elsevier Science Publishers (Biomedical Division)
Ocular Immunology Today. M. Usui, S. Ohno and K. Aoki, editors.

CHARACTERIZATION OF ANTIGEN REACTIVE T CELLS IN MICE WITH P815 INDUCED ANTERIOR CHAMBER ASSOCIATED IMMUNE DEVIATION(ACAID)

YASUHARU BANDO, BRUCE KSANDER, AND J.WAYNE STREILEIN
Department of Microbiology and Immunonogy, University of Miami, Miami, FL, U.S.A.

INTRODUCTION

The injection of P815 tumor cells, which is minor histoincompatible with BALB/c mice, into the anterior chamber(AC) of the eyes of BALB/c mice elicits a deviant form of immunity - Anterior Chamber Associated Immune Deviation (ACAID). In animals with ACAID the intraocular tumor grows progressively. These animals have suppressed delayed type hypersensitivity(DTH) against P815.   However, their sera contain anti-P815 antibodies, and their spleen and lymph nodes(LN) contain high frequencies of precursors of cytotoxic T cells(1).   These results imply that some, but not all, types of P815 reactive lymphocytes are activated in mice with ACAID. Recently, Mossman reported that among CD4(+) T cell clones, at least two functionally distinct subpopulations exist; TH1 cells, which mediate DTH and secrete IL2, but not IL4; and TH2 cells, which help antibody production and secrete IL4, but not IL2(2). Since absence of DTH and presence of antibody in ACAID   coincides with the features of TH2 cells, we have formed the tempting hypothesis that TH2' cells are preferentially activated in ACAID.   In mice with ACAID,   we 1) assayed lymphocyte proliferative responses against P815 to test if any antigen activated cells are present and 2) conducted limiting dilution analysis of the frequency of IL2/IL4 producing cells to test if there are more IL4 than IL4 producing cells.

MATERIAL AND METHODS

Lymphocyte proliferation Assays

Animals.   P815 cells(2×10^5) were injected into the anterior chamber (AC) or subconjunctival space (SC) of the right eyes of adult male BALB/c mice.   Animals were sacrificed on days 3,8,14 post inoculation.   Their right cervical LN and spleens were removed for in vitro assays.

Cell cultures. Lymphocytes from LN and spleens (5×10^5 cells/well) were cultured with 10000R irradiated P815 cells (3×10^4 cells/well) in RPMI1640 supplemented with 10% fetal calf serum.   48 hours later each well was pulsed with ^{3}H-thymidine (0.5uCi). 24 hours later cultures were harvested and assayed in beta-counter.

Limiting dilution analysis of IL2/IL4 secreting cells.

Animals. Same as above except P511, which is a HAT sensitive clone of P815, was injected in the eyes instead of P815. LN and spleens were assayed on day 14.

Cell Cultures. Limiting dilution cultures were set up with serially diluted responder lymphocytes(80000-625 cells/well) and 10000R irradiated P511(3x10^4/well) with 2000R irradiated normal syngeneic splenocytes(2x10^5/well) in RPMI1640 supplemented with 10% fetal calf serum, 15% growth factor(murine ConA sup), and 2%HAT. HAT was necessary to prevent the growth of metastasized P511 among LN and spleen cells. 14 days later, cultures were washed and restimulated with P511 and syngeneic splenocytes without exogenous growth factor. 24 hours later, supernatants were harvested and tested for IL2 and IL4 in CTLL bioassay(3) with anti-IL4 mAb(11B11) and anti-IL2 mAb(S4B6), respectively. In CD4/CD8 depletion experiments, responder lymphocytes were treated with anti-CD4 mAb(RL172) and/or anti-CD8 mAb(HO2.2) followed by low toxicity complement before limiting dilution cultures were set up.

Statistics. The frequencies of IL2/IL4 producing cells were estimated statistically by single hit poisson distribution.

RESULTS

Lymphocyte proliferation assay

In LN, AC showed vigorous proliferation although its peak in time course was later than SC. In spleens on day 8, AC showed even higher response than SC. These results confirmed the presence of antigen activated cells in LN and spleen of ACAID animals as well as of SC animals(Fig.1A,1B).

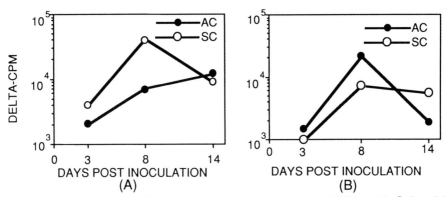

Fig. 1 Lymphocyte proliferation response against P511 in LN(A) and in Spleen(b) delta cpm = mean cpm of cultures with P815 - those without P815, standard deviations were less than 20% of the mean cpm of the quadruplets, delta cpm of naive animals < 2000

Limiting dilution analysis of IL2/IL4 secreting cells

LN of SC recipients of P511 showed a large expansion of IL2 producing cells as expected, and a modest number of IL4 producing cells. Contrary to our hypothesis, animals with ACAID also showed a large expansion of IL2 producing cells, but no IL4 producing cells(Fig.2A). The same pattern was observed in spleens(Fig.2B). Considering the possibility that some populations of lymphocytes are masking the IL4 producing cells either by taking up IL4 or suppressing IL4 producing cells, we depleted CD4 and/or CD8 subpopulation of lymphocytes before setting up the limiting dilution cultures from LN. In IL2 assay of both AC and SC, CD4 depletion alone or CD8 depletion alone partially reduced the frequency whereas depletion of both CD4 and CD8 at the same time removed the positive cells completely. This shows that both CD4(+) and CD8(+) IL2 producing cells were expanded in both AC and SC animals(Fig.3). In normal control animals, a small frequency(9.5/10⁶) of CD4(+) IL2 producing cells was detected, but no CD8(+) IL2 producing cells were observed (data not shown). In IL4 assay, after depletion, CD4 depletion removed the small numbers of positive cells in non-depleted group of SC, whereas CD8 depletion remarkably unmasked a high frequency of CD4(+) IL4 producing cells in SC animals, but not in AC animals(Fig.4). This clearly demonstrates IL4 producing cells are present in SC animals but not in animals with ACAID.

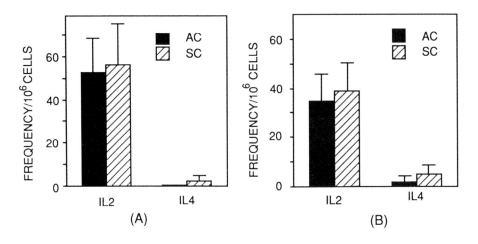

Fig.2 Frequency of IL2 / IL4 producing cells in LN (A) and spleen (B).
Frequency in naive animals; LN IL2 9.5, IL4<0.6, spleen IL2 7.1, IL4<1.2

266

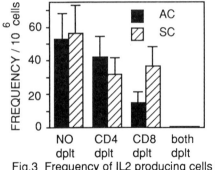

Fig.3 Frequency of IL2 producing cells in LN CD4 CD8 depletion. Frequency in naive animals: no dplt<9.5, CD4 dplt<0.6, CD8 dplt<10

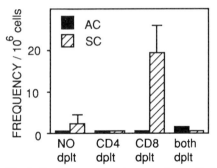

Fig.4 Frequency of IL4 producing cells in LN CD4 CD8 depletion. Frequency in naive animals <0.6 in all groups

DISCUSSIONS

The results of these studies confirm that antigen-reactive T cells are activated in the lymphoid organs of mice with ACAID. However, the data refute the hypothesis that P815-induced ACAID results from the preferential activation of IL4-secreting CD4+ T cells - so-called TH2 cells. Instead, antigen-specific T cells activated in these mice are IL2-secreting, and some display CD8 on their surface. To explain this pattern of results, we take note of several recent reports that suggest that memory T cells are of the IL4-secreting variety(4,5,6,). Moreover, Hauser and Katz have claimed that Langerhans cells preferentially activate IL4-producing T cells in vitro(7). Since the normal AC lacks conventional antigen presenting cells(8), and since co-injection of Langerhans cells with P815 into the AC results in delayed hypersensitivity, rather than ACAID(9), we conclude that the immune defect in ACAID is a failure to activate IL4-producing memory T cells. We further suggest that the lack of conventional antigen presenting cells in the tissues surrounding the AC are the cause of this defect.

REFERENCES

1. Streilein JW (1987) FASEB J 1;199-208
2. Mosmann TR et al (1986) J Immunology 136:2348-2357
3. Mosmann TR et al (1989) J Immunological Methods 116:151-158
4. Powers GD et al (1988) J Immunology 140:3352-33574.
5. Hayakawa K and Hardy RR (1989) J Exp Medicine 169:2245-2250
6. Powell TJ and Streilein JW (1990) J Immunology 144:854-859
7. Hauser C et al (1989) Eur J Immunology 19:245-251
8. Williamson JSP and Streilein JW (1989) Transplantation 47:519-524
9. Williamson JSP and Streilein JW (1989) Immunology 67:96-102

© 1990 Elsevier Science Publishers (Biomedical Division)
Ocular Immunology Today. M. Usui, S. Ohno and K. Aoki, editors.

ANALYSIS OF THE WAVELENGTH OF LIGHT RESPONSIBLE FOR THE SUPPRESSION OF THE IMMUNE RESPONSE FOLLOWING ANTERIOR CHAMBER INJECTION OF ANTIGEN

THOMAS A. FERGUSON AND HENRY J. KAPLAN

Washington University School of Medicine, Department of Ophthalmology, St. Louis, Mo. USA

INTRODUCTION

Injection of 2,4,6,-trinitrophenol (TNP)-coupled spleen cells (TNP-Sp) into the anterior chamber (AC) of the eye results in the induction of suppressor T-cells (Ts-cells) for systemic delayed type hypersensitivity (DTH).(1,2) We have previously demonstrated (3) that light entering the eye establishes the conditions necessary for the induction of suppressed DTH by influencing the intraocular T-cell reactions that initiate suppression. In order to examine further the effect of light on the eye, we sought to determine an action spectrum. By using narrow, variable wavelength filters we show the wavelength responsible for suppression is 510 ± 3nm. Using C3H/HeJrd/rd mice greater than six months of age we found that the effect of light is identical to that of animals with normal retinas. We also show that the minimum amount of light required to induce suppression is 2 lux and that the pineal gland has no influence on the observed results. These studies have important implications for understanding intraocular immune regulation and determining the molecular mediators which regulate intraocular immune responses.

MATERIALS AND METHODS

Construction of Box for Wavelength Determinations.

Two x two inch filters covering the visible spectrum from 450-650 nm were purchased from Oriel Corp. (Stratford, CT). Neutral density filters were purchased from Kodak Co. (Rochester, NY). The light source was a halogen beam automobile headlight (Western Auto, Fenton, MO) powered by a standard 12 volt power source equipped with a rheostat. The power source is connected to a timer switch so that the appropriate wavelength is delivered on a 12 hr light/12 hr dark cycle. The light was focused through the 2 x 2 inch filters fitted in the top of a box and the light illuminated a cage containing five mice. The amount of light was adjusted by the rheostat on the power source.

Mice.

Balb/cJ and C3H/HeJ mice were purchased from Jackson Labs (Bar Harbor, ME). Balb/c mice that are neonatally pinealectomized or sham operated mice were purchased from Taconic Farms (Germantown, NY) when they are 4-6 weeks of age.

Delayed-Type Hypersensitivity Response.

The induction of DTH to TNP has been previously described (1).

Anterior chamber inoculations

Cells are delivered to the AC in .005 ml volume using a Hamilton Microliter syringe (Hamilton Co., Reno, NE) fitted with .25 ml syringe and a 33 ga needle as described (1).

RESULTS

In order to further explore the effect of light on the induction of suppressed DTH following AC injection, we sought to determine the amount of light required to produce the effect. Groups of five Balb/c mice were injected in the AC with TNP-spl and immunized with TNBS. They were immediately placed in the described boxes fitted with various neutral density filters which reduce the amount of light by specific amount, while letting through the entire visible spectrum.

TABLE I

AMOUNT OF LIGHT

% Reduction[a]	AC Injection[b]	Ear Swelling(units ± SE)[c]
None	–	16.89 ± 2.8
None	+	3.73 ± 0.4*
50	+	2.72 ± 0.3*
90	+	3.61 ± 0.5*
99	+	14.33 ± 7.1
100	+	13.06 ± 2.5

a. % Reduction in light vs 20 lux in control group A.
b. Balb/c mice were AC injected and immunized as described (1).
c. 1 unit = 10^{-3} cm. Represents the right ear (challenged) minus the left ear (unchallenged)·
* Significant suppression vs control group A.

Starting with a maximum amount of light of 20 lux (lumens/meter^2, light was reduced 50%, 90%, and 99%. The results in Table I indicate that a 99% reduction in light is required to abolish suppression.

Our previous results indicated that the important wavelengths of light to support the induction of suppression following AC injection were in the visible range (3). In order to determine more precisely the wavelengths responsible for suppression, an apparatus was constructed to deliver narrow wavelengths through narrow band filters. Using 450, 500, 550, 600, and 650nm filters with the amount of light adjusted to 2 lux, we performed a preliminary experiment and determined that only the 500 ± 10nm filter supported suppression (data not shown).

Further experiments were performed 490, 500, 510 and 520nm filter which transmit light at these wavelengths ± 3nm. These results are presented in Table II and show that light at 510nm supports the induction of suppression.

TABLE II

WAVELENGTH OF LIGHT

Filter[a]	AC Injection[b]	Ear Swelling(units ± SE)[c]
Mylar	–	10.50 ± 0.6
Mylar	+	5.80 ± 1.9*
490	+	13.12 ± 4.9
500	+	9.46 ± 3.5
510	+	5.80 ± 0.7*
520	+	11.50 ± 0.4

a. Wavelength of filter used.
b. See footnote, Table I.
c. See footnote, Table I.
* Significant suppression.

Since the optimal wavelength from the induction of suppressed DTH is close to 510nm, a possible candidate for the absorption of light by the eye in this range is rod rhodopsin (4). Thus, we next sought to determine the possible role of the retina in this system. To do this, we purchased C3H/HeJ rd/rd mice from Jackson Labs (Bar Harbor, ME) that were 6 or 20 wks of age. These rd mice have been shown to have severely degenerated rods by six weeks and are completely devoid of rods by 20 weeks (5). Mice were injected in the AC, immunized, and placed in normal lighting for the remainder of the experiment.

TABLE III

ROLE OF THE RETINA

Age[a]	AC Injection[b]	Ear Swelling(units $\pm$ SE)[c]
6 wks	–	8.22 $\pm$ 0.9
6 wks	+	1.12 $\pm$ 0.2*
20 wks	–	6.31 $\pm$ 0.5
20 wks	+	1.90 $\pm$ 0.1*

a. Age of C3H/HeJ rd/rd mice.
b. See footnotes Table I.
c. See footnotes Table I.
* Significant suppression.

The result in Table III show that even C3H/HeJ rd/rd mice that are 20 weeks of age develop suppressed DTH.

Recent studies have suggested that the pineal gland is a light sensitive organ that is associated with light detection by the retina (6). Melatonin is synthesized in this organ and this compound has been shown to have potent immunoregulatory properties. To determine the role of the pineal gland we purchased pinealectomized Balb/c mice from Taconic Farms (Germantown, NY). The results in Table IV show that both pinealectomized and sham operated display suppression of DTH.

TABLE IV

EFFECT OF THE PINEAL GLAND

Operation[a]	AC Injection[b]	Ear Swelling(units $\pm$ SE)[c]
None	–	11.90 $\pm$ 1.1
Sham	–	11.00 $\pm$ 1.0
Sham	+	4.10 $\pm$ 0.5*
pn1x	–	14.09 $\pm$ 0.4
pn1x	+	5.56 $\pm$ 0.3*

a. 6 wk old sham operated or Pinealectomized Balb/c mice
b. See footnote, Table I.
c. See footnote, Table I.
* Significant suppression

DISCUSSION

The link between the induction of suppressed DTH following AC injection and light still remains mystery. There are several possibilities that have to be considered. First, the wavelength of light required for suppression may induce the formation of oxygen reactive compounds. The presence of superoxide and hydrogen peroxide have been reported in the eye, as well as compounds which neutralize their effects (ascorbate, etc) (7). These compounds have been shown to effect lymphocytes (8). Second, several neuropeptides with immunoregulatory properties [vasoactive intestinal peptide (VIP) and substance-P] have been shown to fluctuate in the eye in response to light and dark (9-10). Perhaps these compounds are induced by light in the 510nm range. Third, compounds such as dopamine, serotonin, melatonin, and histamine which have potent effects on lymphocytes are produced in the eye and vary in response to light and dark (11). Studies need to be performed to determine the production of these molecules in the eye in response to 510nm light.

It is still not clear what is the initial, light absorbing event in the eye leading to suppressed systemic DTH. Since the wavelength responsible for the observed effects corresponds closely to the absorbance of rhodopsin, we were surprised that this effect was not linked to retinal rhodopsin. One possibility might be the existence in rodents of a cone pigment still remaining in 20 wk old rd mice. It is also possible that there is rhodopsin in the anterior segment of the eye of mice that might mediate the observed effects. This presence of rhodopsin in the mouse iris has been suggested by some recent studies (Adolph Cohen, personal communication). Studies are currently underway to determine the specific role of light in ocular immune responses and the role of these processes in ocular inflammation and disease.

REFERENCES

1. Ferguson TA, Kaplan HJ (1987) J Immunol 139:346
2. Ferguson TA, Waldrep JC, Kaplan HJ (1987) J Immunol 139:352
3. Ferguson TA, Hayashi JD, Kaplan HJ (1988) FASEB J 2:3017
4. Saari JC (1989) In: Moses RA, Hart WM Jr (eds) Adler's Physiology of the Eye: Clinical Application. The CV Mosby Co, St Louis, pp 356-372
5. Cohen AI (1967) Am J Anat 120:319
6. Mochizuki M, Kuwabara T, Gery I (1988) Graefes Arch Klin Exp Ophthalmol 226:346
7. Giblin FJ, McCready JP, Kodama T, Reddy VN (1984) Exp Eye Res 38:87
8. Niwa Y, Sakane S, Shingu M, Yokoyama MM (1983) J Clin Immunol 3:228
9. Payan DG, Goetzl EJ (1985) J Immunol 135(suppl):783s
10. Stone RA, Laties AM, Raviola E, Wiesel TN (1988) Neurobiology 85:257
11. Nowak JZ, Nawrocki J, Malinski C (1985) Agents and Actions 16:80

© 1990 Elsevier Science Publishers (Biomedical Division)
Ocular Immunology Today. M. Usui, S. Ohno and K. Aoki, editors.

IDENTIFICATION OF A NEW PATHOGENIC SITE FOR EAU IN HUMAN S-AG

DALE S. GREGERSON*, WESLEY F. OBRITSCH*, CARMEN F. MERRYMAN#, AND LARRY A. DONOSO+

*Department of Ophthalmology, University of Minnesota, Minneapolis, MN, U.S.A., 55455, #Department of Biochemistry and Molecular Biology, Thomas Jefferson University, and +Wills Eye Hospital, Research Division, Philadelphia, PA, U.S.A., 19107

ABSTRACT

Evidence for a proliferative site unique to the human S-Ag-specific R17 T cell line was previously reported. A 20 residue synthetic peptide, residues 343-362, corresponding to this site was found to be actively uveitogenic in LEW rats. A 13 residue peptide from this region was also pathogenic, eliciting severe EAU at 50 µg doses and less with onset of EAU as early as 10 days. Two T cell lines were made to this site adoptively transfered EAU to LEW rats, confirming the pathogenicity of this site. This may be the major pathogenic site in human S-Ag.

INTRODUCTION

In previous reports using the LEW rat model for S-Ag-induced EAU we have identified pathogenic and proliferative T cell recognition sites in bovine S-Ag (BSAg) and human S-Ag (HSAg), and raised several T cell lines[1-7]. Although a T cell line raised to HSAg (R17) displayed a modest proliferative response to BSAg, its response to CB123, which contained the known uveitogenic sites, was weak. Since the R17 line is highly uveitogenic, we suspected the presence of an additional pathogenic site in HSAg. We recently screened the R17 and R9 (raised to BSAg) T cell lines for proliferative responses to synthetic peptides spanning the lengths of BSAg and HSAg[7]. Proliferative T cell sites were mapped to four regions of S-Ag, sites A,B,C, and D[7]. A proliferative site unique to the R17 line and located near the C-terminus (site D) was found. In this study we report that a 20 residue synthetic peptide, residues 343-362 in site "D", was immunopathogenic. Smaller peptides from this region were tested to define the minimal pathogenic site. T cell lines were made to this site which adoptively transfer EAU to LEW rats, confirming the pathogenicity of this site.

MATERIALS AND METHODS

Animals and immunizations. Specific pathogen-free (SPF) female LEW rats, 125g, were purchased from Charles River Laboratories, (Wilmington, MA). They were given a single subcutaneous immunization with peptides or S-Ag emulsified in complete Freund's adjuvant so that each animal received the indicated amount of antigen in 50 µl of emulsion containing 2.5 mg/ml M. tuberculosis H-37Ra (Difco Laboratories, Detroit, MI).

Antigen and peptide preparation. BSAg and HSAg were isolated as described[1]. Synthetic peptides were made by solid phase techniques as described[3,5]. The amino acid sequences of the peptides are shown in the Tables. Peptides are denoted by the origin of their sequence, whether BSAg or HSAg, followed by numbers indicating the positions of the first and last residues of the peptides.

Lymphocyte proliferation assays. Single-cell suspensions of lymph node cells were cultured in 96-well plates at 2×10^6 cells per well in RPMI 1640 supplemented with 2% rat serum, 2 mM glutamine, 1 mM pyruvate, 0.1mM non-essential amino acids, 5 x 10^{-5} M 2-mercaptoethanol and antibiotics in 7% CO_2. Cell cultures were incubated for 72 h, labeled with 0.5 µCi per well of ^{3}H-thymidine for 6 h and harvested. Assays of line cells were done as described[1,2].

T cell lines. The R610 line was made from an animal immunized with BSAg352-364 by repeated *in vitro* selection with BSAg352-364 as described[1,2]. Two other peptide-specific lines, R17-578(35) and R17HS-16, were made by *in vitro* sub-selection of the R17 line with either peptide BSAg343-362 or HSAg315-333, respectively. The peptide-specific sublines were maintained by propagation on the peptides. The R9 line and R17 lines were prepared using BSAg or HSAg, respectively, as described[1,6]. The lines are CD4+ and class II MHC restricted. The uveitogenic activity of the R9 and R17 lines and their responses to peptides have been reported[1,2,6,7]. Peptides were used at concentrations of 1 to 1.25 µM in culture.

Histopathology. The eyes were processed, numerically coded, stained with hematoxylin and eosin for examination, and graded from 0 to 5+. The slides were decoded and the scores were averaged to give a single score for each group.

RESULTS

Identification of a new pathogenic site. A larger peptide, residues 343-362, containing the proliferative site at residues 352-362[7], was highly pathogenic (Table 1). EAU was elicited at doses of BSAg343-362 as low as 0.5 µg per animal and onset of EAU was observed as early as day 8 in animals receiving high doses (Table 1).

TABLE 1. PRESENCE OF A PATHOGENIC SITE WITHIN AMINO ACID RESIDUES 343-362

| Peptide | Dose, µg | Sequence | Induction of EAU | | |
			Incidence	Onset, days	Histopathology
BSAg343-362	100	TSSEVATEVPFRLMHPQPED	2/2	9	3.8
	50		12/12	11	3.5
	25		5/5	15	2.4
	5		3/3	11	2.1
	1		2/2	19	2.0
	0.5		2/2	22	1.0

Smaller peptides were assessed for uveitogenicity (Table 2). The minimal uveitogenic site was defined at its N-terminus by the proline at position 352 which appeared essential for induction of severe EAU. At the C-terminus, residues 363 and 364 were required when short peptides were tested, but were not essential as the 343-362 sequence was highly uveitogenic. The smallest peptide capable of eliciting severe EAU was thirteen residues in length and included residues 352-364.

Proliferative responses to site D peptides. Lymph node (LN) cells from animals immunized with either BSAg or peptide BSAg343-362 were tested for proliferation. S-Ag-sensitized LN cells gave moderate proliferative responses to peptide BSAg343-362 (Table 3), showing that some

TABLE 2. LOCALIZATION OF THE PATHOGENIC SITE

			Induction of EAU	
Peptide	Dose, μg	Sequence	Incidence	Histopathology
BSAg351-364	50	VPFRLMHPQPEDPD	3/3	3.2
BSAg352-364	100	PFRLMHPQPEDPD	2/2	4.0
	50		3/3	2.5
	25		2/2	1.8
	15		3/3	1.7
BSAg352-362	100	PFRLMHPQPED	0/3	0
BSAg353-372	100	FRLMHPQPEDPDTAKESFQD	2/6	0.2
BSAg353-363	100	FRLMHPQPEDP	1/6	0.2

responsiveness to site D peptides is present in LN cells from these animals. Cells recognizing this site may play a role in EAU induced by BSAg; however, the proliferative response to this site was rapidly lost on *in vitro* propagation of the R9 line. Conversely, responsiveness of R17 line cells to this region increased with *in vitro* propagation (data not shown). Further testing showed that the site elicited by immunization with BSAg343-362 or intact BSAg was not same as that elicited by immunization with HSAg or peptide BSAg352-364. As shown in Table 3, the R17 line responded

TABLE 3. SPECIFICITY OF THE PROLIFERATIVE RESPONSES TO PEPTIDES FROM SITE D

		Proliferation, cpm x 10^{-3}					
		Lymph node cells[a]		T cell lines			
		BSAg343		R9	R17	R610	R17-578(35)
Peptide/antigen	Sequence	-362	BSAg	4X[b]	19X[b]	3X[b]	4X[b]
BSAg		4	149	112	-[c]	5	-
HSAg		-	-	-	312	11	4
BSAg339-355	LGELTSSEVATEVPFRL	1	-	-	1	-	1
BSAg343-362	TSSEVATEVPFRLMHPQPED	31	13	6	271	104	12
BSAg353-372	FRLMHPQPEDPDTAKESFQD	3	3	8	302	110	5
BSAg363-382	PDTAKESFQDENFVFEEF	-	3	-	1	-	-
BSAg352-362	PFRLMHPQPED	-	-	-	317	144	4
BSAg352-364	PFRLMHPQPEDPD	-	-	-	-	199	3
BSAg354-370	RLMHPQPEDPDTAKESF	-	-	-	364	25	-
BSAg356-370	MHPQPEDPDTAKESF	-	-	-	81	6	-
control		1	5	8	1	3	1

[a]Lymph node cells from BSAg343-362 or BSAg sensitized animals.
[b]Number of *in vitro* cycles of selection of the R9, R17, R610, and R17-578(35) lines on BSAg, HSAg, BSAg352-364, and BSAg343-362, respectively.
[c](-), not determined.

equally well to peptides BSAg343-362 and BSAg353-372 while LN cells from BSAg or BSAg343-362 immunized animals responded well to BSAg343-362 only. LN cells raised to peptide BSAg343-362 were only moderately responsive to BSAg. The responsiveness of S-Ag-specific T cell lines was unique to the human specific R17 line, not being found in any line raised to BSAg. The N-terminus of the proliferative site defined by the R17 and R610 lines differed from that of the uveitogenic site in that residues 352 to 354 were not required, and some responsiveness to a peptide lacking residue 355 was still present. These findings show that the critical residues of the proliferative site are nested within the uveitogenic site.

T cell lines and adoptive transfer of EAU. T cell lines specific for this site were prepared. *In vitro* selection of the R17 'parental' line was begun after the R17 line had undergone seven cycles of propagation on HSAg. Three parallel sets of cultures were carried, one was selected with BSAg343-362, another with HSAg315-333, and one with HSAg. Peptide HSAg315-333 is a non-pathogenic, proliferative peptide from site C. The subline selected with BSAg343-362 was designated R17-578(35) and showed an increased proliferative response to BSAg343-362 (Table 4) while losing responsiveness to HSAg315-333.

TABLE 4. SELECTION OF PEPTIDE-SPECIFIC LINES

					Proliferative response, cpm x 10^{-3}		
In vitro selection					BSAg peptides		
Line Cells	Selective Antigen	Number of cycles	Media	HSAg	303-322	313-332	343-362
R17	HSAg	7	1.5	72.0	1.3	64.9	12.9
R17-578(35)	BSAg343-362	4	1.4	9.2	1.2	2.8	20.1
R17HS-16	HSAg315-333	6	2.0	25.7	2.4	69.8	2.2

The R17-578(35) subline adoptively transferred EAU (Table 5). The converse was true of the R17HS-16 subline which was selected on HSAg315-333 and lost responsiveness to BSAg343-362 (Table 4) and lost the ability to transfer EAU (Table 5). This result shows that uveitogenic subpopulations are not maintained in lines unless their antigen is present in accord with previous observations[7]. The R17 line maintained on HSAg has retained pathogenicity through 22 cycles. A T cell line specific for the minimal uveitogenic peptide, BSAg352-364, was prepared from an animal immunized with this peptide followed by *in vitro* propagation on BSAg352-364. This line, R610, was able to transfer severe EAU with onset as early as day 4 post-transfer (Table 5). The fine specificity of the proliferative response of the line was similar to that of the R17 and R17-578(35) lines, but lacked responsiveness to intact HSAg (Table 3).

DISCUSSION

The proliferation and pathogenicity data demonstrate the presence of a new region in S-Ag which contains pathogenic and proliferative sites in close proximity. Our previous inability to detect these sites can be explained by the presence of a methionine residue at position 356, which is in the minimal sequence and serves as a cleavage site in the CNBr reaction. Only when synthetic peptides spanning this region were tested was it found to contain a potent uveitogenic site.

TABLE 5. ADOPTIVE TRANSFER OF EAU USING LINE CELLS RAISED TO PEPTIDES FROM SITE D

Line cells	# of cells	Incidence	Severity
R17-578(35)	5-20 x 10^6	5 / 5	2.3
R610	5-10 x 10^6	4 / 4	3.1
R17HS-16	5-10 x 10^6	0 / 7	0

Dissociation of proliferative and pathogenic sites has also been observed in the LEW rat model of myelin basic protein (MBP)-induced experimental autoimmune encephalomyelitis (EAE) where the proliferative and pathogenic sites of MBP were found to be overlapping[8-10] or 'nested'[11]. Our previous study of dissociated sites in S-Ag[7] found one pair of proliferative and pathogenic T cell epitopes to be overlapping but spatially distinct, while another pair were directly adjacent. The consistent appearance of this motif suggests that the association might be functional rather than coincidental in the rat EAE and EAU models.

ACKNOWLEDGEMENTS

This work was supported by NIH grants EY-05417 and EY-05095 and Research to Prevent Blindness. We thank Marcella Isaac for histology.

REFERENCES

1. Gregerson DS, Obritsch WF, Fling SP, Cameron JD (1986) J Immunol 136:2875

2. Gregerson DS, Obritsch WF, Fling SP (1987) Eur J Immunol 17:405

3. Donoso LA, Merryman CF, Shinohara T, Dietzschold B, Wistow G, Craft C, Morley W, Henry RT (1986) Curr Eye Res 5:995

4. Donoso LA, Yamaki K, Merryman CF, Shinohara T, Yue S, Sery TW (1988) Curr Eye Res 7:1077

5. Donoso LA, Merryman CF, Sery TW, Shinohara T, Dietzschold B, Smith A, Kalsow CM (1987) Curr Eye Res 6:1151

6. Gregerson DS, Fling SP, Obritsch WF, Cameron JD (1989) In: Secchi A, Fregona IA (eds) Modern Trends in Immunology and Immunopathology of the Eye. Masson, Milano, pp 20-25

7. Gregerson DS, Fling SP, Obritsch WF, Merryman CF, Donoso LA (1989) Cell Immunol 123:427

8. Mannie MD, Paterson PY, U'Prichard DC, Flouret G, (1985) Proc Natl Acad Sci USA 87:5515

9. Offner H, Hashim GA, Chou YK, Celnik B, Jones R, Vandenbark AA (1988) J Immunol 141:3828

10. Mannie MD, Paterson PY, U'Prichard DC, Flouret G (1989) J Immunol 142:2608

11. Sakai K, Sinha AA, Mitchel DJ, Zamvil SS, Rothbard JB, McDevitt HO Steinman L (1988) Proc Natl Acad Sci USA 85:8608

© 1990 Elsevier Science Publishers (Biomedical Division)
Ocular Immunology Today. M. Usui, S. Ohno and K. Aoki, editors.

ANTIGEN PROCESSING IN IRBP INDUCED EAU: RECOGNITION OF A NON-DOMINANT PEPTIDE DETERMINANT *IN VIVO* BUT NOT *IN VITRO*

W. LIPHAM, T.M. REDMOND, H. TAKAHASHI, B. WIGGERT, J. BERZOFSKY, G.J. CHADER, AND I. GERY.

National Eye Institute and National Cancer Institute, NIH, and Howard Hughes Medical Institute, Bethesda, MD 20892 U.S.A.

INTRODUCTION

IRBP (interphotoreceptor retinoid binding protein) is a glycoprotein of 1264 residues (bovine) which localizes in the retina and induces uveoretinal inflammation in the eyes of immunized animals. This inflammatory process is referred to as experimental autoimmune uveoretinitis (EAU). EAU is a model for certain human uveitic conditions that are believed to have an autoimmune etiology (e.g. Vogt-Koyanagi-Harada syndrome, birdshot choroidoretinopathy, and sympathetic ophthalmia) (1,2). In addition to IRBP, it has been demonstrated that IRBP-derived synthetic peptides are capable of inducing EAU in Lewis rats (3-5). In recent studies we have focused on two immunopathogenic peptides designated "R4" and "W10", which occupy sequences 1158-1180 and 1179-1191, respectively, of bovine IRBP . W10 was capable of inducing EAU at doses far lower than those of R4. This superior activity of W10 was associated with its being an immunodominant epitope of IRBP in Lewis rats. Immunodominant epitopes are the small number of peptide determinants of a protein that dominate the immune response to the whole protein; the majority of the peptides are non-dominant and are not involved in this response.

Recently we have observed that Lewis rats immunized with the non-dominant peptide, R4, develop EAU, but lymph node cells obtained from these animals are incapable of recognizing intact IRBP in culture (3,4). In addition, an R4 specific T-cell line is capable of inducing EAU in naive recipient rats, but fails to respond (proliferate) to whole IRBP in culture (6). The aim of this study, therefore, is to understand how R4 sensitized T-cells recognize IRBP in vivo (as evidenced by their capacity to induce disease) yet fail to respond to whole IRBP in culture.

MATERIALS AND METHODS

<u>Antigens</u>. The peptides used in this study were derived from the sequence of IRBP as reported by Borst et al (7) and included R4 (sequence 1158-1180; HVDDTDLYLTIPTARSVGAADGS) and W10 (1179-1191: GSSWEGVGVVPDV). IRBP was purified as described in detail (8). Digestion of IRBP (1µg/ml) with the endoproteinasesV-8, Asp-N and Lys-C (Mannheim Boehringer) was carried out for 16 hours in darkness, as described by the manufacturer's manual.

<u>Lymphocyte Proliferation Assay</u>. T-cell lines specific to each of the peptides were derived and their proliferative responses were measured as described elsewhere (6).

RESULTS AND DISCUSSION

We have examined two hypothetical explanations for the dissociation observed between recognition of IRBP by R4-sensitized cells in vivo and in vitro: (a) It is possible when IRBP is processed in vitro, immunodominant epitopes compete with R4 and inhibit its interaction with the MHC molecules on the antigen processing cells (APC). This explanation would assume that both of the peptides are restricted by the same MHC molecule if they are to directly compete for binding. The second explanation (b) proposes that the R4 epitope is not generated from IRBP by the APC in culture, whereas enzymes in the local environment digest IRBP molecules, to be processed in such a way that R4 antigenicity is generated.

To examine the first explanation, we determined the MHC restriction for each of the peptides. Responses to both R4 and W10 were inhibited by antibodies to I-A (OX-6) but not by antibodies to I-E (OX-17). This implies that both peptides are restricted by I-A (data not shown). Therefore, we tested whether the immunodominant peptide, W10, could compete with and successfully displace R4, the non-dominant peptide, from the I-A molecule. One would infer that competition for MHC binding would occur at relatively equivalent doses of peptide. It was observed, however, that W10 required a far greater dose than that of R4 to successfully inhibit a R4 specific T-cell line from proliferating (Fig.1).

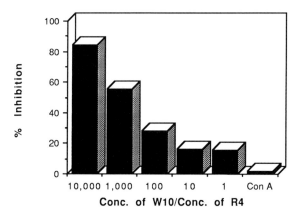

Fig. 1. Competition studies: W10 competes with and inhibits the specific response of line cells toward R4, but only at exceedingly high concentration ratios. The competitor peptide, W10, was added at the concentration of 1μM, while that of R4 was decreased in increments by a factor of 10. W10 did not, however, inhibit non-specific Con A (0.5μg/ml) proliferative responses.

In light of these findings, we could rule out the possibility that R4 sensitized cells do not recognize IRBP in vitro because of the competition by immunodominant peptides: peptide W10 was inhibitory only at exceedingly high concentration ratios.

To test our second hypothetical explanation, we digested IRBP with a number of endoproteinases prior to its being added to the test cultures. The fragments that could be produced by digestion with the tested enzymes are shown in Fig. 2.

Lys-C DIGEST

1158   H V D D T D L Y L T I P T A R S V G A A D Ⓖ Ⓢ *S W E G V G V V P D V*   1191

V-8 DIGEST

H V D D TD L Y L T I P T A R S V G A A D Ⓖ Ⓢ *S W E G V G V V P D V*

Asp-N DIGEST

H V D DT D L Y L T I P T A R S V G A A D Ⓖ Ⓢ *S W E G V G V V P D V*

Fig. 2. Cleavage sites by the endoproteinases in the region of IRBP containing R4 and W10. Residues that comprise R4 are in normal type, italics indicate W10 and outlined type indicates a two amino acid overlap. Arrows are at sites of enzyme cleavage. (Note that Lys-C cuts outside of the domain illustrated).

We found that R4 sensitized lymphocytes proliferated in vitro when stimulated with IRBP that had been previously digested with the endoproteinases Asp-N and V-8. In contrast, these line cells did not respond to either native IRBP or Lys-C digested IRBP (Fig. 3).

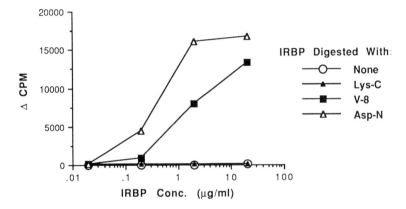

Fig. 3. An R4 specific line recognizes IRBP only after digestion with the endoproteinases V-8 and Asp-N. The data are expressed as Δ cpm. These line cells responded to the peptide R4 (1μM) with a peak Δ cpm of 24,487.

Since proteolytic degradation of IRBP permits R4 sensitized lymphocytes to recognize IRBP in culture, we propose that a similar process may play a role in R4 specific recognition of this antigen in vivo; IRBP degradation in vivo could be produced by local tissue proteinases. This study, therefore, describes a putative antigen processing mechanism that allows lymphocytes sensitized to a non-dominant determinant to induce an autoimmune disorder in spite of their incapacity to recognize the native antigen in culture.

280

SUMMARY

This study examined possible explanations for the finding that lymphocytes sensitized against the IRBP-derived peptide, R4, which are uveitogenic and, therefore, recognize IRBP in vivo, do not recognize this protein in vitro. One explanation could be that the response to the non-dominant peptide, R4, is inhibited by immunodominant peptides, which compete with R4 for the MHC interaction site. This was ruled out: only exceedingly high concentrations of a dominant peptide, W10, inhibited the response to R4. The study supports, however, another explanation, that IRBP is digested in vivo by tissue proteinases, to yield fragments with R4 antigenicity. IRBP digested by endoproteinases (V-8 or Asp-N) stimulated an R4 specific cell line to proliferate. It is proposed that a similar breakdown of IRBP occurs in vivo and enables recognition of the protein and, consequently, EAU induction.

REFERENCES

1. Faure, J.-P. (1980) Curr Top Eye Res 2:215
2. Gery, I., Mochizuki, M., and Nussenblatt, R.B. (1986) Prog Retinal Res 5:75
3. Sanui, H., Redmond, T.M., Hu, L.-H., Kuwabara, T., Chader, G.J., and Gery, I. (1988) Curr Eye Res 7:727
4. Sanui, H., Redmond, T.M., Kotake, S., Wiggert, B., Hu, L.-H., Margalit, H., Berzofsky, J.A., Chader, G.J., and Gery, I. (1989) J Exp Med 169:1947
5. Donoso, L.A., Merryman, C.F., Sery, T.W., Vrabec, T., Arbizo, V., and Fong, S.-L. (1988) Curr Eye Res 7:1087
6. Hu, L.-H., Redmond, T.M., Sanui, H., Kuwabara, T., McAllister, C.G., Wiggert, B., Chader, G.J., and Gery, I. (1989) Cell Imm 122:251
7. Borst, D.E., Redmond, T.M., Elser, J.E., Gonda, M.E., Wiggert, B., Chader, G.J., and Nickerson, J.M. (1989) J Biol Chem 264:1115
8. Redmond, T.M., B. Wiggert, F.A. Robey, N.Y. Nguyen, M.S. Lewis, L. Lee, and G. J. Chader. (1985) Biochem 24:787

© 1990 Elsevier Science Publishers (Biomedical Division)
Ocular Immunology Today. M. Usui, S. Ohno and K. Aoki, editors.

ANALYSIS OF THE IMMUNODOMINANT AND HIGHLY UVEITOGENIC EPITOPE OF INTERPHOTORECEPTOR RETINOID-BINDING PROTEIN (IRBP)

S. KOTAKE, M.D. DE SMET, H. SANUI, B. WIGGERT, T.M. REDMOND, G.J. CHADER, and I. GERY.

National Eye Institute, NIH, Bethesda, MD, U.S.A.

INTRODUCTION

Interphotoreceptor retinoid-binding protein (IRBP), a major component of the interphotoreceptor matrix, induces experimental autoimmune uveitis (EAU) in a variety of animals. We have previously shown that peptide "R14", which comprises the sequence 1169-1191 (PTARSVGAADGSSWEGVGVVPDV) of bovine IRBP, is the immunodominant epitope of this protein in Lewis rat, i.e., it dominates the response to whole IRBP, as depicted by its being recognized by lymphocytes sensitized against the intact protein (1). Peptide R14 is highly uveitogenic, inducing EAU in Lewis rats at doses as low as 0.024 nmol/rat (1).

This study was aimed at identifying the R14 residues which are pivotal for the immunological activities of this determinant.

MATERIALS AND METHODS

All procedures of antigen preparation, immunization and disease assessment were described in detail in ref 1. The lymphocyte proliferation assay was performed as detailed in ref 2, except that the medium was supplemented with 1% normal rat serum and 2-mercaptoethanol at 5×10^{-5}M. The cell line against peptide 1181-1191 was established and tested for proliferation as described in ref 3.

RESULTS

The shortest sequence within determinant 1169-1191 to exhibit immunodominance and uveitogenicity was determined by testing truncated forms of the original peptide. The two activities were found in the nonapeptide 1182-1190, but not in 1181-1189, 1183-1191, or any of the shorter peptides.

To determine the role played by each residue of sequence 1182-1190 in the immunological activities of this determinant, we examined the activities of nine analogs of peptide 1181-1191 in which residues 1182-1190 were individually substituted by alanine. Table 1 summarizes the uveitogenicity of the analogs. A correlation was observed in general between the uveitogenicity and immunogenicity of the analogs, i.e., their capacity to initiate immune response in Lewis rats. Thus, no immune responses were detected in rats immunized with analogs A(1182) or A(1190), while the other peptides initiated various levels of immune response, measured by the lymphocyte proliferation assay (data not shown). It is noteworthy that the responses were always higher toward the immunizing analogs than toward the original peptide 1181-1191.

TABLE 1

Immunopathogenic properties of alanine-substituted analogs of peptide 1181-1191

Analog injected	Dose (n mol/rat)	EAU		
		Incidence	Onset day(mean)	Severity(mean)
1181-1191 (SWEGVGVVPDV)	200	4 / 4	10.0	1.5
	20	4 / 4	10.5	1.8
A(1182) (SAEGVGVVPDV)	200	0 / 4	-	-
A(1183) (SWAGVGVVPDV)	200	4 / 4	11.5	1.0
	20	0 / 4	-	-
A(1184) (SWEAVGVVPDV)	200	4 / 4	9.5	1.8
	20	4 / 4	10.8	1.3
A(1185) (SWEGAGVVPDV)	200	4 / 4	12.0	1.0
	20	0 / 4	-	-
A(1186) (SWEGVAVVPDV)	200	4 / 4	10.5	1.0
	20	4 / 4	11.5	1.0
A(1187) (SWEGVGAVPDV)	200	4 / 4	10.8	1.0
	20	3 / 4	13.3	1.0
A(1188) (SWEGVGVAPDV)	200	4 / 4	10.3	1.0
	20	4 / 4	12.0	1.0
A(1189) (SWEGVGVVADV)	200	4 / 4	11.8	1.0
	20	1 / 4	14.0	1.0
A(1190) (SWEGVGVVPAV)	200	1 / 4	15.0	1.0
	20	0 / 4	-	-

To determine the contribution of each of the residues to the immunodominance of sequence 1182-1190, we tested the capacity of the nine analogs to be recognized by line cells specific toward the natural immunodominant site, 1181-1191 (Fig 1). Three of the analogs, A(1182), A(1188) and A(1189), were not recognized by the line cells and did not stimulate any detectable proliferation response, whereas the other six peptides stimulated moderate to high responses. It is of note that analogs A(1188) and A(1189), which were inactive in this assay, were found to be uveitogenic and immunogenic (see above). On the other hand, analog A(1190), which was poorly uveitogenic and non-immunogenic, did stimulate good responses by the line cells, albeit only at the high tested concentrations (Fig 1).

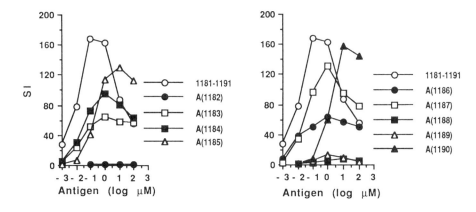

Fig 1. Recognition of the alanine-substituted analogs by a lymphocyte cell line sensitized against peptide 1181-1191. The recognition was determined by the proliferation assay and the data are expressed as the stimulation index values (SI=mean cpm in cultures with antigen / mean cpm in control cultures without stimulant).

DISCUSSION

Using truncated forms of peptide 1169-1191 ("R14") we have shown here that the exceedingly strong immunological capacity of this determinant of bovine IRBP (1) resides in sequence 1182-1190. Our experiments with the alanine-substituted analogs have identified four of the nine residues of 1182-1190 to be particularly important: 1182 (W), 1188 (V), 1189(P) and 1190(D). A finding to be underscored is that of these four residues only 1182 was essential for all immunological activities of 1182-1190, whereas the other three residues played pivotal roles in only some of these activities. Thus, residue 1190 was necessary for the strong uveitogenicity and immunogenicity of the site, while residues 1188-1189 were essential for its immunodominance, as determined by the capacity to stimulate lymphocytes sensitized against 1181-1191 (Fig 1), or whole IRBP (data not shown here). These two different patterns of activities suggest that residues 1188 and 1189 are involved in the interaction of the peptide with the receptor of the responding T-lymphocytes, while residue 1190 is essential for an efficient interaction of the peptide with the major histocompatibility complex product on the antigen presenting cell (APC). The assumption concerning residues 1188 and 1189 is supported by our finding that analogs A(1188) and A(1189) compete well with the native peptide 1181-1191 and inhibit its recognition by the line cells (data not shown). The proposed activity of residue 1190 is in line with the finding that analog A(1190) was antigenic in culture only at the high tested concentrations (Fig 1). As to residue 1182, it seems that the tryptophan at this position is pivotal for an effective interaction of the peptide with APC: analog A(1182) showed no activity in the competition assay (data not shown).

SUMMARY

The immunodominance and exceedingly potent immunological activities in Lewis rats of the IRBP-derived peptide 1169-1191 ("R14") were found to reside in sequence 1182-1190. Four of these nine amino acids, 1182 (W), 1188(V), 1189(P) and 1190 (D), were found to be pivotal for the immunological activities of the peptide. It is noteworthy, however, that different residues were essential for different immunological activities of the peptide determinant.

REFERENCES

1. Sanui H, Redmond TM, Kotake S, Wiggert B, Hu L-H, Margalit H, Berzofsky JA, Chader GJ, Gery I (1989) J Exp Med 169: 1947
2. Mochizuki M, Nussenblatt RB, Kuwabara T, Gery I (1985) Invest Ophthalmol Vis Sci 26: 226
3. Hu L-H, Redmond TM, Sanui H, Kuwabara T, McAllister CG, Wiggert B, Chader GJ, Gery I (1989) Cell Immunol 122: 251

© 1990 Elsevier Science Publishers (Biomedical Division)
Ocular Immunology Today. M. Usui, S. Ohno and K. Aoki, editors.

CELLULAR IMMUNE RESPONSES TO FRAGMENTS OF S-ANTIGEN IN PATIENTS
WITH UVEITIS

M. D. DE SMET, B. WIGGERT, G. J. CHADER, M. MOCHIZUKI*, I. GERY, and R. B.
NUSSENBLATT

Laboratory of Immunology, National Eye Institute, NIH, Bethesda, MD 20892, USA
*Tokyo University Branch Hospital, Tokyo, Japan

INTRODUCTION

Cellular mechanisms are known to play a pivotal role in the induction of experimental
autoimmune uveitis (EAU) in susceptible animals. Helper T cells sensitized to S-Antigen (S-Ag) or
its fragments are capable of causing uveitis by adoptive transfer into naive recipients, while disease
induction is not possible in athymic animals, or following treatment with Cyclosporine.
T cells recognize an antigen only after internal processing by antigen-presenting cells (APC).The
resulting fragments are then re-expressed on the cell surface of the APC in association with an
appropriate histocompatibility molecule. Two fragments of S-Ag, peptides M and N, have been
found to be uveitopathogenic in Lewis rats (1).

Cellular responses to bovine S-Ag have been documented in patients suffering from various
endogenous posterior uveitis (2,3). Bovine M peptide was recently found to cause *in vitro*
proliferation in about 50% of responders to S-Ag while N peptide was recognized by a minority of
patients (4). However neither of these determinants generates a proliferative response comparable
to S-Ag itself. The immunodominant determinants of S-Ag have yet to be established. In order to
ascertain the sites on human S-Ag which participate in cellular immunity, and possibly identify the
immunodominant determinant, forty overlapping fragments of human S-Ag were prepared and
tested in patients suffering from uveitis affecting the posterior pole.

MATERIAL AND METHODS
Subjects

Patients carrying a diagnosis of Behçet's disease, Vogt-Koyanagi-Harada, sympathetic
ophthalmia and Birdshot retinochoroidopathy were selected from the uveitis clinic of the NEI. All
patients had evidence of past or present disease affecting the retina. All patients gave informed
consent prior to their participation in this study. Normal volunteers were taken from the nursing
staff and NEI allied staff not involved in the study of S- Antigen.

Cellular Proliferation Assay.

Lymphocytes from 40 mls of peripheral venous blood were isolated on an Isolymph gradient.
Cultures were set up in triplicate in flat bottom wells. 2×10^5 cells were used per well and cultured

for 5 days in 0.2 ml of RPMI-1640 supplemented with HEPES, 20% heat inactivated human AB (+) serum, and antibiotics. The data recorded here were obtained with the antigens at a concentration of 100 μg/ml.

Antigens:

Forty overlapping fragments, each measuring 20 amino acids in length, except for the last fragment measuring 15 amino acids, were based on the sequence of human S- Antigen as reported by Yamaki et al (5). Each fragment overlapped the previous sequence by 10 amino acids. The exact sequence of each fragment will be published in a forthcoming article. All fragments as well as human M and N peptides were synthesized by solid phase chemistry using t-butyloxycarbonyl derivatives of the amino acids and were purified by Applied Biosystems Inc., Foster City, CA. As many antigens as were available at the time of study were simultaneously studied.

Thirty one of the forty fragments had been synthesized and tested in thepresent study.

RESULTS AND DISCUSSION

Twenty six patients (11 male and 14 female) and ten normal individuals (4 male and 6 female) were studied. All patients and controls showed strong proliferative responses to PHA, used as a control. While both groups were capable of lymphoproliferative responses to some of the fragments, the patients tended to have stimulation indices which were higher than those of the normal subjects (Fig.1). The response profile to all fragments tested is shown in Figures 2 and 3. Of particular interest is the fact that both patients and normal subjects are capable of responding to multiple epitopes of S-Ag, a phenomenon which has previously not been described in uveitis and has not been seen in EAU. Current concepts of T cell activation suggest that a response is generally specific to a few fragments and, as with IRBP, is usually restricted to one epitope. The basis for the enhanced capability is not entirely known but at least 2 mechanisms are probably involved. It was recently shown that lymphocytes from mice infected with HSV-1 are able to recognize multiple epitopes of a coat protein from the surface of the infecting herpes virus (6) while immunization with the same protein generates only one immunogenic epitope. It suggests that in situations of intense inflammation as is seen in uveitis, a very broad based T cell response is generated against several epitopes of S-Ag but also to other autoantigens such as IRBP (Fig. 3).

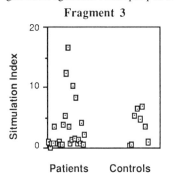
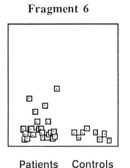

Fig. 1. Proliferative Responses of patients and controls subjects to fragments 3 and 6. The response is given as a stimulation index (cpm of fragment / cpm of contol culture).

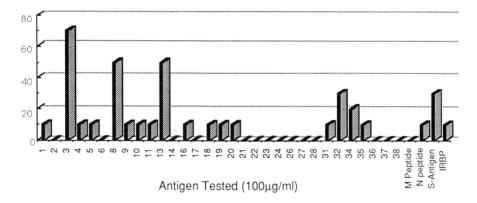

Fig. 2. Percentage of controls subjects showing a stimulation index of 2.0 or more in a 5 day proliferation assay (n = 10 subjects for each antigen tested). IRBP refers to interphoto-receptor retinoid binding protein and was tested at a concentration of 50 µg/ml.

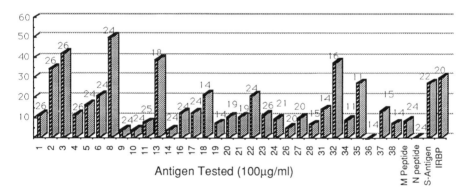

Fig. 3. Percentage of patients showing a stimulation index of 2.0 or more in a 5 day proliferation assay (number of patients tested is shown above each column). IRBP refers to interphotoreceptor retinoid binding protein and was tested at a concentration of 50 µg/ml.

There is thus a fundamental difference in the mechanism of naturally induced disease which makes the emergence of immunodominant epitopes less probable and might explain at least in part the presence of numerous sites of response in patients as compared to the controls. Another recent discovery in human T cell lines from multiple sclerosis patients suggests that human class II molecules are capable of presenting and inducing proliferation of lymphocytes to several different epitopes of myelin basic protein, a behavior which was not seen in their normal controls (7). It suggests that human class II antigens are more permissive than the rat or murine counterpart in their interactions with peptide determinants and also that this ability is enhanced in patients suffering from autoimmune diseases.

In addition to the overall pattern of responses, it is interesting to note the frequency of response of some of the fragments tested. M and N peptides which are uveitopathogenic in Lewis rats and in other animal species, do not appear to play a role in this patient population since they rarely generate a stimulation index above 2.0. The frequency of response to these peptides was also quite low in the population of patients studied by Yamamoto et al and reported in this symposium (4). Several other fragments, particularly near the amino terminal end of the molecule of S-Ag appear to be stimulatory in a large number of patients. While the controls did respond to several of the same fragments, the degree of response was usually much less than that of the patients. It is not possible to conclude from these studies that a response to a given fragment predisposes to disease, but it is clear that a response to a portion of the S-Ag molecule is found in a large number of patients even in cases where a response to S-Ag was not found. It suggests that we should further analyse the response to these fragments in terms of different disease entitites.

SUMMARY

We have shown that the response of patients to fragments of human S-Ag is very diverse with many epitopes being recognized simultaneously. No given epitope appears to be immunodominant. This pattern of response may be related to differences in the mode of disease induction as compared to the existing experimental model but an inherent difference in the ability of human class II antigens to present antigens is likely to also be present. It is interesting to note that both M and N peptides which are immunopathogenic in rats do not seem to ellicit much of a response in humans further indicating that there are major differences between the experimental model and human disease. It is hoped that by studying the responses in patients with different diagnoses, a differential pattern of response will become evident and possibly help in diagnosis or therapy.

REFERENCES
1. Shinohara T, Donoso L, Tsuda M, Yamaki K, Singh VK (1989) Prog Retinal Res 8:51-651.
2. Nussenblatt RB, Gery I, Ballintine EJ, Wacker WB (1980) Am J Ophthalmol 89:173-179
3. Nussenblatt RB, Mittal KK, Ryan S, Green WR, Maumenee AE (1982) Am J Ophthalmol 94:147-158
4. Yamamoto JH, Mochizuki M, Wiggert B, Chader GJ, Shinohara T, Gery I, Nussenblatt RB (1990) In: Proceedings of the 5th International Symposium on the Immunology and Immuno-pathology of the Eye. Elsevier, Amsterdam
5. Yamaki K, Tsuda M, Shinohara T (1988) FEBS Lett 234:39-43
6. Yamashita K, Heber-Katz E (1989) J Exp Med 170:997-1002
7. Humanou YK, Vainiene M, Whitham R, Bourdette D, Chou CH-J, Hashim G, Offner H, Vandenbark AA (1989) J Neurosci Res 23:207-216

© 1990 Elsevier Science Publishers (Biomedical Division)
Ocular Immunology Today. M. Usui, S. Ohno and K. Aoki, editors.

HORMONAL AND NEURAL MODULATION OF SECRETORY COMPONENT PRODUCTION BY LACRIMAL GLAND ACINAR CELLS

ROBIN S. KELLEHER, LOUANE E. HANN, JOAN A. EDWARDS AND DAVID A. SULLIVAN

Department of Ophthalmology, Harvard Medical School and Immunology Unit, Eye Research Institute, Boston, MA, USA

INTRODUCTION

The extensive interaction between the immune, endocrine and nervous systems is especially evident in mucosal tissues, wherein hormones and neuropeptides influence many parameters of secretory immune function [1,2]. In the ocular immune system, it has been demonstrated that steroid hormones regulate secretory immunity [2]. Specifically, androgens control the production of immunoglobulin A (IgA) and secretory component (SC) by the lacrimal gland and increase the concentration of IgA antibodies and SC in tears. This hormone action appears to be dependent upon other endocrine and neural factors, because androgen effects are significantly diminished in both diabetic and hypophysectomized animals [3,4]. To advance our understanding of the regulation of the ocular secretory immune system, this study was designed to reveal the extent of neural and endocrine modulation of SC synthesis by acinar cells from the lacrimal gland.

MATERIALS AND METHODS

Materials

Animals: Six-week old male Sprague-Dawley rats were purchased from Zivic-Miller Laboratories and housed for a period of one day or more before use.

Hormones and peptides: Vasoactive intestinal peptide, substance P, somatostatin, α-endorphin, ß-endorphin, methionine-enkephalin, leucine enkephalin, human chorionic gonadotropin, oxytocin and arginine vasopressin were purchased from Boehringer-Mannheim. Insulin, 8-bromoadenosine- 3'5'-cyclic monophosphate (cAMP), 8-bromoguanosine- 3'5'-cyclic monophosphate (cGMP), 5α-dihydrotestosterone (DHT), α-melanocyte stimulating hormone, carbamyl choline, phenylephrine, melatonin, and 3-isobutyl-1- methyl xanthine (IBMX) were obtained from Sigma. Adrenocorticotrophic hormone, isoproterenol, neuropeptide Y, and cholera toxin were purchased from Calbiochem-Behring. Calcitonin gene-related peptide was purchased from Cambridge Research Biochemicals. Growth hormone and prolactin were obtained from the National Hormone Pituitary Program.

Methods

Cell culture. Male rats were euthanized by CO_2 asphyxiation. Lacrimal glands were removed and acinar cells were isolated as previously described [5]. Acinar cells (2×10^6 per 35mm plate) were cultured (n=5/group) for 4 days on reconstituted basement membranes

(Matrigel, Collaborative Research) in serum-free media containing defined supplements and specified factors, hormones, or peptides [6,7,8].

SC analysis. Media was removed from above cells after 4 days in culture. Levels of SC in the media were measured by radioimmunoassay [9].

RESULTS

Experiments were conducted in vitro to determine the influence of a variety of hormones and neuropeptides on SC synthesis by lacrimal gland acinar cells . Acinar cells (2 x 10[6]) were cultured on Matrigel for 4 days in defined, supplemented media. Cells cultured in the presence of the androgens, testosterone or DHT, synthesized significantly more SC (2- to 4-fold) compared to untreated cells (6, Table I). This hormone effect was specific for androgens. Treatment of cells with other steroids, such as dexamethasone, aldosterone, estrogen and progesterone, had no effect on SC output (6, Table I).

TABLE I. Effect of Steroids on SC Synthesis by Lacrimal Gland Acinar Cells.

Treatment	Secretory Component Synthesis
Dexamethasone	—
Aldosterone	—
Testosterone	↑
Dihydrotestosterone	↑
Estradiol	—
Progesterone	—

Acinar cells were cultured in the presence or absence of specified steroid hormones (10^{-6}M). Arrows (↑) indicate significantly ($p < 0.0005$) higher SC output than control (no treatment); Dashes (—) indicate no significant difference from control values. Data from (6).

The magnitude of the androgen effect was significantly enhanced by the addition of certain hormones and factors to the culture media (7,8). As shown in Table II.1, the ß-adrenergic agonist, isoproterenol, as well as insulin, but not a variety of other peptide hormones, substantially increased basal or androgen-stimulated SC synthesis. Certain neuropeptides and neurotransmitters, or their analogues, also had effects on SC production. Vasoactive intestinal peptide caused a marked stimulation of basal and androgen-induced SC output (Table II.2). In contrast, the cholinergic agonist, carbamyl choline, inhibited SC synthesis by untreated and DHT-treated cells (Table II.2).

Given that insulin, isoproterenol, and vasoactive intestinal peptide are all known to exert effects through the second messenger, cAMP, it was of interest to determine whether cAMP stimulated aciner cell SC output. It was found that cAMP, IBMX (a phosphodiesterase inhibitor), and cholera toxin (an irreversible activator of adenylate cyclase), all caused increased basal or androgen-enhanced SC output (Table II.3). However, inclusion of cGMP in the culture media had no effect on SC output.

Table II. Effects of Various Endocrine Factors on Basal and Androgen-stimulated SC Synthesis.

Treatment	Secretory Component Synthesis	
	Basal	DHT-stimulated
1.Peptide Hormones and Hormone Analogues		
Adrenocorticotrophic Hormone	—	—
Arginine Vasopressin	—	—
Oxytocin	—	—
Prolactin	—	—
Growth Hormone	—	—
Insulin	↑ *	↑
Isoproterenol	—	↑
α-Melanocyte Stimulating Hormone	—	—
Melatonin	—	—
Human Chorionic Gonadotropin	—	—
Bovine Pituitary Extract **	—	—
2. Neuropeptides/Transmitters/Opioids/Analogues		
Calcitonin Gene-Related Peptide	—	—
Carbamyl Choline	↓	↓
α-Endorphin	—	—
ß-Endorphin	—	—
Leucine-Enkephalin	—	—
Methionine-Enkephalin	—	—
Neuropeptide Y	—	—
Phenylephrine	—	—
Somatostatin	—	—
Substance P	—	—
Vasoactive Intestinal Peptide	↑	↑
3. Secretagogues/Second Messengers/Lymphokines		
Cyclic AMP ^	↑	↑
Cyclic GMP ^	—	—
IBMX ~	—	↑
Cholera Toxin †	↑	↑
Gamma-Interferon	—	—

Acinar cells (n = 5 cultures/group) were cultured in the presence or absence of DHT (10^{-6}M). The arrows indicate significantly ($p < 0.05$) higher (↑) or lower (↓) SC output than control or DHT cell cultures; dashes (—) indicate no significant difference from control values. Hormones were added to the media at a final concentration of 10^{-6} M except as indicated. *If added as insulin, transferrin and selenous acid; ** 25 ug/ml; ^ 2 x 10^{-4}M; ~ 10^{-3} M; †10 μg/ml. Data from (7,8).

DISCUSSION

The present results demonstrate that treatment of lacrimal gland acinar cells in vitro with insulin, isoproterenol or vasoactive intestinal peptide causes a significant increase in constitutive or androgen-stimulated SC synthesis. The mechanism underlying this stimulation may relate to effects of these hormones on intracellular cAMP levels, because cAMP also increased acinar cell SC output. In contrast, carbamyl choline inhibited basal and androgen-induced SC production. These findings indicate that a combination of neural and endocrine factors may play an important role in the regulation of SC production and subsequent IgA transport in the lacrimal gland. This contention is supported by the fact that the lacrimal gland is innervated by cholinergic, adrenergic and peptidergic neurons [10]. Future studies will further analyze the mechanism of action of these hormones in this system. Results of such studies should contribute to a better understanding of the nature of neural and endocrine influence on the ocular mucosal immune system.

ACKNOWLEDGEMENTS

This research was supported by NIH grants EY05612 and EY07074.

REFERENCES

1. Stead RH, Bienenstock J, Stanisz AM (1987) Immunol Rev 100:333-359

2. Sullivan DA (1990) In Freier S (ed) The Neuroendocrine Immune Network. CRC Press, Boca Raton, FL, pp.199-237

3. Sullivan DA (1988) J Steroid Biochem 30:429-433

4. Sullivan DA and Hann LE (1989) J. Steroid Biochem 34:253-262

5. Hann LE, Tatro J, Sullivan, DA (1989) Invest Ophthalmol Vis Sci 30:145-158

6. Sullivan DA and Hann LE (1990) Submitted

7. Hann LE, Kelleher RS, Sullivan DA (1990) Submitted

8. Kelleher RS, Hann LE, Edwards JA, Sullivan DA (1990) Submitted

9. Sullivan DA, Wira CR (1983) J Immunol 130:1330

10. Dartt DA (1986) Current Eye Research 8:619-636

© 1990 Elsevier Science Publishers (Biomedical Division)
Ocular Immunology Today. M. Usui, S. Ohno and K. Aoki, editors.

ADOPTIVE TRANSFER OF EXPERIMENTAL AUTOIMMUNE DACRYOADENITIS

S. H. LIU and R. A. PRENDERGAST
The Wilmer Institute, The Johns Hopkins University School of Medicine, Baltimore, Maryland, USA

INTRODUCTION

Severe chronic inflammatory reactions in the lacrimal gland (LG) lead to decreased tear flow and dry eye, an important clinical element in Sjögrens syndrome. The pathogenesis of these lesions is unclear. The development of experimental animal models may help to elucidate the pathogenesis of some of these human disease processes which are thought to be of autoimmune origin. Recently we have succeeded in producing severe dacryoadenitis in Lewis rats by immunization with autologous LG extracts (1). This rat model has permitted the isolation and characterization of an organ-specific autoantigen involved in experimental autoimmune dacryoadenitis (EAD) (2). The present studies were designed to assess the possible roles of cell-mediated or humoral immunity by adoptive transfer experiments. Lymphoid cells or serum from donor rats with active disease were used to induce lacrimal gland pathology in naive recipients.

MATERIALS AND METHODS

In vitro activation of donor cells with LG antigen (LG-Ag) and interleukin 2 (IL-2).

Donor Lewis rats were immunized by injection of 200 µg LG-Ag in CFA as previously described (1,2). Single cell suspensions were prepared from donor spleens 12 to 14 days later and cultured at a concentration of 2×10^6 cells/ml for 72 hr in complete medium (3,4). LG-Ag (20 µg/ml), partially purified IL-2 (10 U/ml), or both LG-Ag and IL-2 were added at the beginning of culture. After culture, the lymphoblast numbers were determined by hemacytometer counts.

Percoll gradient centrifugation.

Cultured cells depleted of B cells by panning were fractionated into the blast and the small lymphocyte fraction on Percoll gradient (4). 5×10^7 of each cell fraction was injected i.v. into recipient rats. All recipients were sacrificed 12 days after cell transfer, and the severity of EAD was evaluated histologically as previously reported (1,2).

Passive transfer with antiserum.

Serum was obtained from a group of 6 rats immunized three times at biweekly intervals with 200 µg LG-Ag emulsified in CFA. Each of 4 recipients received 2 ml of antiserum i.p. on 2 consecutive days. The animals were sacrificed 7 days after antiserum transfer.

RESULTS

Adoptive transfer of EAD with donor cells cultured with LG-Ag and IL-2.

EAD transfer activity of immune spleen cells cultured with antigen or with IL-2 or the combination of both antigen and IL-2 is summarized in Table I. Unseparated donor cells following in vitro activation with LG-Ag elicited minimal dacryoadenitis upon transfer of $5x10^7$ cells per recipient. However, separation of these cells on Percoll gradient resulted in a blast cell-enriched population that was capable of inducing severe EAD in naive recipients. Three of the 4 recipients receiving $5x10^7$ lymphoblasts demonstrated in disease comparable in severity to that obtained after active immunization.

Unseparated immune spleen cells cultured with IL-2 were not activated sufficiently to transfer EAD. Nevertheless, lymphoblasts from these cell cultures induced demonstrable EAD following transfer. Half (2/4) of the recipients receiving $5x10^7$ lymphoblasts developed moderately severe dacryoadenitis.

Sensitized donor cells cultured with LG-Ag plus IL-2 resulted in a substantially better yield of lymphoblasts and an increased capacity to transfer EAD to naive recipients. All 4 recipients receiving $5x10^7$ dual-activated lymphoblasts developed moderate to severe disease. This suggested that those cells in the immune spleen cell population proliferating in response to LG-Ag were responsible for EAD transfer. The data also suggest that IL-2 might serve to expand these actively proliferating effector cells.

The antigenic specificity of these lymphoblasts was essential for disease development after adoption transfer. For example, ovalbumin-immune spleen cells cultured with both OA and IL-2 resulted in a great yield of lymphoblasts, but these cells were devoid of the ability to transfer EAD (Table I).

TABLE I

ADOPTIVE TRANSFER OF EAD WITH IMMUNE SPLEEN CELLS CULTURED WITH LG-Ag AND IL-2

Donor	LG-Ag immune donor cells cultured with			OA immune donor cells cultured with
	LG-Ag	IL-2	LG-Ag+IL-2	OA+IL-2
% blasts after cell culture	13±3	5±2	22±3	35±4
EAD after cell transfer				
lymphoblasts	3/4	2/4	4/4	0/4
small lymphocytes	0/4	0/4	0/4	0/4

Adoptive transfer of EAD with antiserum.

The attempt to transfer EAD with immune serum to naive recipient rats was completely negative. Each animal received a total of 4 ml antiserum containing 1.5 mg of anti-LG-Ag antibodies, as determined by ELISA. No evidence of lacrimal gland inflammation was seen.

DISCUSSION

In the present studies, we have developed a reliable protocol for adoptive transfer of EAD in naive recipients. The major requirements are: 1) the donors must be immunized with a relevant autoantigen; 2) the immune lymphoid cells must be activated in vitro with both autoantigen and/or IL-2; and 3) lymphoblasts containing the effector cell population must be transferred.

Our results demonstrated that in vitro activation is obligatory. Nonspecific activation of the sensitized cells with IL-2 can substitute for autoantigen-specific activation provided the donors are sensitized with LG-Ag. However, dual activation with LG-Ag plus IL-2 results in marked enhancement of their ability to transfer EAD.

Very similar results have been reported for adoptive transfer of experimental allergic encephalomyelitis (EAE) where donor cells activated in vitro with both antigen and IL-1 or IL-2 exhibit maximum EAE transfer activity (3,5).

Enrichment of lymphoblasts by Percoll gradient enhances the development of EAD following adoptive transfer. When donor cells are activated in vitro with LG-Ag plus IL-2 and fractionated on Percoll gradient, it is the lymphoblasts that are active in transferring EAD; small lymphocytes are ineffective. These findings are in agreement with those obtained in EAE where lymphoblasts generated during culture are responsible for disease transfer (4). Furthermore, IL-2 has been shown to affect only activated blast cells (6). This effect of IL-2 probably accounts for the enhanced ability of dual-activated cells to transfer EAD, a major advantage in generating sufficient numbers of effector lymphocytes. With the present system it should be possible to further clarify the immunologic mechanisms that contribute to the pathogenesis of EAD.

ACKNOWLEDGEMENTS

These studies were supported by USPHS Grants EY-04444 and EY-03521 from the National Institutes of Health.

REFERENCES

1. Liu SH, Prendergast RA, Silverstein AM (1987) Experimental autoimmune dacryoadenitis: I. Lacrimal gland disease in the rat. Invest Ophthalmol Vis Sci 28:270-275.

2. Liu SH. Experimental autoimmune dacryoadenitis: Purification and characterization of a lacrimal gland autoantigen (In preparation).

3. Ortiz-Ortiz L, Weigle WO (1982) Activation of effector cells in experimental allergic encephalomyelitis by interleukin 2. J Immunol 128:1545-1550.

4. Holda JH, Welch AM, Swanborg RH (1980) Autoimmune effector cells: I. Transfer of experimental allergic encephalomyelitis with lymphoid cells cultured with antigen. Eur J Immunol 10:657-659.

5. Mannie MD, DiNarello CA, Paterson PY (1987) Interleukin 1 and myelin basic protein synergistically augment adoptive transfer activity of lymphocytes mediating experimental autoimmune encephalomyelitis in Lewis rats. J Immunol 138:4229-4235.

6. Larsson EL, Coutinho A, Martinez C (1980) A suggested mechanism for T lymphocyte activation: Implications on the acquisition of functional reactivities. Immunol Rev 51:61-91.

© 1990 Elsevier Science Publishers (Biomedical Division)
Ocular Immunology Today. M. Usui, S. Ohno and K. Aoki, editors.

OCULAR COMPLEMENT DECAY-ACCELERATING FACTOR IN HEALTH AND DISEASE

JONATHAN LASS[1], ELIZABETH WALTER[2], MELVIN ROAT[3], TERRY BURRIS[4], HANS GROSSNIK-LAUS[1,2], DEBRA SKELNIK[5], LAURE NEEDHAM[2], MILTON SINGER[4], AND M. EDWARD MEDOF[2]

From the Division of Ophthalmology[1] and the Institute of Pathology[2], Case Western Reserve University, Cleveland, OH; The Eye and Ear Institute of Pittsburgh,[3] Pittsburgh, PA; Corneal Research Laboratory, Devers Eye Institute,[4] Portland, OR; and the Department of Ophthalmology, University of Minnesota,[5] Minneapolis, MN

INTRODUCTION

Decay accelerating factor (DAF) is cell-associated glycoprotein which functions intrinsically in cell surface membranes to inhibit autologous complement activation on the surfaces of cells in contact with complement (1). It is distributed extravascularly as well as intravascularly and is present on epithelial surfaces (2). A hydrophobic form of the regulatory protein is present in adjacent body fluids (2). Deficiency of DAF in paroxysmal nocturnal hemoglobinuria, a rare, acquired hematologic disorder, leads to excessive uptake of C3b onto affected blood cell surfaces (1). DAF inhibits autologous complement activation by binding to C4b and C3b, thereby competitively preventing the interaction between C2 and Factor B with the bound activation fragments (3). This DAF activity interferes with the assembly of C3 and C5 convertases.

The regulation of complement activation in ocular tissues has received little attention. Serum complement regulators, C1 inhibitor (C1INH) and C3b inactivator (Factor I), are detectable in cornea and aqueous humor (4), but the levels of both proteins are insufficient to be functionally significant. Lactoferrin, which is present in tears, is known to inhibit the formation of the classical C3 complexes (5), but has no known role in complement regulation in the vascular space. Moreover, undirected C3 convertase inhibition by lactoferrin in ocular fluids could in principle be counterproductive, since it would dampen complement interaction with targets.

Based on the hypothesis that epithelial cell DAF may play a protective role analogous to blood cell DAF (2), ocular tissues and fluids, as well as the lacrimal gland, were examined to determine if DAF functions similarly in these tissues.

MATERIALS AND METHODS

Methods for immunohistochemical studies, the immunradioimmunometric assay for DAF, flow cytometric studies, phosphatidylinositol-specific phospholipase C (PI-PLC) digestion studies, biosynthetic analysis, western blotting, immunoprecipitation, and the hemolytic assay (7), as well as methods for culturing conjunctival epithelium and fibroblasts (8), corneal epithelium (9), and corneal endothelium (10) have been previously described. Non-stimulated tears were collected from normal subjects using a 50 μl pipette placed in the inferior fornix of the unanesthetized ocular surface and filled by capillary action. Stimulated tears were

collected in similar fashion; however, stimulation was induced by smelling onions.
0.15 ml of aqueous humor was collected from subjects at the time of cataract surgery. 2 ml of vitreous humor was collected from eye bank eyes. Murine anti-E[hu]
DAF monoclonal antibodies (mAbs) IA10, IIH6, and VIIIA7 were obtained as described (6) and used in all studies.

RESULTS

Immunohistochemical detection of DAF in ocular tissues

Immunopathologic changes were most prominent on ocular surface cells, retina,
and lacrimal acinar cells. Staining of the corneal epithelium was noted with intensity increasing towards the superficial layers. The conjunctival epithelium
showed a similar staining pattern. No staining of the stromal keratocytes was
noted. The corneal endothelium stained weakly. Interestingly the inner layers
of the retina stained, but not as intensely as the ocular surface cells. Finally,
the lumens of the lacrimal acinae and apices of the acinar epithelium stained intensely, indicative of DAF secretion by the adjacent epithelium.

Analysis of DAF in cultured conjunctival and corneal cells

Flow cytometric analyses of anti-DAF or control monoclonal-stained cultures of
conjunctival and corneal cells showed that all cell types expressed DAF on their
surfaces. The conjunctival and corneal epithelia exhibited high surface DAF concentrations, whereas the corneal endothelium and conjunctival fibroblasts showed
lower concentrations (Figure 1).

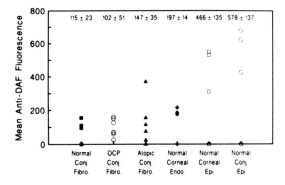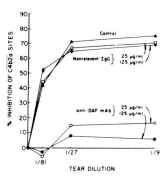

Fig. 1 (right). Inhibition of C4b2a hemolytic activity by tears and > 90% loss of
effect with addition of anti-DAF mAbs. Fig. 2 (left). Scatter plot of individual average anti-DAF fluorescence intensity of cultured conjunctival (conj.) fibroblasts from normals, patients with active ocular cicatricial pemphigoid and
atopic dermatitis, as well as normal corneal endothelium (endo.), corneal epithelium (epi) and conjunctival epithelium (conj. epi). Average values for entire
group are shown above. (Presented in part in Ref. 7)

Characterization of ocular surface DAF protein

SDS-PAGE analyses of anti-DAF immunoprecipitates of extracts of[35]S-cysteine, biosynthetically labeled corneal endothelial cells revealed a DAF species of an apparent Mr of 75k, similar to HELA cell DAF. Incubation of conjunctival epithelium with PI-PLC, an enzyme which cleaves glycoinositolphospholipid (GPL) membrane anchors, released about 70% of the conjunctival surface DAF protein, similar to leukocyte surface DAF protein.

Detection of DAF antigen in ocular fluids

Non-stimulated tears from normal subjects (n=12), aqueous humor from cataract surgery patients (n=10), and vitreous humor from eye bank eyes (8 donors, 12 eyes), were analyzed for DAF antigen by two site radioimmunometric assay. The average tear DAF concentration, 325 ng/ml, was 15x higher than the average vitreous concentration (22ng/ml) and 65x higher than the average aqueous concentration (5 ng/ml). Five normals also had simultaneous body fluids analyzed, showing the average tear DAF concentration, 216 ng/ml, was the highest concentration of DAF in any of the body fluids examined, being approximately 4x as high as urine, and as much as 7x as high as plasma.

Characterization of ocular fluid DAF

Western blot analysis of pooled, non-stimulated tears demonstrated two DAF species, one of 72k corresponding in size to soluble DAF in other body fluids, as well as a larger, previously undescribed, 100k species. The proportion of the 100k species increased in a pooled sample of stimulated tears, suggesting that the 100k form derives from the lacrimal gland.

Effects of ocular DAF on complement activation

The ability of tears to regulate C3 convertase activity was determined by an assay employing EAC14. Untreated tears markedly inhibited the formation of C3 convertase site-forming units on these intermediates (Figure 2). In the presence of anti-DAF mAbs, similar concentrations of tears had minimal or no effect. This suggests that tear DAF proteins constitute a major source of the convertase inhibitory activity in tears.

Analysis of DAF in cultured conjunctival fibroblasts in ocular cicatricial pemphigoid and atopic dermatitis

Flow cytometric studies of anti-DAF monoclonal-stained cultures of conjunctival fibroblasts from patients with active ocular cicatricial pemphigoid (n=8) and atopic dermatitis (n=6) showed a similar average surface DAF concentration as stained cultures of normal conjunctival fibroblasts (n=4)(Figure 1). The average anti-DAF fluorescence intensity of these three groups was significantly lower than the average values for normal corneal epithelium and conjunctival epithelium (p < 0.01), but similar to normal corneal endothelium.

DISCUSSION

These studies demonstrate that 1) DAF protein is present in high concentrations on the ocular surface, lacrimal acinar cells, and tears, 2) ocular DAF protein is synthesized de novo and resembles blood cell DAF protein in size and GPL anchoring, 3) tear DAF consists of two molecular forms, one with an apparent Mr of 72k, and one with an apparent Mr of 100k, the latter likely derived from the lacrimal gland, and 4) tear DAF proteins comprise at least 90% of the convertase inhibitory activity in tears. In preliminary studies from patients with active ocular cicatricial pemphigoid and atopic dermatitis expression of DAF on cultured conjunctival fibroblasts was unaffected. Since after multiple passages these cells may have lost some of their in situ characteristics, we are continuing these studies and are developing a quantitative impression cytologic technique which will be potentially more reflective of differences in in situ DAF surface expression.

ACKNOWLEDGEMENTS

Supported in part by grants from the ACS, AHA, NIH AI23598, P01DK38181, and EY06186, the Ohio Lions Eye Research Fund, and Oregon Lions Sight and Hearing Foundation.

REFERENCES

1. Pangburn MK, Schreiber RD, Muller-Eberhard HJ (1983) Proc Natl Acad Sci USA 80:5430

2. Medof ME, Walter EI, Rutgers JL, Knowles DM, Nussenzweig V (1987) J Exp Med 165:848

3. Medof ME, Knoshita T, Nussenzweig V (1984) J Exp Med 160:1558

4. Mondino BJ, Sumner H (1984) Invest Ophthalmol Vis Sci 25:483

5. Kijlstra A, Jeurissen SHM, Koning KM (1983) Br J Ophthalmol 67:199

6. Kinoshita T, Medof ME, Silber R, Nussenzweig V (1985) J Exp Med 162:75

7. Lass JH, Walter EI, Burris TE, Grossniklaus HE, Roat MI, Skelnik DL, Needham L, Singer M, Medof ME (1990) Invest Ophthalmol Vis Sci In press

8. Roat MI, Sossi G, Lo C-Y, Thoft RA (1989) Arch Ophthalmol 107:1064

9. Ebato B, Friend J, Thoft RA (1988) Invest Ophthalmol Vis Sci 28:1450

10. Skelnik DL, Lindstrom RL, Mindrup EA (1985) In: Brightbill FS (ed) Corneal Surgery. CV Mosby, St. Louis, pp 620-627

© 1990 Elsevier Science Publishers (Biomedical Division)
Ocular Immunology Today. M. Usui, S. Ohno and K. Aoki, editors.

PREDICTIVE VALUE OF CELLULAR AND HUMORAL IMMUNE RESPONSES TO CORNEAL ANTIGENS IN CORNEAL TRANSPLANTATION PATIENTS

M.J. JAGER[1], H.J. VÖLKER-DIEBEN[2], A. VOS[3], L. BROERSMA[3], R. VAN DER GAAG[3]

1. Dept. of Ophthalmology, Academic Medical Center, Amsterdam; 2. Diaconessenhuis Leiden; 3. Dept. of Ophthalmo-Immunology, the Netherlands Ophthalmic Research Institute, Amsterdam, the Netherlands.

INTRODUCTION

Studies concerning the survival of corneal grafts in man indicate that there are a variety of factors, which have a negative influence on corneal graft survival. These include retransplantation and vascularization of the recipient cornea (Sanfilippo 1986, Völker-Dieben 1989). Immunological rejection of the transplanted tissue is one of the causes for failure and a cellular immune response against cornea-specific antigens has been associated with this (Stark 1980). Since cornea-specific antibodies can be found in many patients without any sign of rejection, there is no indication that they are relevant to the outcome of a transplantation (Nelken 1965). Previous studies have, however, only focussed on either antibodies or cellular reactions and it may well be that they function complementary. We therefore determined the presence of a humoral and cellular immune response against the cornea in a series of patients undergoing corneal transplantation, in order to test the hypothesis that a systemic humoral and/or cellular immune response correlate with known risk factors or graft rejection.

MATERIALS AND METHODS

Subjects

Heparinized and clotted blood samples were obtained from 55 patients before corneal transplantation. Clinical diagnosis, degree of vascularization, number of previous transplants were registered.

Cellular immune response

The cellular immune response was measured in a two step migration inhibition assay (van der Gaag 1989) against the Major 54 kd Corneal Protein (Kruit 1986). Peripheral blood mononuclear cells were isolated by density gradient centrifugation on Ficoll-Paque (Pharmacia Fine Chemicals, Uppsala, Sweden). After washing in phosphate buffered saline the cells were incubated overnight with the 54 kd protein, and the supernatant was tested in a migration inhibition assay using monocytoid U937 cells. A migration lower than 80% of a control supernatant (without inhibitory capacity) was regarded as indicating a positive cellular response against the 54 kd protein. In order to obtain the major soluble corneal protein, corneal epithelium was scraped from bovine eyes, homogenized, and extracted in a 3M KCl 0.1M EDTA buffer, pH 7.4. The 54 kd corneal antigen was purified by anion exchange chromatography.

Humoral response

The presence of circulating antibodies against corneal epithelium was determined with an indirect immunofluorescence technique on frozen sections of rabbit corneas ().

RESULTS

A positive cellular response was not seen in controls, but was present in patients with a great variety of corneal diseases (Table 1). There was no association with recipient vascularization, or with the number of previous transplants (data not shown). The occurrence of rejection during the first three months after transplantation was not related to a positive cellular response before transplantation (Table 2).

Table 1. Positive cellular immune response in patients with different diseases of the cornea.

Disease	Number positive	Diseases	Number positive
graft failure	0/6	trauma	3/5
keratoconus	3/12	keratitis	4/7
secondary decompensation	3/10	herpes	2/4
rejection	4/6	controls	2/30

Anti-corneal antibodies were present in many patients, but were also observed in 25% of normal controls (data not shown). The presence of anti-cornea antibodies was not related to the degree of vascularization, or the number of previous transplantations. Rejections were limited to patients who had anti-corneal antibodies before transplantation.

Table 2. Numbers of individuals with clinical problems in the first three months after transplantation versus anti-cornea immune responses before transplantation.

Complications	cellular reactivity before transplantation		humoral reactivity before transplantation	
	-	+	-	+
no	24	13	24	11
fibrinoid reaction	0	2	0	2
thickened graft	4	1	2	3
rejection	5	1	1	5

DISCUSSION

A humoral and a cellular immune response against the cornea can be measured in a great variety of patients with corneal disease for whom a corneal transplantation is necessary. Healthy individuals without any ocular disease only rarely demonstrate such reactivity (van der Gaag 1989), while the development of such a response was quite common in all groups of patients tested. Patients with a graft failure not due to rejection did not show any reactivity. It may be that an anterior chamber inflammatory response, e.g. due to keratitis or rejection, leads to sensitization of the patient against the cornea. The absence of an association between an immune response and any clinical parameters decreases the importance of the in vitro findings. However, it may be that some patients had immunoreactive memory T-cells but no active cell population, and that the test method was not made to detect those cells. It may therefore be more relevant to test the patients after transplantation and to determine whether a previously dormant reaction becomes activated due to the transplantation. One reason to assume that the pre-transplantation cellular reaction may be false negative is that rejection of the graft was seen in patients who did not show a positive cellular anti-cornea immune response before transplantation, but had anti-corneal antibodies. Previous sensitization must therefore at some time have taken place in these patients. Since our results demonstrate that the presence of anti-corneal antibodies prior to transplantation is associated with a higher risk of graft rejection, it may be worthwhile to consider matching for the HLA class I antigens in patients positive for such antibodies in order to decrease the risk for rejection.

REFERENCES

1.   Gaag R van der, Broersma L, Rothova A, Baarsma S, Kijlstra A. Immunity to a corneal antigen in Fuchs' heterochromic cyclitis patients. Invest. Ophthalmol. Vis. Sci. 30, 443-448, 1989.

2.   Kruit PJ, Gaag R van der, Broersma L, Kijlstra A. Autoimmunity against corneal antigens. I. Isolation of a soluble 54 kd corneal epithelium antigen. Curr. Eye Res. 5, 313-320, 1986.

3.   Nelken E, Nelken D. Serologic studies in keratoplasty. Brit. J. Ophthalmol. 49, 159, 1965.

4.   Sanfilippo F, MacQueen JM, Vaughn WK, Foulks GN. N. Engl. J. Med 315, 29, 1986.

5.   Stark WJ, Transplantation immunology of penetrating keratoplasty. Tr. Am Soc. 88, 1079-1117, 1980.

6.   Völker-Dieben HJ. Corneal transplantation: state of the art. Transplant. Proc. 21, 3116-3119, 1989.

© 1990 Elsevier Science Publishers (Biomedical Division)
Ocular Immunology Today. M. Usui, S. Ohno and K. Aoki, editors.

THE ROLE OF NEUROPEPTIDES IN OCULAR IMMUNE MECHANISMS

R. MALATY, R. M. FRANKLIN AND N. S. OESCHGER

LSU Eye Center, 2020 Gravier Street, Suite B, New Orleans LA 70112 USA

INTRODUCTION

The lacrimal gland (LG) contains a high proportion of IgA producing plasma cells; however, the mechanisms leading to their accumulation are not well defined. The sequence of events leading to IgA committed B-cells and their maturation to plasma cells may involve T-cells retained in the LG by an adherence mechanism (1,2). Other systems have shown the binding of lymphocytes to epithelial cells (3,4) as well as modulation of lymphocyte adherence to nonlymphoid cells by various cell factors (5,6).

The LG has been shown to contain Substance P (SP) and vasoactive intestinal polypeptide (VIP), neuropeptides already demonstrated to have effects on lymphocyte function (7). More specifically, VIP, SP, and somatostatin have been shown to have direct T-cell effects responsible for alterations in IgA production (8). Because of these interesting observations on IgA regulation by neuropeptides and the presence of neuropeptide containing nerves in the LG, it was decided to explore a relationship between the adherence of lymphocytes to lacrimal gland epithelial cells (LGEC) and to examine any possible role for neuropeptides in modulating the IgA plasma cells within the gland or the adherence of lymphocytes to the glandular epithelium.

MATERIALS AND METHODS

In Vivo Studies

Female BALB/c mice weighing 14-16 grams were used in this study. Unilateral sensory denervation by ablation of the trigeminal ganglion (TG) was achieved by electrocautery (9) following general anesthesia. Sympathetic denervation was accomplished by surgical removal of the superior cervical ganglion (SCG). At necropsy the LG and the TG (in sensory denervated animals) were removed and studied by light and electron microscopy, and LG were examined by immunohistochemistry for IgA producing plasma cells using a fluorescein conjugated goat anti-mouse IgA serum (Kirkegaard-Perry, Gaithersburg MD). Stained cells were counted in 15 microscopic fields in each of ten sections per gland using a Zeiss microscope with an epifluorescent attachment. In other studies, LGs were directly injected with 3 microliters of 10^{-5}M SP on one side. After one and four weeks, mice were sacrificed and IgA plasma cells were counted in four fields per section at 400x in each of 12 tissue sections per LG.

In Vitro Studies

The exorbital LGs of BALB/c mice (13-16 grams) were digested with EDTA, then with a collagenase II/hyaluronidase mixture, then with Dispase. Washed cells were then allowed to adhere to a plastic tissue culture dish precoated with a basement membrane gel (Matrigel, Collaborative Research, Bedford MA).

Lymphocytes were isolated from the spleen (spl), Peyer's patches (PP), and LGs and then separated into T or B-cells with nylon wool columns or specific antisera.

The LGEC were cultured for four days, then 10^6 T or B-cells labeled with a supravital DNA stain (Hoechst 33342, Calbiochem) were added. After overnight incubation, the cultures were washed to remove unattached lymphocytes and the plates examined with a Zeiss IM 35 fluorescence microscope to determine the attachment of labeled lymphocytes to LGEC.

The effects of tumor necrosis factor (TNF), Interferon/gamma (IFN) and VIP were tested in this system by exposing four day cultures of LGEC for four hours then incubating with labelled T-cells. After overnight incubation, T-cells attached to LGEC were counted and compared to attachments to untreated LGEC.

RESULTS

TG ablation resulted in LGEC swelling, vacuolation and loss of secretory granules. The trigeminal nerve and the nerves within the LG showed axonal degeneration with myelin abnormalities.

IgA plasma cell members were higher in SCG denervated LG than in controls (410 and 284, n=3; p=0.4) four weeks post denervation. With trigeminal denervation, the numbers were slightly lower than controls one week post denervation (280 and 308, n=6; p=0.14) and were lower still (259 and 314, n=6; p=0.01) at four weeks.

Injection of SP into the LG had no effect on acinar morphology. IgA plasma cells were higher than controls after one week (10.1 ± 0.15 and 8.1 ± 0.14, n=4, p=0.0001) and reversed after four weeks. Control untreated animals however, showed no differences between right and left LGs (11.7 ± 0.2 and 11.5 ± 0.2, n=6, p=0.07).

T-cells from the LG showed a 67% and 54% increase in attachment in LGEC culture, over T-cells from spl or PP respectively. Depletion of T-helper cells reduced the attachment by 60% using spl T-cells. The attachment of B-cell enriched preparations was consistently below 10% of the T-cell attachment rate. Addition of TNF to either LGEC or T-cells did not significantly change the degree of attachment. When LGEC were preincubated with IFN or VIP, attachment increased to 50% or 82%, respectively.

DISCUSSION

In this series of experiments, we examined whether neuropeptides or cell factors might participate in the lymphocyte migration to and lodging in the mouse LG. In our in vivo studies, sensory denervation resulted in axonal degeneration of the trigeminal nerve and nerves within the gland and alteration of the architecture of the acinar cells. The IgA plasma cell numbers decreased when compared to controls. With sympathetic denervation, there were no morphological changes, however, the IgA plasma cell numbers increased. When the LG was exposed to SP, the IgA plasma cell content increased at one week. These findings can be interpreted in the context of previous studies in ocular tissues which have shown decreased neuropeptide levels and destruction of SP immunoreactive nerves following sensory denervation (10). Also, trigeminal nerve stimulation resulted in an increase in concentration of SP (11). Sympathetic denervation caused an increase in SP levels and density of immunoreactive nerve fibers (12). Therefore, in the present studies, sensory denervation may have decreased SP levels with a resultant decrease in IgA plasma cell numbers. Sympathetic denervation may have increased SP levels leading to the increases of IgA plasma cells which was also seen following direct injection of SP into the LG. Whether the effects of neuropeptides on lymphocytes led to increased proliferation of cells (8) or to an increase in lymphocyte homing receptors (13) cannot be directly answered from these studies.

The above observations could lead to an increased number of IgA plasma cells in the LG but might not be sufficient to explain the predominance of IgA plasma cells in LG. The migratory lymphocytes could be restrained by cellular interactions between lymphocytes and nonlymphoid cells of the LG. Such interactions have been described in other systems (3) and extracellular factors such as IFN and TNF have been shown to alter the T-cell attachment to nonlymphoid cells. For instance, epidermal keratinocytes

308

bind T-cells via an IFN-induced intracellular adhesion molecule (4,5), and TNF stimulates the adhesion of T-cells to cultured human umbilical vein endothelial cells (6). In our in vitro experiments, we examined whether neuropeptides and various cytokines could alter the attachment of lymphocytes to cultured LGEC. It was found that T-cells, probably T-helper cells, were the predominant binding cell type. In addition, TNF was without effect on these cell interactions, however, pretreatment of LGEC with IFN or VIP resulted in an increase in attachment of the T-cells. Since the LG contains nerve fibers containing various neuropeptides (7), and since our studies suggest an inducible intracellular adhesion molecule in the LGEC for T-helper cells, it is possible that such a mechanism exists in the LG to explain the accumulation of a subgroup of T-helper cells specific for IgA production. Although the details of this mechanism have yet to be demonstrated, the present experiments demonstrate that at least parts of such a mechanism are present within the LG and can lead to further studies to examine more critically this possibility.

ACKNOWLEDGMENTS

This study was supported in part by NIH grants EY 03028 and EY 07213.

REFERENCES

1. Mestecky J and McGhee JR (1987) Adv in Immunol 40: 153-245

2. Franklin RM, McGee DW and Shepard KF (1985) J Immunol 135: 95-99

3. Singer KH, et al (1986) Proc Natl Acad Sci USA 83: 6588-6592

4. Dustin ML, Springer TA (1988) J Cell Biol 107(1): 321-31

5. Bierer BE and Burakoff SJ (1988) FASEB J 2: 2584-2590

6. Cavendar D, Saegusa Y and Morris Z (1987) Immunol 139: 1855-1860

7. Nikkinen A, et al. (1984) Histochemistry 81: 23-27

8. Stanisz AM, Befus D, Bienenstock J (1986) J Immunol 136: 152-156

9. Schimmelpfennig B and Beuerman R (1982) Graefe's Arch Clin Exp Ophthal 218: 287-293

10. Stone RA, Kuwayama Y, and Laties AM (1987) Experientia 43: 791-900

11. Bill A, et al. (1979) Acta Physiol Scan 106: 371-373

12. Tervo K, et al. (1982) Exp Eye Res 34: 577-585

13. Ottaway CA (1984) J Exp Med 160: 1054-1069

© 1990 Elsevier Science Publishers (Biomedical Division)
Ocular Immunology Today. M. Usui, S. Ohno and K. Aoki, editors.

IMMUNOHISTOCHEMICAL STUDY OF SCLERITIS

MAITE SAINZ DE LA MAZA, C.STEPHEN FOSTER, LYE PHENG FONG AND
BEVERLY A. RICE

Immunology Service, Massachusetts Eye and Ear Infirmary, Harvard Medical
School, Boston, Massachusetts, USA

INTRODUCTION

Necrotizing scleritis is the most severe and destructive form of scleritis (1).
The well documented association with systemic autoimmune disorders, response
to immunosuppressive therapy, histopathologic evidence of vasculitis and vascular
non-perfusion on anterior segment fluorescein angiography all suggest an autoimmune vasculitic process, possibly mediated by immune-complexes (2-4). However,
direct evidence of immune-complex vasculitis has not been previously reported.

We studied scleral and/or conjunctival biopsies from patients with necrotizing
scleritis and recurrent non necrotizing scleritis by histopathologic and immunopathologic techniques. The findings have both diagnostic and therapeutic implications.

MATERIAL AND METHODS

We reviewed the records of the patients with necrotizing scleritis and with
recurrent non necrotizing scleritis seen in the Immunology Service at the
Massachusetts Eye and Ear Infirmary Hospital between January 1983 and August
1988 in whom scleral and/or conjunctival biopsies had been performed. All
patients had been treated elsewhere with topical and systemic steroidal and/or
non steroidal antiinflammatory drugs.

Historical features, a comprehensive review of systems, a complete clinical
examination and results of laboratory evaluation were obtained for each patient.

Under local anesthesia and operating microscope control, necrotic and inflammed
conjunctival and scleral tissues were carefully resected. In cases of major scleral
loss, scleral homografting was used for structural support (5). The specimens
were processed for histopathology (HP), immunofluorescence (IF) and immunoperoxidase (IP) studies. Healthy individuals undergoing cataract surgery provided
normal conjunctival tissue used as controls. Normal scleral specimens came from
eye bank eyes. The presence of vasculitis, defined as neutrophil invasion with
fibrinoid necrosis or as immunoreactant deposition in the vessel wall seen by
HP or IF respectively, and the detection of specific cell types by IP were evaluated.

Patients with scleritis associated with a specific systemic vasculitic disease
received systemic immunosuppressive therapy (6).

RESULTS

Twenty-eight patients (32 eyes), 23 with necrotizing scleritis and five with recurrent non necrotizing scleritis, form the basis of this report, including 14 males and 14 females, with a mean age of 61 years (range 37-87 years). The mean follow-up period was 3.07 years (range 1.25-6.33).

Biopsy evaluation through light microscopy demonstrated a vasculitic process in 50% of the conjunctival and 71% of the scleral specimens obtained. Biopsy evaluation through immunofluorescence microscopy showed immune-complex deposition in the vessel walls in the 82% of the conjunctival and 93% of the scleral specimens obtained. The immunoperoxidase studies with monoclonal antibodies showed as a predominant finding a dramatic increase of inflammatory cells with a high helper/suppressor ratio in conjunctival and scleral tissues. Conjunctival epithelium showed increased numbers of T helpers, macrophages and B cells. All epithelial cell membranes in the scleritis patients stained intensely for HLA-DR glycoproteins. Normal epithelium did not show this intense staining pattern. Scleral specimens showed large numbers of dendritic cells, T cells, T helpers, T cytotoxic/suppressors, B cells, natural killer cells and macrophages.

Underlying systemic autoimmune disease was present in 24 of the 28 patients (86%), including rheumatoid arthritis (eight patients), suspected Wegener´s granulomatosis (incomplete syndrome, six patients), classic multi-system Wegener´s granulomatosis (complete syndrome, three patients), relapsing polychondritis (four patients), ulcerative colitis (one patient), Reiter s syndrome (one patient) and juvenile rheumatoid arthritis (one patient). Local ocular diseases, such as herpes simplex infection and bacterial periorbital cellulitis, were diagnosed in two patients. The remaining patients were classified as idiopathic (two patients).

Twenty-three of the 28 patients (82%), all of them with evidence of vasculitis at the biopsy, required immunosuppressive therapy for halting progression of the disease.

Circulating immune-complexes were measured by either Raji cell assay and/or by C1q binding assay in serum obtained from 20 patients at the time of biopsy. The Raji cell assay was more sensitive to detecting circulating immune-complexes (78% of 18 samples with levels above normal). Circulating immune-complexes were detected in 80% of the ten patients with confirmed vasculitis, as defined by both histopathology and immunofluorescence positivity.

DISCUSSION

The immunopathologic response in necrotizing scleritis or recurrent non necrotizing scleritis refractory to conventional treatment appears to be integrally related to abnormalities in the vasculature. The findings of immune-complex deposition, neutrophil infiltration and fibrinoid necrosis of the vessel walls in the majority of our patients, suggest that immune-complex mediated vasculitis plays a pivotal role in these types of scleritis. Its demonstration in ocular tissue is helpful in the diagnostic pursuit of potentially lethal systemic vasculitic diseases which can be treated with systemic immunosuppression. Either conjunctiva or sclera may provide adequate information for detection of vasculitis if both histopathologic and immunofluorescence techniques are used although sclera is better tissue if only histopathologic evaluation is available. Immunofluorescence technique increases the sensitivity for detection of vasculitis in either tissue.

Circulating immune-complexes were elevated in 80% of ten patients with confirmed vasculitis. It is not unreasonable to postulate that immune-complexes are deposited in scleral vessels and that necrotizing scleritis represents a classic Gell and Coombs type III hypersensitivity reaction. The increased numbers of macrophages, T, T helper and B cells and the high helper-suppressor ratio can explain the complex network of cellular interactions leading to B cell development into plasma cell and eventual immunoglobulin secretion. Interplay between antigen and surface immunoglobulin receptors and between T helper cells and macrophages result in the expression of receptors for and in the release of specific growth factors respectively such as B cell growth factor (BCGF) which causes proliferation of B cells (7-8). Also released from T helper cells are the B cell differentiation factors (BCDF) which cause a differentiation of B cells into immunoglobulin secreting plasma cells (9-10). It is known that interferon gamma is one of the commonest procucts of T cell clones, of both helper and suppressor or cytotoxic phenotypes. Work with human tonsillar B cells has confirmed the role of interferon gamma as a B cell differentiating factor, indicating a synergistic effect of interferon gamma with interleukin-2 for proliferation and immunoglobulin production (11-12). Thus, although interferon gamma alone does not suffice for B cell differentiation, it appears to be an obligatory, late acting factor that synergizes with earlier acting stimuli.

Interestingly, it has been shown that synthesis of types I and III collagen by rheumatoid synovial cells in culture is inhibited by interferon gamma; this is associated with decreases in types I and III procollagen in messenger RNAs in these cells (13). Interferon gamma also induces HLA-DR antigens, dramatically increased in our conjunctival and scleral specimens. This may enhance antigen presentation, not only by immune cells, but also by non immune cells such as epithelial, endothelial, retinal pigment epithelium and corneal stromal cells. Recent studies with interferon gamma have demonstrated aberrant expression of MHC class II antibodies in ocular tissue and spontaneous uveitis in animal models.

Furthermore, anti-MHC class II antibodies have been shown to abrogate experimental autoimmune uveitis inflammation (14-15). The pivotal role of HLA-DR expression in the initiation and perpetuation of inflammatory and autoimmune processes is the basis for the provocative suggestion by Bottazzo et al. (16) that aberrant expression of HLA-DR is instrumental to the activation of T helper cells and the initiation of the immune response leading to autoimmune disorders.

REFERENCES

1. Watson PG, Hayreh SS (1976) Brit J Ophthalmol 60:163-191

2. Rao NA, Marak GE, Hidayat AA (1985) Ophthalmology 92:1542-48

3. Calthorpe CM, Watson PG, McCartney ACE (1988) Eye 2:267-77

4. Latina M, Flotte T, Crean E, Sherwood ME, Granstein RD (1988) Arch Ophthalmol 106:95-9

5. Sainz de la Maza M, Tauber J, Foster CS (1989) Ophthalmology 96:306-10

6. Foster CS (1983) Int Ophthalmol Clin 23(1):183-96

7. Howard M, Paul WE (1983) Annu Rev Immunol 307-33

8. Ambrus JL Jr, Jurgensen CH, Brown EJ, Fauci AS (1985) J Exp Med 162:1319-35

9. Paul WE (1983) In: Yanamora Y, Tada T eds. Fifth International Conference Immunology. Academic Press, Tokio pp 727-31

10. Sakane T, Ueda Y, Suzuki N, Niwa Y, Hoshino T, Tsunematsu T (1985) Clin Exp Immunol 62:112-20

11. Lethi BT, Fauci AS (1986) J Clin Invest 77:1173-79

12. Nakagawa T, Hirano T, Nakagawa N, Yoshizaki K, Kishimoto T (1985) J Immunol 134:959-66

13. Stephenson ML, Krane SM, Amento EP, McCroskery PA, Byrne M (1985) FEBS Lett 180:43-50

14. Wetzig R, Hooks JJ, Percopo CM, Nussenblatt R, Chan CC, Detrick B (1988) Curr Eye Res 7:309-18

15. Attala L, Israeli L, George F, Marin J, Steinman L, Rao NA (1988) Invest Ophthalmol Vis Sci 29 (Suppl):268

16. Bottazzo G, Pumol-Borrell R, Hanafusa T (1983) Lancet 2:1115-9

© 1990 Elsevier Science Publishers (Biomedical Division)
Ocular Immunology Today. M. Usui, S. Ohno and K. Aoki, editors.

313

COMPLEMENT ALLOTYPING IN ANTERIOR UVEITIS: ASSOCIATION WITH C4B2 AND HLA B27

DENIS WAKEFIELD, PETER McCLUSKEY, ELIZABETH TOMPSETT AND JOHN CHARLESWORTH.

Laboratory of Ocular Immunology, School of Pathology. UNSW, PO Box 1, Kensington NSW, 2033, Australia.

INTRODUCTION

The complement components, factor B, C2 and C4 are coded by genes in the HLA region on the short arm of chromosome 6[1]. Codominant allelic genes occur at each locus with factor B and C2 being controlled by a single gene and C4 by two closely linked genes, C4A and C4B, both of which show a high degree of structural and functional polymorphism[2].

Anterior uveitis is a common inflammatory eye disease associated with seronegative arthropathies and the HLA B27. The HLA B27 antigen is believed to be directly involved in susceptibility to ankylosing spondylitis, Reiter's syndrome and anterior uveitis[3]. We have previously reported the association between anterior uveitis and the C4B2 allotype[4]. In our previous study, we examined complement allotypes in patients with a variety of inflammatory eye diseases, including subjects with anterior uveitis, posterior uveitis and retinal vasculitis. Only patients with AU showed an association with a particular complement allotype. In our preliminary study of 18 subjects, the increased frequency of C4B2 occurred in those subjects with AU who were HLA B27-positive[4]. In order to further examine this association we have studied a separate, larger population of patients with AU to define the relationship between this genetic marker and other HLA B27 related disease.

MATERIALS AND METHODS

Thirty seven consecutive patients referred to the Uveitis research clinics at Sydney Eye Hospital, Prince of Wales and St Vincents hospitals, Sydney, were investigated over a six month period. There were 23 males with a mean age of 48 years (SD 18) and 14 females with a mean age of 47 years (SD 14). All patients were examined by an ophthalmologist and a physician. Etiological investigations for uveitis performed according to our previously published protocols[5].

Complement (C4) allotyping was performed by the method of Mauff and colleagues[6]. A haemolytic overlay technique was used to distinguish C4A and C4B loci. Heterogeneous null alleles were defined, where necessary, by two dimensional electrophoresis using the same anti-C4 antibody for the second stage. Null alleles were not considered in the final analysis as family members were not available for confirmatory studies.

A group of 288 normal adult Australian subjects were C4 allotyped using the above method served as the control population for this study. HLA typing for the HLA B27 antigen was performed by the NSW Red Cross blood transfusion service using the modified NIH microlymphocytotoxicity test.

Chi squared analysis was used to compare the frequency of C4 allotypes in patients and controls. The p values were corrected for the number of tested antigens[7]. Relative risks were calculated by Woolf's method.

RESULTS

Twenty-eight patients with anterior uveitis had idiopathic disease. Nine male patients with AU had ankylosing spondylitis (AS) (all were HLA B27-positive).

The results of C4 allotyping are summarised in table 1. The C4B2 allotype was increased in the group of patients with AU (p_c<0.005). Although all ten patients with C4B2 were also HLA B27-positive, this allotype was not increased in this group when compared to the non-HLA B27 group of patients with AU (ie. p_c>0.05). Comparison of uveitis patients, with and without AS did not show a difference in the frequency of C4B2.(Pc=0.08)

TABLE 1

Complement allotypes in anterior uveitis

ALLOTYPE	PATIENTS (%) N=37	CONTROLS (%) N=288	RELATIVE RISK	Pc
C4A 1	2 (5.4)	4 (1.4)	4.1	
2	3 (8.1)	20 (6.9)	1.2	
3	35 (94.6)	238 (82.6)	3.7	
4	5 (13.5)	18 (6.3)	2.3	
6	1 (2.7)	3 (1.0)	2.6	
C4B 1	36 (97.3)	258 (89.6)	4.2	
2	10 (27.0)	14 (4.9)	7.3	<0.005
3	0 (0.0)	4 (1.4)		
5	0 (0.0)	1 (0.3)		

DISCUSSION

This study confirms and extends our previous observation that this is an increased frequency of C4B2 allele in patients with AU (4). The data indicate that there is an increase in the frequency of C4B2 in HLA B27 positive patients with anterior uveitis. All ten patients with C4B2 allotype were HLA B27. However, when we compared HLA B27 positive AU patients with those who were HLA

B27 negative, the difference in the prevalence of the C4B2 allotype failed to reach statistical significance (p_c=O.08).

Previous studies in patients with AS and their families failed to show a relationship between HLA B27 and complement allotypes[8]. This is consistent with the present study where patients with HLA B27 AU and AS had an increased frequency of C4B2 although this did not occur in patients with AS alone. Thus, the C4B2 allotype is associated selectively with AU, it is not increased in HLA B27 subjects or patients with AS when compared with non HLA B27 subjects and those who do not have AS.

Previous studies have documented in increased frequency of the C4B2 allotype in patients with pauciarticular juvenile arthritis[9]. This rheumatic disease is often associated with chronic AU. Hence it has a similar genetic profile to that observed in adult subjects with AU. The increase in C4B2 in patients with AU may be related to the pathogenesis of AU. Complement proteins play an important role in inflammatory reactions, viral neutralisation and the dissolution of immune complexes. Immune complexes and autoantibodies have been implicated in the pathogenesis of AU, particularly where there is no association with HLA B27[5]. Circulating immune complexes and hypocomplementaemia have been reported in patients with uveitis[10]. Vargani et al[11] reported increased serum levels of C3d, a marker of complement activation, in 11 of 15 patients with idiopathic uveitis, 13 of whom had circulating immune complexes containing complement. Thus activation of complement, possibly triggered by uveal deposition of immune complexes, may have an important role in the pathogenesis of uveitis.

The C4B2 allelic marker observed in our patients with uveitis may form part of a supratype associated with this disease, which is linked to the HLA B27 antigen. Such an association has been recognised in other autoimmune diseases, such as SLE and pauciarticular juvenile arthritis, and further studies are required to define such supratypes in patients with inflammatory eye disease.

REFERENCES

1. Wakefield D, Breit SN, Clark P, Penny R. Immunogenetic factors in inflammatory eye disease. Arth Rheum 1982;25:1432.

2. Porter RR. The complement components coded in the major histocompatability complexes and their biological activities. Immunol Rev 1985; 87: 7.

3. Brewerton DA, Caffrey M, Nicholis A, Walters D, James DCO. Acute anterior uveitis and HLA B27. Lancet 1973;i:994.

4. Wakefield D, Buckley R, Golding J, Mc Cluskey P, Abi-Hanna D, Charlesworth J. and Pussell B. Association of complement allotype C4B2 with anterior uveitis. Hum Immunol 1989; 21: 233-7.

5. Wakefield D, Easter J, Robinson JP, Penny R. Immunological features of HLA B27 anterior uveitis. Aust J Ophthalmol 1983; 11: 15.

316

6. Mauff G, Bender K, Giles CM, Goldman S, Opferkuch W, Wachauf B. Human C4 polymorphism : pedigree analysis of qualitative, quantitative and functional parameters as a basis for phenotype interpretations. Human Genet 1984; 65: 362.

7. Svejgaard A, Jersild C, Staub-Nielsen L, Bodmer WC. HLA antigens and disease, statistical and genetical considerations. Tissue antigens 1974;4:95.

8. Gran JT, Teisberg P, Olaissen O, Thorsby and Husby G. HLA B27 and allotypes of complement components in ankylosing spondylitis. 1984 J Rheum. 11:3 324-326.

9. Hall PJ, Burman SJ, Laurent MR, Briggs DC, Venning HE, Leak AM, Bedford PA, Ansell BM. Genetic susceptibility to early onset pauciarticular juvenile chronic arthritis: a study of HLA and complement markers in 158 British patients. Ann Rheum Dis 1986;45: 464.

10. Corwin JM, Baum J. Iridocyclitis in two patients with hypocomplementemic cutaneous vasculitis. Am J Ophthalmol 1982; 94: 111-3.

11. Vergani S, Di Mauro E, Davies ET, Spinelli D, Mieli-Vergani G, Vergani D. Br J Ophthalmol 1986; 70:60-3.

© 1990 Elsevier Science Publishers (Biomedical Division)
Ocular Immunology Today. M. Usui, S. Ohno and K. Aoki, editors.

PHOSPHOLIPID AUTOIMMUNITY IN THE PATHOGENESIS OF VASCULAR RETINOPATHY

AMJAD RAHI, SWARN RAHI & JUGNOO RAHI*

Ministry of Health, P.O. Box 3112, Dammam 31471, Saudi Arabia & Dept.Ophthalmology
Hospital for Sick Children, London.

Inflammation and/or thrombosis of retinal vasculature is a feature of several
inflammatory systemic diseases including Behcets syndrome, sarcoidosis, systemic
lupus erythematosus, polyarteritis nodosa and other connective tissue disorders.
Inflammation of retinal vessels, however also occurs as an isolated event (ie.
idiopathic); it may also accompany other eye diseases such as intermediate uveitis,
sympathetic ophthalmitis, Vogt-Koyanagi syndrome and lens-induced inflammation.
Idiopathic or isolated retinal vasculitis is a well recognised clinical syndrome
occuring predominantly in young people , characterised by cells in the vitreous,
disc oedema, periphlebitis as evidenced by sheathing, and frequent occurence of
macular odema (1). Histologically there is perivascular cuffing by lymphocytes
which may be associated with retinal degeneration. In later stages reduced
perfusion leads to retinal neovascularisation and vitreous haemorrhage. Connective
tissue diseases such as systemic lupus erythematosus although do not produce
characteristic sheathing are, however, associated with retinal microinfarcts
characterised by cotton wool exudates and intraretinal haemorrhages (2). Since
there is no obvious significant inflammatory component (such as cells in the
vitreous or vascular sheathing) SLE is not regarded as a cause of retinal
vasculitis. This is because the term retinal vasculitis traditionally focusses
attention on the vessel wall and tends to ignore the vascular endothelium which
acts as an important interface between the components of the blood and the vessel
wall. In this presentation we propose that factors working at the level of this
interface alone may play a significant role in the pathogenesus retinal vascular
disease which may or not be associated with obvious cellular infiltrates. Recent
studies suggest that vascular endothelium can bind inflammatory immune-complexes,
and can also behave as antigen-presenting cell by expressing on its surface
class II (eg HLA-DR) histocompatibility antigens (3). Inflammatory cells have to
negotiate with the vascular endothelium before entering the vessel wall and
in this event inter-cellular adhesion molecules (ICAM) such as fibronectin, human
leukocyte function antigens such as LFA-1, and receptor for third component of
complement (CR-3) play an important role (4). Phospholipid is an integral
component of vascular endothelial membrane; recent studies suggest that autoimmune
response to phospholipids particularly cardiolipin may be of pathogenetic
significance in a variety of clinical disorders including unexplained venous
or arterial thrombosis, myocardial infarction in   young patients, SLE, thrombo-
cyteopenia and recurrent abortion (5,6). Although the precise mechanism by

which anti-phospholipid antibody can produce vascular damage is not known, it is plausible that it may cause an imbalance between intrinsic pro-coagulant and anti-coagulant factors thus tipping the balance in favour of thrombosis. Thrombosis of retinal or systemic vasculature may thus be regarded as an auto-immune disease initiated by endotheliitis. It is of relevance in this context, that using umblical vein endothelial cell culture, it has been possible to demonstrate anti-endothelial cell antibody in SLE, rheumatoid arthritis, progressive systemic selerosis, IgA nephropathy (Bergers disease) haemolytic uraemic syndrome, thrombotic thrombocytopenic purpura and Kawasaki disease (7,8). The damage to the blood vessel may be brought about by complement mediated or K-cell dependent machanisms.

MATERIAL AND METHODS

Twenty out of 58 patients with SLE seen in Ministry Health Hospitals in the Eastern Povince had characteristic retinal lesion. Serum from these 20 patients along with another 28 patients with systemic lupus erythematosus but without retinal involvement were tested for antiphospholipid antibody. Serum from another 7 patients with idiopathic retinal vasculitis was also tested for the presence of this antibody. Blood from 37 healthy adults matched for age and sex was also tested to obtain the reference range. IgG & IgM anti-cardiolipin antibodies were estimated by solid phase ELISA (cheshire Diagnostic, England). The results were expressed as units of IgG phospholipid antibody (GPL) or IgM phospholipid antibody (MPL) per ml of serum. One unit of antibody (GPL or MPL) is defined as cardiolipin binding activity of 1 ug/ml of affinity purified anticardiolipin antibody.

RESULT

The upper limit of anticardiolipin antibody (GPL & MPL) in normal Saudi population was taken as 10 U/ml. As shown in Tables I & II 50 % of patients with SLE had anticardiolipin antibody of either G or M type. However in those patients in whom the disease was associated with vascular retinopathy the antibody was present in 85 % cases. In idiopathic retinal vasculitis, however, only 42 % cases had significant levels of anticardiolipin antibody.

TABLE I ANTICARDIOLIPIN ANTIBODY IN SLE

NO: PATIENTS POSITIVE = 24/48

IgG TYPE	IgM TYPE
6 (25%)	6
0	6 (25%)
12 (50%)	0
18	12

TABLE II ANTICARDIOLIPIN ANTIBODY IN VASCULAR RETINOPATHY

	G + M TYPE	G-TYPE	M-TYPE	% POSITIVE
VAS.RETINOPATHY + SLE (20 PATIENTS)	4	10	3	85
IDIOPATHIC VAS.RETINOPATHY (7 PATIENTS)	-	3	-	42

DISCUSSION

The aetilogy of isolated retinal vasculitis and that associated with systemic disease is unknown but it has been suggested that it may result from deposition of immune-complexes (9). These authors have noted circulating immune complexes as well as auto-antibody to soluble retinal antigen in about 50 % of such cases. It was found, however, that if isolated retinal vasculitis was associated with reduced perfusion (due to capillary closure) rather than increased vascular permeability immune-complexes were demonstrable in less than 25 % cases, but almost 90 % patients showed auto-immunity to retinal photorceptors. Since in systemic vasculitides, apart from immune-complexes, antiphospholipid antibody antiendothelial antibody as well as antibody to neutrophil cytoplasmic antigens including myeloperoxidose appear to play a pathogenetic role (10,11) it is conceivable that similar machanisms may operate in the retina. Furthermore venous or arterial thrombosis associated with phospholipid autoimmunity may not overtly appear inflammatory in the conventional sense but it appears to be initiated by auto-immune damage to the vascular endothelium. Since 85 % patients with vascular retinopathy due to systemic lupus erytheatosus had raised levels of either IgG or IgM anti-cardiolipin antibody, it is possible that vascular occlusion leading to micro-infarcts in the retina was due to autoimmune damage to the retinal vasculature. It is of interest that 3 of the 7 (42 %) cases with idiopathic retinal vasculitis also had raised levels of anticardiolipin antibody.

CONCLUSION

Autoimmune response to phospholipid seems to play a significant pathogenic role in a variety of systemic diseases associated with either arterial or venous thrombosis. Although this may not be associated with overt inflammatory changes in the vessel wall, the disease may be regarded as inflammtory in which the auto-immune insult operates at the level of the vascular endothelium which acts as an intraface between the vessel wall & the circulating blood. It is not surprising, therefore, that vascular retinopathies with microinfarcts in association with SLE or retinal vasculitis of unknown origin show strong to moderate association with phospholipid auto-immunity. Since anticardiolipin antibodies appear to cross react with antigens recognised by anti-endothelial antibodies it is possible that the auto-antibody detected in our patients

320

were also directed to against the endothelial cells of the retinal vasculature.

REFERENCES

1. Stanford, M, Graham, E, Kasp, E et. al. (1987) Eye 1, 69

2. Graham, E, Spalton, D, Barnard, R et. al. (1985) Ophthalmology 92, 444

3. Nunez, G, Ball, E, Stastny, P (1983) J.Immunol 131, 666

4. Brown, K, Mccarthy, D, Bull, M et. al. (1989) Clin.Exp.Immunol 77, 356

5. Harris, E, Gharavi, A, Hughes, G (1985) Clin.Rheum.Dis 11, 591.

6. Gharavi, A, Mellors, R, Belkon, K (1989) Clin.Exp.Immunol 78, 233

7. Heurkens, A, Hiemstra, P, Lafeber, G et. al. (1989) Clin.Exp.Immunol 78, 7.

8. Ferraro, G, Meroni, P, Tincani, A et. al. (1990) Clin.Exp.Immunol 79, 47.

9. Graham, E, Spalton, D, Sanders, M (1981) Trans.Ophthal.Soc.UK 101, 12.

10. Van Der Woud, F, Daha, M, Van Es. L (1989) Clin.Exp.Immunol 78, 143.

11. Lee, S, Adu, D, Thompson, R (1990) Clin.Exp.Immunol 79, 41.

© 1990 Elsevier Science Publishers (Biomedical Division)
Ocular Immunology Today. M. Usui, S. Ohno and K. Aoki, editors.

INFLUENCE OF NEURAL INNERVATION ON THE EXPRESSION OF THE SECRETORY IMMUNE SYSTEM OF THE LACRIMAL GLAND

DAVID A. SULLIVAN, LOUANE E. HANN, LYDIA YEE, CYNTHIA SOO, JOAN A. EDWARDS AND MATHEA R. ALLANSMITH
Department of Ophthalmology, Harvard Medical School and Immunology Unit, Eye Research Institute, 20 Staniford Street, Boston, MA, USA 02114

INTRODUCTION

A complex, regulatory interaction is known to exist between the nervous and immune systems (1,2). Neuropeptides and neurotransmitters directly modulate lymphocyte migration, localization and function (3,4), whereas lymphocytic signals exert a significant impact on neural activity (1,2). Recently, the influence of this neural-immune interrelationship has been shown to extend to the secretory immune system (3), which is designed to protect mucosal surfaces against microbial challenge. Thus, neuropeptides may modulate both the production of IgA (3), as well as secretory component (SC; 5), the IgA antibody receptor. Given this neuroimmunological association, the present study sought to determine whether ocular nerves might be involved in the distribution, density and output of IgA-containing cells in the lacrimal gland. Experiments evaluated the role of the: 1) superior cervical ganglion, which serves as the primary source of sympathetic nerves to lacrimal tissue and reportedly modulates the IgA cell number in this gland (6); 2) sphenopalatine ganglion, which is the origin of peptidergic and parasympathetic nerves to the lacrimal gland; 3) trigeminal ganglion, which may act as a conduit for sensory input from lacrimal tissue and possibly alter IgA-containing cell localization (6); 4) tempero-facial nerve division, which in rats appears to provide innervation to the lacrimal gland (7); and 5) optic nerves, because light has been demonstrated to regulate T cell function both systemically (8) and within the eye (9).

MATERIALS AND METHODS (10)

Adult male Sprague-Dawley rats (6 weeks old) were obtained from Zivic-Miller Laboratories, Inc., and maintained in constant temperature rooms with light/dark intervals of 12 hours duration. Animals underwent one of the following surgical protocols: ablation of the superior cervical ganglion, extirpation of the sphenopalatine ganglion, severance of the major nerve issuing from the trigeminal ganglion, denervation of the tempero-facial nerve division or sectioning of the optic nerve. Ganglionectomies and denervations were conducted on the left side and sham-operations on the right. Additional groups of rats received either bilateral sham or complete optic nerve denervation. All operative procedures were performed by surgeons at Zivic-

Miller Laboratories, Inc. To verify surgical success, examinations included: the presence of ptosis in the ipsilateral lid after superior cervical ganglion removal; the existence of pupillary dilation, lens opacification and/or retinal pathology following optic nerve destruction; and the intensity and extent of acetylcholinesterase and vasoactive intestinal peptide staining in lacrimal tissue after sphenopalatine ganglionectomy.

Tears were obtained from the eyes of etherized rats and IgA levels were quantitated with a specific radioimmunoassay (11). For immunofluorescence studies, lacrimal glands were collected, weighed, then fixed in an ethanol/glacial acetic acid solution (19:1) at 4°C. Following overnight fixation, tissues were dehydrated, embedded in paraffin and cut into 5 μm sections, which were placed on gelatin-coated slides and deparaffinized before staining. When required, lacrimal glands were serially sectioned. The protocol for the immunofluorescent measurement of IgA-containing cells in lacrimal gland sections has been previously described (12). For quantitative analysis of the density of IgA-positive cells, at least 2 sections/tissue and approximately 15 microscopic fields (312.5 x magnification)/ section were examined with a Zeiss Photoscope II fluorescence microscope, equipped with epiillumination and fitted with a xenon lamp, a 460-490 nm excitation filter and a 528 nm barrier filter. To determine the total number of IgA-containing cells in lacrimal tissue, the lymphocyte density/field was multiplied by gland weight (mg) and by an appropriate correction factor (13). Experimental data was analyzed statistically with Student's t test, or, for tests of randomness, chi square goodness of fit.

RESULTS (10)

Location of IgA-containing cells in the lacrimal gland (10)

Evaluation of serial sections of lacrimal glands from non-operated rats showed that significant variations existed in the frequency distribution of IgA-containing cells. Pronounced fluctuations were observed in the: 1) density of IgA-positive lymphocytes in different microscopic fields/section; and 2) number of IgA-containing cells in various sections/gland. Statistical analysis of this heterogenous distribution demonstrated that the topographical location of IgA-positive cells per section or through the gland was not random (p < 0.0001). This distribution of IgA-containing cells did not appear to be modified by surgical interference with neural innervation of the eye.

Influence of ocular nerves on tear IgA levels and the number of IgA-containing cells in the lacrimal gland (10)

To analyze the role of sympathetic innervation in the expression of the secretory immune system of the lacrimal gland, rats (n = 26) underwent unilateral superior cervical ganglionectomy (SCG) and sham-surgery (S) on the opposite side; all ganglionectomized rats had ptosis in the ipsilateral lid.

Interruption of the sympathetic nerve supply to lacrimal tissue for 2 weeks did not influence the level of tear IgA (S = 886 $\pm$ 177 ng IgA; SCG = 887 $\pm$ 151 ng IgA) or the density or total population (S = 3.13 $\pm$ 0.27 x 10^5 cells/gland; SCG = 3.07 $\pm$ 0.20 x 10^5 cells/gland) of IgA-containing cells in the lacrimal gland.

To assess the impact of the trigeminal nerve on lacrimal immunity, rats (n = 17) were subjected to trigeminal denervation (TD) on the left side and sham-surgery on the right. Analysis of tears collected 27 days after surgery demonstrated that nerve severance had no effect on the amount of IgA (S = 1015 $\pm$ 97 ng IgA; TD = 1021 $\pm$ 144 ng IgA). Similarly, neural disruption did not alter either the density or total quantity (S = 1.97 $\pm$ 0.25 x 10^5 cells/gland; TD = 1.51 $\pm$ 0.23 x 10^5 cells/gland) of lacrimal IgA-positive cells.

To determine the possible influence of the temporo-facial nerve division on IgA content in tears and the lacrimal gland, rats (n = 13) were subjected to unilateral tempero-facial denervation (TFD) and sham-surgery (S) on the contralateral side. Tears and lacrimal glands were obtained 4 weeks after surgical operations. Examination of tear IgA levels showed that nerve denervation had no apparent effect (S = 771 $\pm$ 160 ng; TFD = 761 $\pm$ 175 ng). In addition, neural sectioning did not modify either the density (S = 7.40 $\pm$ 0.71 cells/field; TFD = 7.46 $\pm$ 1.70 cells/field) or total number of IgA-containing cells in the lacrimal gland.

To test whether the optic nerve regulates IgA expression in tears or lacrimal tissue, rats (n = 9/treatment group) underwent one of the following surgical procedures: 1) optic nerve denervation on one eye, and sham-surgery on the other; 2) bilateral optic nerve denervation; and 3) bilateral sham-surgery. Results demonstrated that unilateral or bilateral optic nerve disruption or sham surgery exerted no significant impact on either tear IgA levels or the IgA-containing cell number in the lacrimal gland.

Similarly, apparent unilateral extirpation of the sphenopalatine ganglion (n = 15 rats; collections 29 days after surgery) had no influence on the population of IgA-containing cells in lacrimal tissue or the content of tear IgA, relative to levels in controls. However, surgical success of this experimental operation could not be later verified: lacrimal tissue displayed no reduction in the intensity or extent of acetylcholinesterase or vasoactive intestinal peptide staining, compared to that present in control glands. Thus, the effect of the sphenopalatine ganglion on immune expression in the lacrimal gland has yet to be clarified.

DISCUSSION

Our findings indicate that the heterogenous distribution of IgA-containing cells in lacrimal tissue has an apparent organization, because the topographical location of lymphocytes is not random. However, it seems that the sympathetic, trigeminal, tempero-facial or optic nerves do not modulate this cellular distribution. In addition, these neural processes do not appear to control IgA levels in the lacrimal gland or tears. In contrast, the parasympathetic and peptidergic nerves from the sphenopalatine ganglion do influence the secretory immune system of the eye: neuropeptides and transmitters from these neurons exert a significant impact on SC synthesis by acinar cells from the lacrimal gland (5,14). This neural action might result in dramatic alterations in IgA transport into tears. Although our current surgical procedures were insufficient to completely ablate the sphenopalatine ganglion and thereby evaluate its effect on tear and lacrimal gland IgA content, studies are underway in our laboratory to more fully explore the immunological role of this ganglion.

ACKNOWLEDGEMENTS

We wish to express our appreciation to Dr. Elcio H. Sato for his ocular examinations of rats with optic nerve denervations. This research was supported by NIH grants EY02882 and EY05612.

REFERENCES

1. Jancovik BD, Markovic BM, Spector NH (1987) Ann NY Acad Sci 496:1-756
2. Raine CS (1988) Ann NY Acad Sci 540:1-745
3. Stead RH, Bienenstock J, Stanisz AM (1987) Immunol Rev 100:333-359
4. Felten DL, Felten SY, Bellinger DL, Carlson SL, Ackerman KD, Madden KS, Olschowki JA, Livnat S (1987) Immunol Rev 100:225-260
5. Kelleher RS, Hann LE, Edwards JA, Sullivan DA (1989) Invest Ophthalmol Vis Sci Suppl 30:472
6. Franklin R, Malaty R, Amirpahani F, Beuerman R (1988) Invest Ophthalmol Vis Sci Suppl 29:66.
7. Greene EC (1963) Anatomy of the Rat. Hafner Pub Co, NY
8. Maestroni GJ, Conti A, Pierpaoli W (1987) N Y Acad Sci 496:67-77
9. Ferguson TA, Hayashi JD, Kaplan HJ (1988) FASEB J 14:3017-3021
10. Sullivan DA, Hann LE, Yee L, Soo C, Edwards JA, Allansmith MR (1990), submitted.
11. Sullivan DA, Allansmith MR (1984) Immunology 53:791-799
12. Sullivan DA, Colby EB, Hann LE, Allansmith MR, Wira CR (1986) Immunol Invest 15:311-318
13. Allansmith MR, Gudmundsson O, Hann L, Keys C, Bloch K, Sullivan DA (1987) Curr Eye Res 6:921-928
14. Kelleher RS, Hann LE, Edwards JA, Sullivan DA (1990) In Proceedings of the 5th International Symposium on the Immunology and Immunopathology of the Eye, in press

© 1990 Elsevier Science Publishers (Biomedical Division)
Ocular Immunology Today. M. Usui, S. Ohno and K. Aoki, editors.

SEVERE PROTEIN MALNUTRITION:
IMPACT ON TEAR IgA LEVELS DURING DEVELOPMENT AND AGING

DAVID A. SULLIVAN, CYNTHIA SOO AND MATHEA R. ALLANSMITH
Department of Ophthalmology, Harvard Medical School and
Immunology Unit, Eye Research Institute, 20 Staniford Street, Boston,
MA, USA   02114

INTRODUCTION

The integrity of the immune system is critically dependent upon optimal nutrition. Malnutrition generally reduces resistance of the host to bacterial, viral, fungal and parasitic infections and infectious disease exacerbates existing malnutrition (1). Consequently, given recent estimates that over 560 million people suffer from various nutritional deficiencies (2), it is not surprising that protein-calorie malnutrition is the most frequent form of acquired immunodeficiency worldwide (3).

Protein malnutrition significantly impairs both cell-mediated and humoral immunity (1,4). Thus, in malnourished animals and humans, lymphocytes exhibit decreased function, reduced lymphokine production, lessened response to antigenic challenge and diminished proliferative capacity (1,4). Moreover, the impact of protein deprivation on systemic immunity appears to be dramatically enhanced in immunologically-compromised individuals, such as very young children and the elderly (1,5,6). Yet, it remains to be determined whether malnutrition and aging synergize to suppress the secretory immune system, which protects mucosal surfaces against invasive and toxic organisms. Therefore, the objective of the present study was to examine the influence of severe protein malnutrition during development and aging on the expression of the ocular secretory immune system.

MATERIALS AND METHODS (7)

Age-matched male Sprague-Dawley rats (n = 9-14/ treatment group) at 21 days (weanling), 3.5 months (adult) and 16.5 months (senescent) of age were fed isocaloric diets ad libitum containing 3.2, 6, 10, 14, 19 or 24% (control) protein levels. Tears were collected immediately before, and 2, 4, 6 and 8 weeks after, initiation of the dietary regimen; the method of tear collection with calibrated microcapillary pipets followed reported procedures (8). At experimental termination, lacrimal glands, as well as saliva (by pilocarpine-induction), intestinal secretions (by saline lavage) and serum (by cardiac aspiration), were obtained as previously described (9). Mucosal samples were centrifuged at 10,000 x g and supernatants were stored at -20°C until experimental analysis. Lacrimal tissues were transferred to St. Marie's fixative (19 parts 100% ethanol: 1 part glacial acetic acid) at 4°C. After fixation, glands were dehydrated using ethanol and xylene, embedded in paraffin and cut into 5 μm sections. Sections were placed on gelatin-coated slides, then deparaffinized immediately prior to staining.

Techniques for the quantitation of rat IgA and secretory component (SC; primarily free form) by specific, double antibody radioimmunoassays have been published in detail (10,11). The protocol for the indirect immunofluorescent identification of IgA-containing cells in lacrimal gland sections has also been described (9). For numerical analysis of IgA-containing cells, 2-4 sections/tissue and approximately 30 microscopic fields (312.5 x magnification)/gland were examined with a Zeiss Photoscope II fluorescent microscope. To determine the total number of IgA-containing cells in lacrimal tissue, the cell density/field was multiplied by gland weight (mg) and by a correction factor, which compensated for such variables as lymphocyte size, microscopic field volume and gland density (12).

RESULTS (7)

To determine the impact of severe protein malnutrition during development and aging, weanling, adult and senescent rats (n = 9-11/ treatment group) were fed isocaloric diets ad libitum containing 3.2% or 24% (control) protein content. Our results demonstrated that protein deprivation for 8 weeks had no effect on IgA levels in tears, or on IgA-containing cell densities in lacrimal glands, of adult or aged rats, as compared to those of control animals. In contrast, the low 3.2% protein diet dramatically curtailed the development of mucosal immunity in eyes of weanling rats (Table 1). Following 2 weeks of exposure to the 3.2% protein diet, total tear IgA content in the young rats was 28-fold less than that measured in controls. By 8 weeks of protein malnutrition, tear IgA levels had undergone a precipitous decrease, such that IgA antibodies could not be detected in tears. This response was associated with a marked and significant decline in tear SC content, the number of IgA-containing cells in lacrimal tissue, as well as the levels of SC and/or IgA in saliva, intestinal secretions and serum.

To evaluate whether the impact of protein malnutrition on weanling animals was dose-dependent, 21 day old rats (n = 14/treatment group) were fed isocaloric diets containing 24%, 19%, 14%, 10%, 6% or 3.2% protein. After 4 weeks of this dietary regimen, total tear IgA levels (ng) equaled 834 $\pm$ 135 (24%), 1055 $\pm$ 175 (19%), 1032 $\pm$ 176 (14%), 249 $\pm$ 49 (10%), 141 $\pm$ 39 (6%) and 25 $\pm$ 11 (3.2%). Thus, the influence of protein deprivation was dose-dependent: maintenance of weanling rats on 3.2%, 6% or 10% protein diets considerably impaired the establishment of ocular mucosal immunity.

Table 1. Influence of severe protein malnutrition on tear IgA levels in weanling, adult and aged rats

| Group | Total Tear IgA (ng) | | | |
| | Control | | Protein Deficient | |
	Day 0	Week 4	Day 0	Week 4
Weanling	122 $\pm$ 48	1489 $\pm$ 275 [*]	132 $\pm$ 34	6 $\pm$ 6 [†]
Adult	1823 $\pm$ 370	1779 $\pm$ 355	1482 $\pm$ 327	1457 $\pm$ 195
Aged	1976 $\pm$ 425	1791 $\pm$ 378	1564 $\pm$ 322	2099 $\pm$ 546

Rats (n = 9-11/group) at 21 days (weanling), 3 months (adult) and 16.5 months (aged) of age were fed isocaloric diets containing either 3.2% (protein deficient) or 24% (control) protein. Tears were collected prior to (Day 0), and 4 weeks after (Week 4), the initiation of the diet. Numbers equal the mean $\pm$ SE. [*] Significantly (p < 0.0001) higher than Day 0 value; [†] Significantly (p < 0.005) less than Day 0 amount. Data from (7).

DISCUSSION

Our results demonstrated that severe protein malnutrition for 2 months during development, but not adulthood or senescence, exerts a tremendous impact on the expression of the secretory immune system of the eye. Protein deprivation almost completely suppressed the maturation of ocular mucosal immunity in weanling animals. Similarly, protein starvation also curtailed the development of intestinal and salivary immunity. These findings indicate that dietary nutrients play a major and determinant role in the imunological health and well being of the eye.

328

ACKNOWLEDGEMENTS
This research was supported by NIH Grant EY02882

REFERENCES
1. Scrimshaw NS, Taylor CE, Gordon JE (1968) WHO Monograph Series No. 57. WHO, Geneva
2. Chandra RK (1983) J Pediatric Gastroenterology Nutrition 2 (Suppl 1): S181
3. Watson RR, Safranski D (1981) CRC Handbook on Ageing 4:125
4. Watson RR, McMurray DN (1979) CRC Crit Rev Food Sci Nutr 12:113
5. Makinodan T, James SJ, Inamizu T, Chang MP (1984) Gerontology 30:279
6. Neumann CG, Lawlor GJ. Stiehm ER, Swendseid ME, Newton C, Herbert J, Ammann AJ (1975) Amer J Clin Nutr 28:89
7. Sullivan DA, Soo C, Allansmith MR (1990) submitted
8. Sullivan DA, Bloch KJ, Allansmith MR (1984) J Immunol 132:1130
9 Sullivan DA, Colby E, Hann LE, Allansmith MR, Wira CR (1986) Immunol Invest 15:311
10. Sullivan DA, Allansmith MR (1984) Immunology 53:791
11. Sullivan DA, Wira CR (1983) J Immunol 130:1330
12. Allansmith MR, Gudmundsson OG, Hann LE, Keys C, Bloch KJ, Sullivan DA (1987) 6:921

© 1990 Elsevier Science Publishers (Biomedical Division)
Ocular Immunology Today. M. Usui, S. Ohno and K. Aoki, editors.

CLINICAL TYPES OF GRAFT REJECTION IN PENETRATING KERATOPLASTY

U. PLEYER, E.G. WEIDLE, H.-J. THIEL
University Eye Hospital Tübingen, F. R. Germany

INTRODUCTION

Experimental studies (1) and clinical experience (2, 3, 4, 5) show that allograft rejection in penetrating keratoplasty occur to individual layers of the graft. The purpose of this work is to analyse incidence, clinical manifestations and relationship between various types of rejection and evaluate their prognostic significance.

PATIENTS AND METHODS

740 penetrating keratoplasties, followed up for at least one year, were assembled in two groups: favorable prognosis (Fig.1a) vs. poor prognosis (Fig.1b). The latter was evaluated in accord with the following criteria: vascularisation > 2/4 of circumference, previous inflammatory disease and/or previous graft rejection. Allograft rejection types are differentiated according to biomicroscopic appearances into:

a. Epithelial rejection   b. Subepithelial ˙infiltration (SEI)
c. Focal endothelial rejection   d. Progredient endothelial rejection

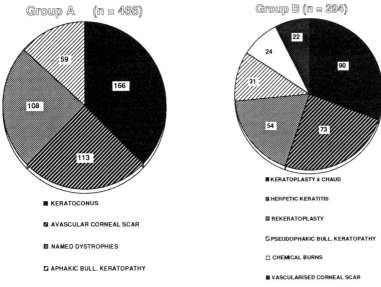

Fig. 1 a/b: Preoperative diagnoses of patients undergoing keratoplasty

Nonpreserved donor material was transplanted with attached donor epithelium in almost all cases. Trephine diameter ranged between 6.8 to 7.8 mm o in 86%. Administration of immunosuppressiva started with intravenous prednisolone(250/150/100/80mg/day), subconjunctival dexamethasone (2mg over 3 days) and topical dexamethasone (0.5% , q6h) in an overlapping regime and continued with flourmetholone 1% (group A) or dexamethasone (group B) gradually tapered during at least 9 months. In some cases, low dose topical steroids were applied for a longer period. Endothelial allograft rejection was treated with topical dexamethasone o.5% (6-8/d). Most cases of progredient endothelial rejection were also administered with oral steroids.

Data of preoperative findings and postoperative survey records were filed and evaluated on computerized printed forms. The data were analayzed using the Statistical Analysis System (SAS / IBM 4381). The chi-square test was used to compare rejection manifestation in both groups and Fisher`s Exact test to compare the relationships between various types of allograft rejections.

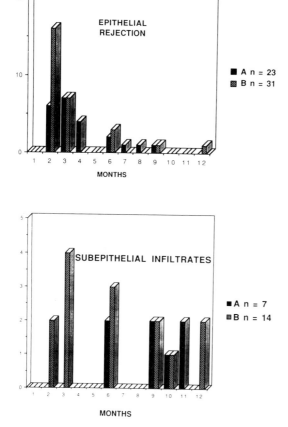

Fig. 2 a/b: Postoperative   interval   to   rejection   episode

RESULTS

The overall frequency of any kind of rejection was 281 (37.9%), occuring predominantly (74%) within the first 6 postoperative months
(Fig.2 a-d). The lower risk group differed significantly from patients
with unfavorable prognosis (p< o.o22). With regard to isolated rejection types marked differences are seen in focal endothelial
(p<o.oo1) and progredient endothelial rejections (p<o.oo1) whereas
epithelial (p<o.227) and subepithelial (p<o.99) types showed no
significant difference in both groups.

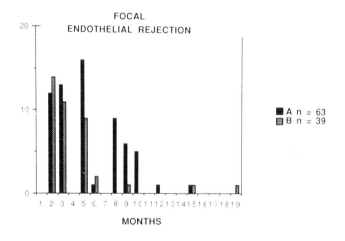

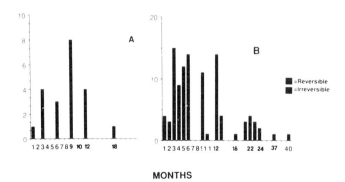

Fig. 2 c/d: Postoperative   interval   to   rejection   episode

332

There seems to be no distinct pattern of relationship between the various types of rejection in group A, whereas in group B focal endothelial manifestation often preceded progredient endothelial (p<o.oo1) allograft rejection as shown in Venn diagrams (Fig. 3 a/b).

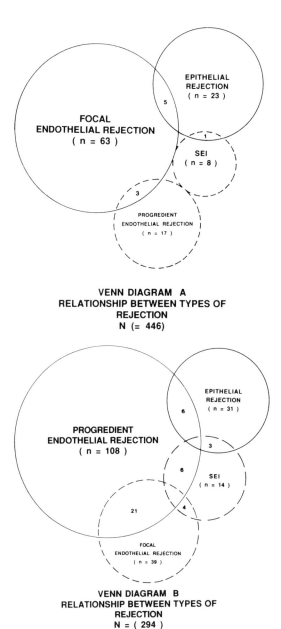

VENN DIAGRAM A
RELATIONSHIP BETWEEN TYPES OF
REJECTION
N (= 446)

VENN DIAGRAM B
RELATIONSHIP BETWEEN TYPES OF
REJECTION
N = (294)

Fig. 3 a/b: Relationship   between   types   of   allograft   rejections

COMMENT

Regarding the preoperative morphological condition, a significant correlation to allograft rejection was clearly noted.Not even in patients with unfavorable prognosis did we find a correlation between "minor allograft rejections" (a./b.) and progredient endothelial manifestations, thus proposing that despite the high expression of HLA class I (A,B,C) and class II (DR) antigens on cornea epithelial cells (6,7), this may not play a major role in triggering more severe rejection types. Since the donor epithelium has not particularly caused immunological disadvantages, its removal can be neglected. The importance of maintained epithelium on healing effects, especially in "risk patients" has to be emphasized.

The majority (74%) of the overall incidence of allograft rejections occurred within the first six postoperative months, yet late manifestations in group B suggest a close monitoring also in the late postoperative period and a prolonged immunosuppression for these patients.

ACKNOWLEDGEMENTS

The authors would like to thank Mrs. B. Pietsch-Breitfeld for statistical analysis and Mr. R. Siedner reviewing the manuscript.

References:

1. Khoudadoust AA, Silverstein A (1969) InvestOphthalmol Vis sci 8:180-195

2. Alldredge OC, Krachmer JH (1981) Arch Ophthalmol 99:599-604

3. Krachmer JH, Alldredge OC (1978) Arch Ophthalmol 96:2234-2237

4. Pleyer U, Weidle EG, et al (1990) Fortschr Ophthalmol 87:14-19

5. Severin M (1986) Klin Monatsbl Augenheilkd 188:200-208

6. Fujikawa LS, Colvin RB, et al (1982) Cornea 1:213-222

7. Pepose JS, Gardner KM, et al (1985) Ophthalmology 92:1480-1484

© 1990 Elsevier Science Publishers (Biomedical Division)
Ocular Immunology Today. M. Usui, S. Ohno and K. Aoki, editors.

IMMUNOREGULATORY PROTEIN(S) IN CILIARY EPITHELIUM AND IRIS EPITHELIUM

TAKASHI YOSHITOSHI and HITOSHI SHICHI

Kresge Eye Institute, Department of Ophthalmology, Wayne State University School of Medicine, Detroit, Michigan 48201, U.S.A.

INTRODUCTION

Histoincompatible grafts transplanted in the anterior chamber of the eye are not rejected (1,2). This phenomenon, called immunological privilege (3), was attributed to a lack of lymphatic drainage from the anterior chamber. Recent studies have shown that immune responses elicited by introduction of intraocular antigens include formation of suppressor T cells (4) and impairment of cell-mediated immunity (5). Although these immune responses indicate the involvement of extraocular immunological sites such as the spleen, the possibility cannot be excluded that some in situ immune regulatory mechanism may exist within the eye tissues surrounding the anterior chamber. As a possible immune regulatory factor, the presence of transforming growth factor beta was recently demonstrated in the aqueous humor (6). Transforming growth factor beta is known to inhibit the proliferation of various cells including T and B lymphocytes (7,8). Bovine vitreous extracts were found to contain a potent inhibitor of lipopolysaccharide-stimulated lymphocyte proliferation (9). The immunosuppressive protein in the vitreous may well originate from the anterior tissues such as the ciliary body and iris. In this work, therefore, we separated ciliary epithelial cells and iris epithelial cells from the porcine eye and investigated whether protein extracts from these cells contain factors which inhibit lymphocyte proliferation in vitro.

MATERIAL AND METHODS
Lymphocyte proliferation assay

Mixed lymphocytes were prepared from rat spleens as described (10). The cells (5×10^5/well) were stimulated by concanavalin A (1.03 µg/well, Pharmacia, Uppsala Sweden) for 48 hours at 37°C in 5% CO_2/95% air. After the addition of [^{3}H]-thymidine (0.5 µCi, NEN/DuPont, Hoffman

Estates, IL) to each well, the cells were cultured for an additional 17 hours, harvested, washed, and subjected to radioactivity measurement.

Separation of iris epithelial cells and ciliary epithelial cells from porcine eye

Porcine eyes were cut along the equator posterior to the lens to collect the anterior cup. After removal of a bulk of vitreous body, lens, and retina, the anterior half was cut in halves and incubated for 15 minutes in 0.02% EDTA in phosphate buffer-saline (PBS, 120 mM, pH 7.4, Sigma) to loosen the cellular contact between the pigmented epithelial (PE) cells and the nonpigmented epithelial (NPE) cells. NPE cells, together with remaining vitreous, were carefully detached from PE cells with a pair of tweezers. PE cells were then separated from the stroma by gentle suction into a pipette and collected as dispersed cells. The pigmented epithelial cells of the iris were collected similarly by gentle suction from the tissue which had been incubated in 0.02% EDTA for 15 minutes.

Extraction and purification of proteins with immunosuppressive activity

The cells were homogenized in PBS containing protease inhibitors [1 μg each per ml of leupeptin, aprotinin, pepstatin and soy bean trypsin inhibitor (Boeringer Mannheim, Indianapolis, IN)] and centrifuged at 12,000 x g for 15 minutes. The supernatant was collected, concentrated, filtered, and applied to a Sephacryl S300 column (1.6 x 32 cm, Pharmacia). The column was eluted with PBS. High performance liquid chromatography (HPLC) was performed with two TSK 3000 SW columns (7.5 x 300 mm, Beckman, San Ramon, CA). Protein was determined according to Smith et al (11).

RESULTS

Gel filtration chromatography of the buffer extract of ciliary PE cells resulted in separation of three major fractions, Fraction 1 containing protein larger than 150×10^3 daltons, Fractions 2 containing protein of 69×10^3 daltons (at the peak of fraction) and Fraction 3 containing 280-nm absorbing components with molecular weights of less than 10×10^3 daltons. As shown in Table I, both Fraction 1 and Fraction 2 contained factors which inhibited lymphoproliferation; Fraction 3 was without effect. HPLC of Fraction 2 separated a sub-fraction of protein with a molecular weight of about 14×10^3 daltons which possessed immunosuppressive activity (data not shown). Chromatography of iris extract on Sephacryl S-300 also separated a high molecular ($> 150 \times 10^3$ daltons) fraction (Fraction 1) which inhibited lymphoproliferation (Table I).

TABLE 1

inhibition of thymidine uptake by concanvalin A-stimulated lymphocytes

Preparation	Concentration (pg/cell)	cpm/well (mean+SD)	% inhibition
Control		13991 ± 689 (n=4)	0
Ciliary PE Fraction 1	6.5	8914 ± 269 (n=4)	36
Ciliary PE Fraction 2	13.6	8223 ± 711 (n=4)	41
Iris PE Fraction 1	7.0	10635 ± 1160 (n=4)	24

DISCUSSION

Immunosuppressive proteins have been extracted from avascular immunologically privileged tissues such as aorta (9,12), seminal plasma (13) and vitreous body (9). The aortic factor has a molecular weight less than 10×10^3 daltons and inhibits proliferation of both concanavalin A-stimulated and lipopolisaccharide-stimulated lymphocytes (9). An immunosuppressive factor in boar seminal plasma has a molecular weight of about 170×10^3 daltons (13). Similar factors found in human seminal plasma (14) and bull seminal plasma (15) have molecular weights of 200×10^3 and 100×10^3 daltons, respectively. The 170×10^3-dalton factor in boar seminal plasma seems to dissociate into smaller components with molecular weights of 30×10^3 and 10^4 daltons during gel-filtration chromatography on Sephacryl S-200. The vitreous factor passes through an Amicon membrane with a molecular weight cutoff of 100×10^3 daltons and treatment of the factor with dithiothreitol or trypsin does not significantly decrease the inhibitory activity of the factor (9). In this work similar factor(s) with immunosuppressive activity were isolated from porcine ciliary epithelial cells and iris epithelial cells. The molecular weight of the immunosuppressive factor in ciliary PE cells was estimated to be over 150×10^3 daltons by Sephacryl S-300 gel filtration. Ciliary PE cells also contained factor(s) with a molecular weight of 69×10^3 daltons. A factor with a molecular weight of about 14×10^3 daltons was separated from this fraction by HPLC. It is not known at the present whether the different molecular weights represent two different factors or the smaller factor is derived from the larger factor. Further studies are in progress to characterize molecular properties of the factor(s) in these epithelial cells and to elucidate their function in the regulation of immune responses in the anterior chamber of the eye.

338

ACKNOWLEDGEMENTS

This work was supported by US Public Health NIH grant EY03807. We thank Debra A. Jones for typing of the manuscript.

REFERENCES

1. Van Dooremaal JC (1873) Albrecht von Graefes Arch Ophthalmol 19:359

2. Zahn FW (1884) Virchow's Arch Pathol Anat Physiol 95:369

3. Barker CF, Billingham RE (1977) Adv Immunol 25:1

4. Wetzig RP, Foster CS, Greene MI (1982) J Immunol 128:1753

5. Streilein JW (1987) FASEB J 1:199

6. Streilein JW, Cousins S (1989) Recent Developments in the Immunopathology of Intraocular Inflammation, Amsterdam,Abstracts p. 63

7. Sporn MB, Roberts AB, Wakefield LM, deCrombrugghe B (1987) J Cell Biol 105:1039

8. Wahl SM, McCartney-Francis N, Mergenhagen SE (1989) Immunol Today 10:258

9. Koker P, Eisenstein R, Schumacher B, Christianson G, Grant D (1985) Curr Eye Res 4:807

10. Tanouchi Y, Shichi H (1988) Immunology 63:471

11. Smith PK, Krohn RI, Hermanson GT, Mallia AK, Gartner FH, Provenzano MD, Fujimoto EK, Goeke NM, Olson BJ, Klenk DC (1985) Anal Biochem 150:76

12. Rabinowitz SG, Eisenstein R, Huprikar J (1980) J Lab Clin Med 95:485

13. Cechova D, Veselsky L, Holan V, Stanek R (1989) Intl J Fertil 34:149

14. Lord EM, Sensabaugh GF, Stites DP (1977) J Immunol 118:1704

15. Prakash C, Coutinho A, Moller G (1976) Scand J Immunol 5:77

© 1990 Elsevier Science Publishers (Biomedical Division)
Ocular Immunology Today. M. Usui, S. Ohno and K. Aoki, editors.

PREVENTION OF EXPERIMENTAL AUTOIMMUNE UVEORETINITIS BY INTRAPERITONEAL INJECTION
OF ANTI-NEUTROPHIL MONOCLONAL ANTIBODY (RP-3)

M. USUI*, T. UTSUMI*, J. SAKAI*, M. TAKEUCH*, S. HIJIKATA*, F. SENDO**

*Department of Ophthalmology, Tokyo Medical College Hospital, Tokyo 160;
**Department of Parasitology, Yamagata University School of Medicine, Yamagata
990-23 (Japan)

INTRODUCTION

It is known that neutrophil infiltration of the uvea and retina is prominent in
the early stage of experimental autoimmune uveoretinitis (EAU) induced by high
doses of retinal S antigen, and neutrophils are thought to have an important role
in the development of the severe inflammatory response seen in EAU (1).

In this study, anti-neutrophil monoclonal antibody (RP-3) was administered to
Lewis rats sensitized by S antigen, and the mechanism of onset of EAU as well as
its prevention were investigated by histopathological and immunological methods.

MATERIAL AND METHODS

Preparation of RP-3

RP-3 was made by hybridization of mouse myeloma cells (P3-X63 Ag 8.653) and
spleen cells of BALB/c mice sensitized with pertoneal neutrophils of WKA/Hok rats
(2).

Animals

Rat EAU model. Lewis rats were sensitized by the injection of 50µg of bovine
retinal S antigen with Freund's complete adjuvant into both hind foot pats and
divided into three groups as follow; Group A: Five rats were given 2ml of RP-3
intraperitoneally 5 times every 24 hours from 10 days after S antigen inoculation.
Group B: Two rats were injected with 2ml of P3-X63 ascites without antineutrophil
antibody in the same manner as in group A. Group C: Three rats were not given any
injections into the peritoneal cavity.

Non-sensitized rats. Four normal Lewis rats were divided into two groups of 2
rats each, one group was given intraperitoneal injections of RP-3 (2ml X 5) and
the other group was left untreated.

Observation of EAU

Inflammatory changes were determined according to a 4-grade scoring system by
daily slit-lamp observation from 9 days after inoculation of S antigen. Rats of
groups B and C were sacrificed 19 days after inoculation and their eyes were
enucleated for histopathological observation. Group A rats underwent enucleation
on day 23 after inoculation except that one eye of one rat was enucleated on day
19.

Peripheral white cell count

The absolute counts and ratios of neutrophils and lymphocytes were determined by the examination of peripheral blood films.

Detection of humoral factors

Serum anti-S IgG antibody titers were determined by enzyme-linked immunosorbent assay (ELISA) (3).

Detection of cellular factors

The kinetics of the peripheral blood lymphocyte subsets were monitored by the indirect monoclonal antibody rosetting (IMAR) method (4).

RESULTS

Onset of EAU

EAU occured at 13.3±1.3 (mean±S.D) days after inoculation of S antigen in group B and at 13.0±0.6 days in group C. However, in rats inoculated with S antigen and treated with RP-3(group A), EAU was observed in one eye on day 19 and in one eye on day 23 i.e. only two eyes out of 10 developed EAU by 23 days after sensitization, Thus, the onset of EAU was delayed from 5 to 11 days compared with groups B and C.

Histopathological examination of groups B and C revealed severe cellular infiltration in the uvea and retina consisting of neutrophils, lymphocytes and monocytes. Subretinal exudate was seen in all eyes from these groups. In contrast, only slight infiltration by lymphocytes was observed in the two eyes of group A that developed EAU, and the others had no inflammatory changes in the uvea or retina.

TABLE I
ONSET OF EXPERIMENTAL UVEORETINITIS INDUCED BY S ANTIGEN

Days after inoculation		10	11	12	13	14	15	16	17	18	19	20	21	22	23
Group A RP3 injection		▼		▼	▼	▼	▼								
R1	R	−	−	−	−	−	−	−	−	−	+1	+1	+1	+1	+1en
	L	−	−	−	−	−	−	−	−	−	−	en			
R2	R	−	−	−	−	−	−	−	−	−	−		−	−	− en
	L	−	−	−	−	−	−	−	−	−	−		−	−	− en
R3	R	−	−	−	−	−	−	−	−	−	−		−	−	+1en
	L	−	−	−	−	−	−	−	−	−	−		−	−	−
R4	R	−	−	−	−	−	−	−	−	−	−		−	−	−
	L	−	−	−	−	−	−	−	−	−	−		−	−	−
R5	R	−	−	−	−	−	−	−	−	−	−		−	−	−
	L	−	−	−	−	−	−	−	−	−	−		−	−	−
Group B P3-X63 injection		▼		▼	▼	▼	▼								
R6	R	−	−	−	+1	+2	+3	+3	+3	+3	+3 en				
	L	−	−	−	+1	+2	+3	+3	+3	+3	+3 en				
R7	R	−	−	+1	+1	+1	+2	+3	+3	+3	+3 en				
	L	−	−	−	−	−	+1	+1	+2	+3	+3 en				
Group C R8	R	−	−	−	−	+2	+3	+3	+3	+3	+3 en				
	L	−	−	−	+1	+2	+3	+3	+3	+3	+3 en				
R9	R	−	−	−	+1	+2	+3	+3	+3	+3	+3 en				
	L	−	−	−	+1	+2	+3	+3	+3	+3	+3 en				
R10	R	−	−	−	+1	+2	+3	+3	+3	+3	+3 en				
	L	−	−	+1	+1	+2	+3	+3	+3	+3	+3 en				

R1~10: Lewis rat examined, en: enucliation
−~+3: severity of EAU,   − : no inflammatory changes
+1: a few cells in the anterior chamber and vitreous
+2: many cells in the anterior chamber and vitreous
+3: fibrin exudates, hypopyon, and synechiae

Neutrophil and lymphocyte counts

The peripheral blood neutrophil count of group A rats was decreased during the administration of RP-3, but increased again after RP-3 injections were ceased. Rats in groups B and C showed no corresponding decrease in the neutrophil count. A similar result to group A was seen in non-sensitized rats given RP-3 injections, while non-sensitized rats without RP-3 approximately followed the pattern of groups B and C. There were no marked differences in the total lymphocyte counts of the three groups at any time.

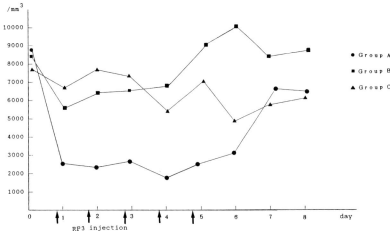

Fig. 1. Numbers of Neutrophils in 3 groups.

Anti-S antibody titer

Anti-S antibody was first defected in the peripheral blood of group A rats on the 9th day after S antigen inoculation and rapidly increased until the 15th, following which a plateau was seen. No marked difference was noted between the antibody titers in groups A and C.

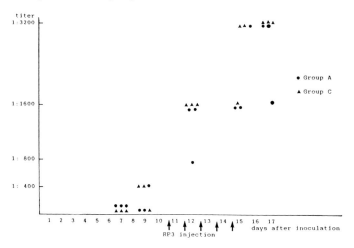

Fig. 2. S antigen antibody titer (ELISA).

Lymphocyte subsets

In 5 normal rats tested separately, the lymphocyte subsets in Lewis rats were as follows; (W3/25 : 51.4±7.1%, OX8 : 27.2±5.3%, and W3/25/OX8 : 1.94±0.39).

At 12 days after inoculation the OX8 positivity rate was higher in group A rats than of 8 days after inoculation or in normal rats. The W3/25/OX8 positivity ratio of group A rats on 12th day was significantly lower compared with group C rats on the same day. The percentage of W3/25 positive cells was not altered at any time after inoculation in groups A and C.

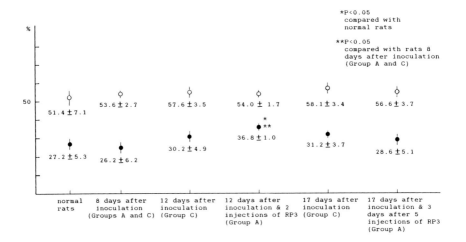

Fig. 3. Parcentage of W3/25(O) and OX8(●) positive peripheral blood lymphocytes

In particular, it did not change at 12 days after inoculation in group A, which was the time when the number of OX8 positive cells increased and the W3/25/OX8 ratio consequently decreased.

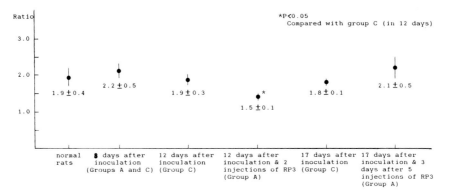

Fig. 4. W3/25/OX8 ratio

DISCUSSION

It is widely known that the principal histological feature of EAU produced by high-dose S antigen immunization in Lewis rats is abundant and temporary infiltration of neutrophils into the retinal lesion (5). However, there has been no definite agreement concerning the role of neutrophils in the immunopathogenesis of EAU.

We showed that the induction of EAU was influence by the selective depletion of neutrophils with the administration of RP-3 being able to completely inhibite EAU.

RP-3 can selectively deplete rat neutrophils without any influence on other white blood cells or anti-S antibody titer. Our findings suggest that neutrophils may not only take part in the retinal inflammatory response but may also have an important role in the induction of EAU.

The percentage of supresser T cells was significantly higher in S antigen treated rats which had undergone depletion of their peripheral blood neutrophils following RP-3 injection. This finding strongly suggested that neutrophils take an important part in the induction of EAU. At the same time, our data also suggests that neutrophils have a major influence on the immune regulation mechanism or lymphocyte recyclation. In this content, Staite report that activated neutrophils inhibited the function of suppresser T cells is also of interest (6).

CONCLUSION

The EAU induced in Lewis rats by S antigen was strongly inhibited by the administration of anti-neutrophil monoclonal antibody. It is therefore possible that the neutrophils infiltrating into the retinal lesions were not just reactive cells but many have taken an important role in the induction of EAU.

We hypothesized that one of the mechanisms concerned in the prevention of EAU might be the induction of suppresser T cells, on the basis of the depletion of neutrophils which we observed.

REFERENCES

1. de Kozak Y, Sakai J, Thillaye B, et al (1981) Curr Eye Res 1:327-337

2. Sekiya S, Gotoh S, Yamashita T, et al (1989) J Leukocyte Biol 46:96-102

3. Sakai J, Takano S, Takamura K, et al (1983) Folia Ophthalmol Jpn 34:1350-1356

4. Usui M, Takamura K, Shima Y et al (1989) In:Secchi AG, Fregona IA (eds) Modern Trends in Immunology and Immunopathology of the eye. Masson, Roma, pp 320-325

5. de Kozak Y, Sainte-laudy J, Benveniste J, et al (1981) Eur J Immunol 11:612-617

6. Staite ND, Messner RP, Zoschke DC (1987) J Immunol 139:2424-2430

© 1990 Elsevier Science Publishers (Biomedical Division)
Ocular Immunology Today. M. Usui, S. Ohno and K. Aoki, editors.

CHEMOTACTIC ACTIVITY OF THE PEROXIDIZED RETINAL LIPID MEMBRANE IN EXPERIMENTAL AUTOIMMUNE UVEITIS (EAU)

HIROSHI GOTO, GUEY-SHUANG WU, LILY R. ATALLA, NARSING A. RAO,

Doheny Eye Institute, 1355 San Pablo Street
Los Angeles, CA. 90033

INTRODUCTION

Inflammation is often regulated by mediators derived from either plasma protein or inflammatory cells. Mediators such as arachidonic acid metabolites and proteolytic enzymes have been implicated in acute and chronic inflammations, including uveitis. These mediators are believed to be associated with amplification and perpetuation of the inflammatory processes. However, it appears that these mediators are not the sole factor in the amplification of the inflammatory process in uveitis.

Recently, oxygen metabolites liberated from inflammatory cells have been shown to cause tissue damage via peroxidation of membrane lipids and to cause amplification of inflammation in various inflammatory conditions involving lung, kidney and uvea (1,2 3). The retinal photoreceptors are known to contain high concentrations of docosahexaenoic acid (22:6), a polyunsaturated fatty acid extremely susceptible to peroxidation.

In this study, we investigated the mechanism of perpetuation and amplification of inflammation by analyzing the chemotactic activity of peroxidized lipids extracted from retinal tissue.

MATERIALS AND METHODS

Induction of EAU

Lewis rats weighing approximately 175 g were given a hind foot-pad injection of 50 μg of bovine S-antigen (4) in complete Freund's adjuvant containing 0.2 mg heat killed Mycobacterium.

Preparation of lipids

Retinas of normal rats and EAU rats were dissected from the globes and membrane lipids were extracted using the method described by Folch et al.(5). An in vitro production of peroxidized retinal lipids was also carried out by isolating the lipids from normal control rats and incubating with a radical-generating system consisting of 200 μM of 2,2'-azobis(2-amidinopropane) hydrochloride (AAPH) dissolved in Hanks' balanced salt solution (HBSS). In addition, commercial methyl docosahexaenoate was used in pure and oxidized form.

Monitoring of lipid peroxidation

To confirm the presence of fatty acid hydroperoxides and hydroperoxide-derived hydroxy fatty acids in the inflamed retinal tissue, thin layer chromatography (TLC) was used. Total lipids extracted from the normal and inflamed retina were transesterified to obtain fatty acid methyl esters. Thin layer chromatography was carried out using precoated silica gel G plates and solvent system consisting of petroleum ether/diethyl ether/acetic acid (70:30:1). The extent of oxidation of authentic methyl docosahexaenoate was also monitored by TLC using the same solvent system.

Chemotaxis assay

Human polymorphonuclear leukocytes (PMNs) were isolated from heparinized peripheral blood utilizing dextran sedimentation and centrifugation of Ficoll-Hypaque gradients. Chemotactic responses were measured in a modified multiwell Boyden chamber. A portion of lipids to be used for chemotactic activity measurement was initially dissolved in 95% ethanol and solvent was then removed by evaporation under nitrogen. The residue was suspended in 200 μl of HBSS and this solution was placed in the lower compartment of the chamber. The suspension of PMNs (2×10^6/ml) in the same buffer containing 0.5% bovine serum albumin was added to the upper compartment. Two chamber wells were divided by a single nitrocellulose filter with a 5.0 μm pore diameter. The chamber was incubated at 37° C in 5% CO_2 for 60 minutes. Filters were removed, fixed in alcohol and stained with hematoxylin and eosin. The chamotactic activity was quantitated as the average number of cells per high power field (x400) migrating through the filter in four different places. All assays were carried out in triplicate.

RESULTS

Detection of Lipid Peroxidation

The formation of fatty acid hydroperoxides in inflamed retinas was monitored by TLC. The total crude lipids isolated from retinas and choroids without prior chemical reduction, were hydrolyzed to release fatty acid moieties and then the fatty acids were converted to methyl esters to facilitate TLC manipulation.

The peroxidized products isolated from inflamed retinas were compared with the autooxidized products obtained from the commercial methyl docosahexaenoate. The major products formed in both cases were fatty acid hydroperoxides that were seen as multiple spots with Rf values ranging from 0.30 to 0.37. These hydroperoxide spots were not recognizable in fatty acid preparation from normal retinas and in unoxidized docosahexaenoate.

Chemotactic activity

Boyden chamber assay revealed that lipids isolated from inflamed eyes (10 mg/ml) were significantly higher chemotactic activity than those from normal eyes under the same condition (p<0.01). Moreover, the same extent of increase was observed in chemotaxis when lipids from the normal eyes were treated with the radical generating system, AAPH. The assays using reduced concentrations of lipids (1 mg/ml) also gave similar extent of increases in chemotaxis. Using only the docosahexaenoic acid as lipid source, chemotactic activity of the air-oxidized fatty acid was found to be 3-fold higher than that of the unoxidized form (p<0.01).

DISCUSSION

As in other inflammatory process, the intraocular inflammation, such as uveitis, appears to proceed with two steps: induction and perpetuation or amplification. In the amplification phase of EAU, some chemotactic factors are produced and these serve to elicit PMNs and other inflammatory cells to the site of inflammation. In EAU induced by S-antigen, infiltration of PMNs and macrophages can be seen not only in the uvea but also in the retina. These phagocytes, once infiltrated, release inflammatory mediators including oxygen metabolites.

In inflammation, several biologically important peptides, protein and lipid molecules such as arachidonic acid metabolites have been implicated as chemotactic factors. In the present study, the total lipids isolated from retinas of EAU animals were found to have chemotactic activities for PMNs. The chemotactic properties in this case could be due to the peroxidized retinal lipids because the lipids isolated from control animals also showed chemotactic activity when they were exposed in vitro to an effective radical generating system, AAPH. This system is a well-known radical initiator; the spontaneous decomposition of this azo compound to a radical is followed raction with oxygen molecules rapidly to yield the peroxyl radical (6). In the outer segment of photoreceptors, the membrane phospholipids contain more than 50 mole percent of docosahexaenoic acid ($22:6_w3$) and only a small percentage of arachidonic acid (7). In our previous study, we have found that in EAU animals the reactive oxygen species released by PMNs oxidize the retinal polyunsaturated fatty acids (3). Lipids possessing chemotactic activity isolated from retinas of EAU animals possibly include a large proportion of oxidized 22:6, in particular during the initial phase of inflammation. The fact that the oxidized 22:6 is chemotactic was proven by the experiment where authentic 22:6 was oxidized and subjected to Boyden chamber assay.

Lipid peroxidation products are known to lead to cell edema and increased vascular permeability (8). We have found that the most abundant polyunsaturated fatty acid in photoreceptor membranes, 22:6, upon subjecting to PMN-mediated peroxidation could be chemotactic. This, undoubtedly, contributes to further elicitation of PMNs and thus amplifies the inflammtory process. In this study, the contribution from other chemotactic membrane lipids was not excluded, the studies are being conducted to refine the system, thus to evaluate the contribution from other chemotactic factors, in particular oxygenated arachidonic products.

ACKNOWLEDGEMENTS

Supported in part by NIH Grant Nos. EY06953 and EY05662.

REFERENCES

1. Halliwell B, Gutteridge JMC: Lipid peroxidation, a radical chain reaction, in Halliwell B, Gutteridge JMC (eds): Free Radicals in Biology and Medicine. Oxford, England, Clarendon Press, 1985, pp. 139-170.

2. Ward PA, Till GO, Hatherill JR, et al: Systemic complement activation, lung injury, and products on lipid peroxidation. J Clin Invest 1985;76: 517-527.

3. Rao NA, Fernandez MA, Cid LL, Romero JL, Sevanian A: Retinal lipid peroxidation in experimental uveitis. Arch Ophthalmol 1987;105:1712-1716.

4. Dorey C, Cozette J, Faure JP: A simple method for isolation of retinal S-antigen. Ophthalmic Res 1982;14:249-255.

5. Folch J, Less M, Soloane Stanley GH: A simple method for the isolation and purification of total lipids from animal tissues. J Biol Chem 1957;226: 497-509.

6. Terao K, Niki E: Damage to biological tissues induced by radical initiator 2,2'-azobis (2-amidinopropane) dihydrochloride and its inhibition by chain-breaking antioxidants. J Free Radicals Bio Med 1986;2:193-201.

7. Stone WL, Fransworth CC, Dratzs EA: A reinvestigation of the fatty acid content of bovine, rat and frog rod outer segments. Exp Eye Res 1979;28: 387-397.

8. Southorn PA, Powis G: Free radicals in medicine. Chemical nature and biological reactions. Mayo Clin Proc 1988;63:381-389.

© 1990 Elsevier Science Publishers (Biomedical Division)
Ocular Immunology Today. M. Usui, S. Ohno and K. Aoki, editors.

OCULAR INFLAMMATION AND PROSTAGLANDINS

MAHIPAL S.SACHDEV, S.P.GARG, L.K.VERMA, S.K.GUPTA, M.R.MEHTA
Dr. Rajendra Prasad Centre for Ophthalmic Sciences, AIIMS, New Delhi - 110029 , INDIA.

INTRODUCTION :

Prostaglandins have long been incriminated in various ocular inflammatory diseases. Prostaglandins are known to effect the iris tissue, ciliary body, intraocular pressure , retinal tissue , conjunctiva etc(1-3). Since, prostaglandins have been thought to be responsible for the manifestation of different diseases, their inhibitors have been used for treatment in clinical conditions.

We, herein, report 3 different clinical studies undertaken to evaluate the role of prostaglandins and their inhibitors,if any, in the probable causation and management of these. These conditions included different clinical types of uveitis, epidemic dropsy glaucoma , and maintenance of pupillary dilatation during extracapsular cataract surgery.

SUBJECTS AND METHODS :

In the first two clinical studies, aqueous was tapped under strict asepsis after obtaining a written informed consent. Care was taken not to have any contamination with blood. A 26 G hypodermic needle was introduced into the anterior chamber and 0.1-0.2 ml of aqueous was withdrawn without touching the iris. Aqueous from thirty cases of uveitis ; 10 each having active anterior uveitis, evidence of recurrent uveitis and 10 of healed uveitis with a history of the last attack being atleast 6 months ago was tapped. The diagnosis of uveitis was confirmed by biomicroscopic examination.

In addition, aqueous was withdrawn from 6 eyes each of cases of epidemic dropsy glaucoma and open angle glaucoma (OAG). These samples were collected at the time of trabeculectomy being performed for the control of their intraocular pressures. The diagnosis of epidemic dropsy glaucoma was confirmed by biochemical tests for the presence of *Sanguinarine* in the serum and urine of the cases, *Argemone* in the cooking oil and the typical clinical presentation of the cases (4,5). These samples were subjected to bioassays for detection of PGE_2 activity by the rat fundus strip method (6).

In the third study, 60 eyes suffering from senile cataract, without any other local or systemic findings were included. They were randomly divided into 3 equal groups of 20 eyes each. Pupillary dilatation was carried out in all using 2% homatropine hydrobromide and 10% phenylephrine hydrochloride drops. All cases received additional drops: thrice at 1 hourly intervals one night prior to surgery followed by the same regimen in the morning of the surgery. The last drop was instilled 15 minutes before the start of the surgery. These cases also received one tablet on the night of the surgery. Both the drops and the tablets were coded and the code was broken at the end of the study.

In Group I (Control), Methylcellulose drops and Multivitamin tablets were given. Group II patients received 1% Indomethacin drops and 25mg of Indomethacin tablet,while Group III cases got 0.03% Flurbiprofen drops and 50mg Flurbiprofen tablet. The pupillary diameters were measured using calipers at the following points during extracapsular cataract extraction : 1)at the start of surgery after retrobulbar; 2)after capsulotomy; 3) after completing the corneoscleral incision; 4) after delivering the nucleus; and 5) after aspiration of cortical lens matter (Table I).

RESULTS :

In comparison of controls from OAG cases elevated levels of PGE_2 activity was found in all the other groups except from healed uveitis group (Table II). This difference was found to be statistically significant (p <0.001).

Details of the pupillary diameters are given in Table I. The pupillary diameters were better maintained at all stages of surgery in both group II and III as compared to the control group i.e.,Group I (p < 0.001). A comparison between flurbiprofen and indomethacin groups revealed that flurbiprofen continued to maintain a better pupillary dilatation even after completion of the incision. This difference though suggestive of a trend was not found to be statistically significant.

TABLE I:
MEAN PUPILLARY DIAMETERS IN mms $\pm$ S.D. AT VARIOUS STAGES OF SURGERY IN DIFFERENT GROUPS.

STAGES :	1	2	3	4	5
GRP. I	8.0 + 0.4	7.2 + 0.5	6.4 + 0.4	5.6 + 0.7	4.6 + 0.8
GRP.II	8.2 + 0.4	7.7 + 0.4	7.3 + 0.6	7.0 + 0.7	6.6 + 0.7
GRP III	8.6 + 0.5	8.0 + 0.4	7.7 + 0.5	7.3 + 0.5	6.9 + 0.5

TABLE II :
MEAN PROSTAGLANDIN E_2 $\pm$ SD(ng/ml) LEVELS IN VARIOUS GROUPS.

CONTROLS OAG (n=6)	ACTIVE UVEITIS(n=10)	RECURRENT UVEITIS(n=10)	HEALED UVEITIS(n=10)	DROPSY Gl(n=6)
2.3 + 1.8	49.0 + 9.0	40.4 + 7.5	3.4 + 2.3	23.3 + 4.3

DISCUSSION :

Prostaglandins have been thought to be responsible for the mediation of various signs and symptoms of several ocular inflammatory diseases. Release of prostaglandins in patients of uveitis is thought to result in ciliary congestion, aqueous flare ,pupillay miosis etc (2). Our studies demonstrated elevated levels of PGE_2 in all the cases of active and recurrent anterior uveitis. In contrast, these levels were near controls in all the cases of healed uveitis. This difference was found to statistically significant ($p < 0.001$).These increased levels therefore suggest that prostaglandin release is an important factor in the manifestation of various signs and symptoms of uveitis.

Epidemic dropsy is an acute toxic disease characterised by an explosive onset of edema feet in a community using cooking oil contaminated with *Argemone mexicana* (4,5). *Sanguinarine* and *dihydrosanguinarine* have been shown to be the toxic etiologic alkaloids in *A.mexicana* oil (7). The study of glaucoma in epidemic dropsy is important because several authors have been able to produce raised IOP in animals with sanguinarine and its related alkaloids(8-11).

In the present study, aqueous bioassays were undertaken to study the role of prostaglandins ,if any, in the pathogenesis of dropsy glaucoma. The near absence of PGE_2 activity in control samples from OAG cases is comparable with previous reports (1). Increased activity of aqueous prostaglandin in epidemic dropsy glaucoma samples could explain the vascular dilatation of ciliary body and iris (12), increased protien levels in aqueous (4,12), and the significantly elevated IOP. In addition, various systemic features ,including cutaneous , gastrointestinal tract, and cardiovascular manifestations of epidemic dropsy can be attributed to prostaglandin release.

It is concluded from the present study that glaucoma in epidemic dropsy is likely to be hypersecretory in nature. This is because of the absence of any demonstrable outflow obstruction (4), the inefficacy of drugs that act primarily on the outflow, and the relative usefullness of drugs that act by decreasing the aqueous production (13). The demonstration of elevated prostaglandins in the aqueous suggest their role in the pathogenesis of dropsy glaucoma.

The study regards the efficacy of prostaglandin synthetase inhibitors in preventing pupillary miosis during surgery also suggests the role of prostaglandins. Both indomethacin and flurbiprofen were found to be useful in maintaining a better dilatation of the pupil as compared from controls ($p < 0.001$). Though, flurbiprofen was found to be better than indomethacin (Table I), this was not statistically significant in this sample size. This study, however, suggests the importance of prostaglandin synthetase inhibitors , even in darkly pigmented iris , during cataract surgery.

Our studies therefore afford sufficient evidence to suggest the role played by prostaglandin release in various ocular diseases. The role of prostaglandin synthetase inhibitors is also highlighted.

REFERENCES :

1. Wyllie AM,Wyllie JH:Prostaglandins and glaucoma.Br Med J 1971;3:615-617.

2. Eakins KE,Whitelocke RAF,Bennett A,et al:Prostaglandin like activity in ocular inflammation. Br Med J 1972 ; 4: 452-453.

3. Spaeth G: Use of YAG laser in performing peripheral iridectomies,in March WF (ed): Ophthalmic lasers:Current Clinical uses.Thorofare,NJ,SLACK Inc,1984,pp 57-58.

4. Sachdev MS,Sood NN,Verma LK,et al. Pathogenesis of epidemic dropsy glaucoma.Arch Ophthalmol 1988;106:1221-1223.

5. Sachdev MS,Sood NN, Sachdev HPS,et al.Optic disc vasculitis in epidemic dropsy.Jpn J Ophthal 1987;31:467-472.

6. Vane JR. The use of isolated organs for detecting active substances in the blood. Br J Pharmacol 1964;23:360-373.

7. Sarkar SN: Isolation from Argemone oil of dihydrosanguinarine and sanguinarine:Toxicity of sanguinarine.Nature 1948;162:265-266.

8. Hakim SAE: Sanguinarine and hypothalamic glaucoma.J All Ind Ophthal Soc 1962;10:83-102.

9. Leach EH: Ocular changes in monkeys fed with sanguinarine and other substances.Eye 1955;75:425-430.

10. Llyod JPF: Argemone oil and sanguinarine poisoning in monkeys.Eye 1955;75:431-433.

11. Lieb WA,Scherf HJ: Papaveraceae-Alkaloide und Augendruck. Klin Monatsbl Augenheilkd 1956;128:686-705.

12. Kirwan EOG: The aetiology of chronic primary glaucoma. Br J Ophthal 1936;20:321-331.

13. Sood NN,Sachdev MS,Verma LK, et al: Pressure dynamics and treatment modalities of epidemic dropsy glaucoma. Glaucoma 1990;12:20-27.

© 1990 Elsevier Science Publishers (Biomedical Division)
Ocular Immunology Today. M. Usui, S. Ohno and K. Aoki, editors.

353

ACUTE PHASE PROTEIN IN PATIENTS WITH ACUTE IDIOPATHIC ANTERIOR UVEITIS

KIRAN TANDON, D.K.SEN, M.D. MATHUR

Guru Nanak Eye Centre, Maulana Azad Medical College, New Delhi, India.

INTRODUCTION

Clinical and experimental data strongly implicate immune mechanisms in the etiology of Acute Idiopathic Anterior Uveitis (AIAU) (1-3). AIAU and its activity have been correlated with circulating immune complexes, complement components, cryoglobulins etc. (4-6). Acute phase response constitutes a part of body's systemic response to inflammation. It consists of increased production by liver of a number of proteins which participate in inflammatory process. Acute Phase Proteins (APP) are dramatic, sharp and reliable indicators of inflammation (7) especially inflammation that is extensive and has a strong immunological basis. Concurrent controls of traumatic uveitis, being of exogenous origin without any immune mechanisms involved, will be most helpful. This study was undertaken to elucidate the role of serum APP in the etiopathogenesis of AIAU.

MATERIAL AND METHODS

This study undertook investigation of selected APP in serum (Haptoglobin, transferrin, alpha-1-antitrypsin, c-reactive Protein, alpha-2-macroglobin, ceruloplasmin and factor B) in AIAU (28 patients), traumatic uveitis (21 patients) and healthy age/sex matched controls (21 nos). The diagnosis of AIAU was established by detailed clinical and laboratory evaluation. APP in serum were estimated by single radial immunodiffusion technique of Mancini et al (1965) (8).

The standard curve was obtained by plotting the concentrations of various APP (in mg/100 ml) of the reference standard on the horizontal scale and the square of the diffusion ring diameter on the vertical scale. The content of the specific APP in 100 ml of serum could be read directly from the standard curve. The results were analysed statistically by the Student's 't' test.

RESULTS

The ESR was increased in comparison with the level in healthy subjects (ESR more than 15 mm in the 1st hour in males and more than 20 mm in the 1st hour in females) in 10 patients with AIAU (35.7%). None of the patients with traumatic uveitis showed increased values.

Serum CRP was not detected in any of the healthy subjects or patients with traumatic uveitis. However, 10 out of 28 patients (35.7%) of AIAU showed significantly raised levels (p< 0.001) of CRP in serum. These patients showed raised values of ESR as well.

Table
Serum Acute Phase Protein Levels in Various Groups (mg/100 ml)

Acute Phase Protein	Control n = 21	AIAU n=28	Traumatic Uveitis n = 21
Alpha-1-antitrypsin	207.2±15.52	340.4±111.89	265.3±49.03
Alpha-2-macroglobulin	201.3±15.17	270.5± 43.47	261.4±46.05
Ceruloplasmin	21.3± 2.18	23.9± 2.25	24.5± 3.40
Factor B	12.4± 1.82	18.6± 5.26	16.0± 3.29
Haptoglobin	168.6±21.39	226.3± 43.67	204.4±33.48
Transferrin	261.7±38.89	240.9± 24.22	249.5±30.62
C-reactive protein	–	7.58± 0.48*	–

* C-reactive protein was detected in only 10 patients of acute idiopathic anterior uveitis (AIAU).

Serum alpha-1-antitrypsin in patients with AIAU was significantly high (p < .001). It was statistically significant (p < .001) in patients with traumatic uveitis as well. The difference in levels of two types of uveitis was also statistically significant (p <.001).

Serum alpha-2-macroglobulin level in patients with AIAU was raised significantly (p < .001). There was statistically significant (p < .001) rise in patients with traumatic uveitis as well. However, no significant difference (p > 0.2) between the two types of uveitis was found.

The raised levels of serum factor B were statistically significant (p< .001) in patients with acute idiopathic anterior uveitis. There was a statistically significant rise (p< .001) in sera of patients with traumatic uveitis as well. Furthermore the difference in levels of two types of uveitis was also statistically significant (p< .025).

Serum ceruloplasmin level in patients with AIAU was significantly raised (p < .001). It was significantly raised (p (p < .001) in patients with traumatic uveitis as well. The difference in levels of two types of uveitis however, was not statistically significant (p> 0.2).

Serum haptoglobin in patients with acute idiopathic anterior uveitis was significantly raised (p< .001). It was also significantly raised (p < .001) in patients with traumatic uveitis. Furthermore, the difference in two types of uveitis was also significant statistically (p < .05).

Serum transferrin in patients with AIAU showed significant fall (p< .01). However, no change was observed in cases of traumatic uveitis (p > 0.1).

CONCLUSIONS

To sum up, all acute phase proteins under study (exc ept transferrin), viz alpha-1-antitrypsin, alpha-2-macroglobulin ceruloplasmin, Factor B, haptoglobin, and CRP, were found to be altered in case of acute idiopathic anterior uveitis as well as traumatic uveitis. This can be explained on the basis of possible immunological role in acute idiopathic anterior uveitis. Furthermore, alpha-1-antitrypsin, factor B and haptoglobin can be considered to be more sensitive for acute idiopathic anterior uveitis as changes were highly significant statistically (p< .001) when compared with traumatic uveitis.

ACKNOWLEDGEMENT

We gratefully acknowledge the help of Mr. G.S.Sarin, Senior Scientific Officer, Guru Nanak Eye Centre for carrying out the Laboratory analysis of this study.

REFERENCES

1. Char, D.H., Stein, P., Masi, R. and Christensen,M (1979)
    Immune complexes in uveitis. Am.J.Ophthalmol. 87 :678-681.

2. O'Connor, G.R.(1983) Factors related to the initiation
    and recurrence of uveitis. Am.J.Ophthalmol. 96 : 577-590.

3. Vergani S., Mauro E.D., Devies I., Spinelli D., Vergani
    G. and Vergani D. (1986) Br.J.Ophthalmol. 70 : 60-63.

4. Sen, D.K., Sarin G.S., Pal, S., and Sharma, V.K.(1985)
    Serum immunoglobulin levels in endogenous uveitis; before
    and after therapy. Ind.J.Ophthalmol. 33 : 167.

5. Sen, D.K., Sarin G.S. and Mathur, M.D. (1986) Serum
    fibrin degradation products in acute idiopathic anterior
    uveitis. Acta Ophthalmol. 64 : 632.

6. Patanjali, F.P., Gupta, A.K., Sarin G.S. and Sharma, U.K.
    (1985) Afro Asian J.Ophthalmol. 4 : 39-41.

7. Pepys, M.B.(1979). In: A.S.Cohen (Ed) : The science
    and practice of clinical medicine : Rheumatology and
    immunology. Grune and Stratton, New York pg. 85.

8. Mancini, G., Carbonara, A.O. and Hermans, J.F.(1965)
    Immunological quantitation of antigens by single radial
    diffusion. Int.J.Immunochem. 2 : 235.

© 1990 Elsevier Science Publishers (Biomedical Division)
Ocular Immunology Today. M. Usui, S. Ohno and K. Aoki, editors.

CELLULAR IMMUNE RESPONSIVENESS OF JAPANESE UVEITIS PATIENTS TO RETINAL ANTIGENS
AND THEIR UVEITOGENIC PEPTIDES

J.H.YAMAMOTO[*],B.WIGGERT[**],G.J.CHADER[**],T.SHINOHARA[**],I.GERY[**],R.B.NUSSENBLATT[**],
M.MOCHIZUKI[*]
* Dept. of Ophthalmol.,Tokyo University Branch Hospital,Tokyo,Japan
** National Eye Institute,NIH,Bethesda,U.S.A.

INTRODUCTION

Autoimmunity has been suggested to play a major role in uveitis. This notion
is partly supported by the findings that retinal specific antigens, such as S-
antigen (1) and interphotoreceptor retinoid-binding protein(IRBP) (2,3) can
induce experimental autoimmune uveoretinitis(EAU), the clinical and histopathological changes of which resemble certain types of uveitis in human. Furthermore,
specific immune responses to these retinal antigens have been demonstrated in
patients with uveitis(4,5,6,7).

Recent advances in molecular biology made it possible to define the amino
acids sequence of the retinal specific antigens, to determine their pathogenic
sites and to synthetize the uveitogenic peptides of the antigens(8,9,10). As
for the retinal S-antigen, two synthetic peptides, M- and N-peptides, were
found to be uveitogenic in animals(8,9), while peptides R-4, R-9 and R-14 for
IRBP(10). Although the immune responses to the retinal specific antigens were
well studied in patients with uveitis(4,5,6,7), those to the uveitogenic peptides
of the retinal antigens have not been examined. Therefore,the present study was
aimed at analyzing the cellular immune responses to IRBP, S-antigen and their
uveitogenic peptides in patients with uveitis.

MATERIALS AND METHODS

Subjects: Seventy four patients with uveitis from the Branch and the Main Hospitals of Tokyo University were studied. The patients were diagnosed for Behcet's
disease(n=37), Vogt-Koyanagi-Harada's disease(VKH) (n=18) and sarcoidosis(n=19).
Their ages varied from 21 to 71 years; 49 were male and 25 female. Most of the
patients had clinical activity, except those with VKH who were convalescent
stage with sunset glow fundus. Clinical activity was defined when active retinitis, uveoretinitis, vasculitis were detected when examined. A group of healthy
controls consisted of 14 males and 10 females at a mean age of 43±20 years.

Lymphocyte proliferation assay: Mononuclear cells from heparinized peripheral
blood were separated by gradient centrifugation and cultured in RPMI-1640 with
HEPES(Gibco,Island,NY), supplemented with penicillin(100U/ml), streptomycin

(100μg/ml), glutamin(2mM) and heat inactivated human AB serum(10%) (Flow Laborat., Inc.,McLean,VA). Cultures were set up according to the procedure described by Hirose(4). All cultures were carried out in triplicate manner in 96 well micro-plate, with or without stimulants. Bovine S-antigen, M-peptide, N-peptide, bovine IRBP, R-4 and R-14 were tested at concentrations 4, 20 and 100μg/ml. The cultures were incubated for 5 or 7 days, at 37°C and 5% CO_2, pulsed for the last 16 hours with tritiated thymidine and the incorporated radioactivity was counted by a liquid scintillation counter. The results were expressed by stimulation index (S.I.=counts per minute in culture wells with antigen/counts per minute in culture wells without antigen). A significant response was considered to be the stimulation index for a given antigen that was above the mean for the respective control by two standard deviations.

RESULTS AND DISCUSSION

Table I shows the antigen specific lymphocyte proliferation in patients with uveitis, as well as in normal volunteers. Normal volunteers exhibited very low cellular response to all antigens tested. Patients with Behcet's disease exhibited high response to S-antigen, M-peptide and IRBP and the difference between the patients and the normal group was significant. On the other hand, patients with VKH or sarcoidosis showed similar levels of cellular response against the antigens to those in control group.

As for the responders to the retinal antigens, responders to S-antigen were found to be 61%, 40%, 57% and 0% in patients with Behcet's disease, VKH, sarcoi-dosis and normal volunteers, respectivaly. The difference in the number of responders between the three uveitis groups and the control group was statisti-cally significant ($p<0.05$). On the other hand, the responders to IRBP were found to be 38%, 8%, 7% and 5% in Behcet's disease, VKH, sarcoidosis and normal volunteers, and only the frequency in Behcet's disease was statistically significant in comparison to control ($p<0.05$).

Among the responders to S-antigen in Behcet's disease, all the patients were also responders to M-peptide but only 20% to N-peptide. In contrast, none of the non-responders to S-antigen were responders to M-peptide, but 20% of them were responders to N-peptide. Therefore, it is suggested that M-peptide seems to be an immunodominant site of S-antigen molecule at least in Behcet's disease. Such correlations were not found in VKH and sarcoidosis.

Among the patients examined in the study, there were five patients with Behcet's disease who responded to multiple antigens, i.e., S-antigen and IRBP and/or their peptides. Four of the five patients had active ocular inflammation when examined. The five patients also had recurrent episodes of uveitis for the last several years. Therefore, it is likely that patients with uveitis are sensi̱ tized to many retinal antigens. Furthermore, the cellular responses to retinal antigens seem to be related to disease activity. This notion was further supported by a finding of the present study that clinical activity in Behcet's disease was found in 91% of patients who responded to at least one of the tested antigens, but in 64% of patients who responded to none of the antigens, and the difference was statistically significant ($p < 0.05$).

The present study demonstrated significant cellular response to retinal specific antigens and their uveitogenic peptides in patients with uveitis. Also shown was the correlation between the disease activity in uveitis and the cellular response to the antigens. Similar findings were observed in a study by de Smet et al. in American patients with uveitis using the same assay methods as we used in the present study (personal communication). Therefore, cellular response to retinal specific antigens and their pathogenic peptides seems to be universal. However, it is difficult to define whether the cellular response to the retinal antigens plays a primary or a secondary role in the pathogenesis of uveitis. Although autoimmunity to retinal antigens may play the primary role in uveitis, a secondary role seems to be more probable, since cellular immune response to retinal antigens was found not only in inflammatory retinal disease as shown here, but also in non-inflammatory retinal diseases, such as retinitis pigmentosa (11,12). Even so, the autoimmunity to retinal antigens may participate in enhancing ocular inflammation or bringing about the chronic and recurrent course of uveitis. Sequence homology of virus, bacterial, fungus proteins to retinal antigens was found to induce immunological cross-reaction (13). Therefore, evaluation of cellular response to the proteins of pathogens having homology to retinal antigens remains for further investigation.

TABLE I

RESPONSES TO RETINAL ANTIGENS AND THEIR PEPTIDES

Clinical Entity	S-antigen (4µg/ml)	M-peptide[@] (100µg/ml)	N-peptide[@] (100µg/ml)	IRBP (20µg/ml)	R-4 (100µg/ml)	R-14 (100µg/ml)
Behcet's Disease	9.5±7.1[**]	6.5±7.9	1.7±2.1[**]	6.9±6.5[**]	4.1±5.0	2.0±3.0
VKH	3.2±2.3	2.5±2.2	1.7±1.1[*]	1.7±2.3	1.6	1.0±0.5
Sarcoidosis	3.9±2.7	3.0±2.9	2.5±4.6	2.2±1.5	2.1±1.2	1.1±0.7
Normal	1.8±0.9	2.0±1.5	0.8±0.3	1.5±1.4	1.6±1.3	0.9±0.5

Stimulation index(mean±SE), * $p < 0.05$, ** $p < 0.01$, @ 7 days culture.
All cultures were incubated for 5 days , except where indicated (see ref. 4 for details).

360

REFERENCES

1. Wacker WB,Donoso LA,Kalsow CM,Yankeelov JAJr,Organisciak DT(1977):Experimental Allergic Uveitis. Isolation, characterization and localization of a soluble uveitopathogenic antigen from bovine retina. J Immunol 6:1949

2. Gery I,Mochizuki M,Nussenblatt RB(1986):Retinal specific antigen and immuno-pathogenic processes they provoke. In Osborne N and Chader J(eds):Prog Retinal Res New York,Pergamon Press,pp 75-109

3. Chader GJ(1989):Interphotoreceptor retinoid-binding protein(IRBP): a model protein for molecular biological and clinically relevant studies.Invest Ophthalmol Vis Sci 30:7

4. Hirose S,Tanaka T,Nussenblatt RB,Palestine AG,Wiggert B,Redmond TM,Chader GJ, Gery I(1988):Lymphocyte responses to retinal-specific antigens in uveitis patients and healthy subjects.Curr Eye Res 7:393

5. Nussenblatt RB,Gery I,Ballintine EJ(1980):Cellular immune responsiveness of uveitis patients to retinal S-antigen.Am J Ophthalmol 89:173

6. Doekes G,van der Gaag R,Rothova A,van Kooyk Y,Broersma L,Zaal MJM,Dijkman G, Fortuin ME,Baarsma GS,Kijlstra A(1987):Humoral and cellular immune responsi-veness to human S-antigen in uveitis.Curr Eye Res 6:909

7. Nussenblatt RB,Mittal KK,Fuhrman S,Sharma SD,Palestine AG(1989):Lymphocyte proliferative responses of patients with ocular toxoplasmosis to parasite and retinal antigens.Am J Ophthalmol 107:632

8. Donoso LA,Merryman CF,Sery TW,Shinohara T,Dietzschold B,Smith A,Kalsow CM(1987): S-antigen:characterization of a pathogenic epitope which mediates experimental autoimmune uveitis and pinealitis in Lewis rats.Curr Eye Res 6:1151

9. Singh VK,Nussenblatt RB,Donoso LA,Yamaki K,Chan CC,Shinohara T(1988):Identifi-cation of a uveitopathogenic and lymphocyte proliferation site in bovine S-antigen.Cell Immunol 115:413

10.Sanui H,Redmond TM,Kotake S,Wiggert B,Hu L-H,Margalit H,Berzofsky JA,Chader GJ,Gery I(1989):Identification of an immunodominant and highly immunopatho-genic determinant in the retinal interphotoreceptor retinoid-binding protein (IRBP).J Exp Med 169:1947

11.Broekhuyse RM,van Herck M,Pinckers AJLG,Winkens HJ,van Vugt AHM,Ryckaert S, Deutman AF(1988):Immune responsiveness to retinal S-antigen and opsin in serpiginous choroiditis and other retinal diseases.Doc Ophthalmol 69:83

12.Chant SM,Heckenlively J,Meyers-Eliott RH(1985):Autoimmunity in hereditary retinal degeneration.I.Basic Studies.Br J Ophthalmol 69:19

13.Singh VK,Yamaki K,Donoso LA,Shinohara T(1989):Molecular mimicry.Yeast Histone H3-induced experimental autoimmune uveitis.J Immunol 142:1512

© 1990 Elsevier Science Publishers (Biomedical Division)
Ocular Immunology Today. M. Usui, S. Ohno and K. Aoki, editors.

IMMUNOCHEMICAL CHARACTERIZATION OF THREE NOVEL RETINA-SPECIFIC ANTIGENS IN HUMANS AND SOME MAMMALS

SERGEI SUCHKOV & ELENA TREBUKHINA

The Immunochemistry Laboratory, Helmholtz Eye Research Institute, 14/19 Sadovaya-Chernogryazskaya Street, P.O. Box 103064, Moscow (The USSR)

INTRODUCTION

The retina is a highly specialized sensory organ which participates in the visual process. Although the function of proteins established to mediate the process, is not yet clear, however, for instance, S-antigen and interphoto-receptor retinoid-binding protein (IRBP), highly uveitopathogenic retinal proteins have recently been shown to play an intimate role in the phototransduction of vision (1,2).

The second point needed to be mentioned is a significance of those particular retinal antigens, e.g. S-antigen or IRBP, which are not only intimately involved in the visual process but are also highly pathogenic for the induction of experimental autoimmune uveitis (EAU), a natural model of the inflammatory diseases of the eye (3-8). The antigens most commonly used for the induction of EAU are S-antigen and IRBP, major components of the retina. A summary of these studies indicates that both proteins are highly efficient for the induction of EAU in many different animal species and thus appear to be of great significance for basic, applied and clinical research (6,10,11).

In this preliminary study, we investigated human and some mammals' retinal antigens using a panel of conventional anti-retina immune sera raised in rabbits and then sequentially absorbed in a stepwise manner. The sera thus obtained were further tested for the presence of the anti-retina antibodies differing in their specificity. The results suggest that there are, at least, three sorts of antigens in the human and mammals' retina, revealing different immunochemical patterns:

(a) broad interorgan specificity antigens found in retina and other common body tissues;

(b) narrow interorgan specificity antigens occurred only in retina and nervous tissue;

(c) retina-specific antigens restricted to retina only.

MATERIALS AND METHODS

Reagents

Reagents used in this work were purchased from Sigma Chemical Co., Difco Laboratories, Pharmacia Fine Chemicals and Bio-Rad Instruments.

Body Tissues

Retinas. Human retinas were dissected from cadaver eyes and used immediately. For developmental studies, fetal human eyes of 8, 12, 18, 22, 25 and 30 weeks gestational age as well as neonatal and adult eyes were used. Bovine and other mammals' eyes were obtained from local sloughterhouses or from the nearest zoological gardens.

Common body tissues. Common body tissues were obtained from local abbatoires and transported to the laboratory on ice.

Preparation of The Body Tissue Soluble Antigens

Retinas were pooled and homogenized in 0.01M Tris-HCl buffer, pH 8.6 containing 1mM EDTA and 0.5% Triton X-100. After centrifugation for 30 min. at 30,000g, the supernatant was used immediately or stored frozen at -70°C.

Immunization Schedule and Preparation of The Anti-Retina Immune Sera

Grey rabbits were injected with the supernatant mixed with complete Freund's adjuvant and then given sequential booster injections once a week. The total protein was 80 μg. Rabbits were bled 1.5-2 weeks after the final challenge. The sera harvested were absorbed in a stepwise manner with a set of pooled donor serum, pooled tissue extracts, brain and, finally, retina extracts.

Anti-S and anti-IRBP sera were the gifts from Dr Igal Gery and Barbara Wiggert, Bethesda, USA.

Immunochemical Analysis

Ouchterlony immunodiffusion was performed as previously published (12). Grabar-Williams's immunoelectrophoresis was done as widely accepted (12). Gel electrophoresis and immunoblotting were performed according to the common procedure (13).

Immunocytochemistry

Immunofluorescent technique and sandwich method were applied as described earlier (12).

RESULTS

Immunochemistry of The Retina-Specific Antigens

Immunoelectrophoretic (IEP) assay. Anti-human-retina and anti-bovine retina immune sera pre-absorbed in the above-mentioned stepwise manner were used successfully in IEP assay to screen the sera and identify retina-specific antigens. The specificity of the sera is illustrated in the schematic IEP pattern presented in Figure 1. Along with broad and narrow specificity antigens, retina-specific antigens could be found in the human retina. The latter defined as organ-specific antigens were termed due to the IEP pattern as alpha$_1$-, beta- and rho-antigens. Neither of these antigens were detected in common body tissues nor in ocular tissues other than the retina.

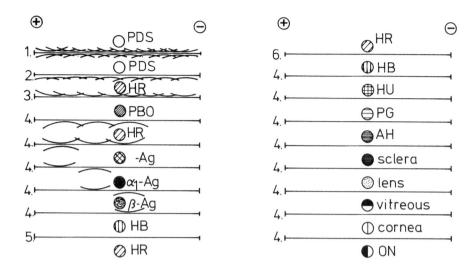

Fig. 1. IEP pattern of the human retinal antigens using a panel of the anti-human-retina immune sera pre-absorbed in a stepwise manner. Wells contain: PDS, pooled donor serum; HR, HU, PBO, HB and PG, human retina, uvea, pooled body organs, brain and pineal gland (total extracts), respectively; AH, aquous humor; alpha$_1$, beta and rho, fractions of the human retina-specific antigens prepared by preparative agarose gel electrophoresis of total retina extract. Longitudinal troughs contain: 1, anti-PDS serum; 2,3,4,5 and 6, anti-human-retina serum pre-absorbed in a stepwise manner with PDS, PDS and PBO, PDS and PBO and HB, PDS and PBO and HB and HR or PDS and PBO and HR, respectively. Running conditions otherwise identical: 0.075 mol/l veronal buffer, pH 8.6, 90 min., 5 V/cm.

Ouchterlony assay. Examples of the comparison Ouchterlony patterns are schematically illustrated in Figure 2.

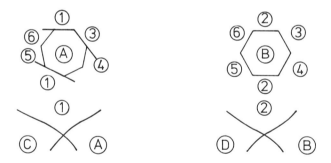

Fig. 2. Comparative immunoprecipitation patterns of the retina-specific antigens in a standard Ouchterlony plate assay.
Wells contain: A,B,C,D, anti-alpha$_1$, anti-rho, anti-S and anti-IRBP sera, respectively; 1-6, electrophoretically eluted human fractions of alpha$_1$- and rho-antigens, exctracts of human, bovine, porcine and horse retinas, respectively.

Partial identity between human and some mammals' alpha$_1$-antigens was observed. On the contrary, rho-antigen was defined as an interspecies one. No crossreactivity was found between $alpha_1$- and rho-antigens on the one hand and S-antigen and IRBP, on the other hand. Such a result has allowed for a conclusion that $alpha_1$- and rho-antigens are fully-confirmed retina-specific antigens other than the previously described (2,4-6).

Ontogeny. In the human fetal retina, $alpha_1$-antigen was observed first in the 22-week stage. Its appearance is coincided with the maturation of first "functional columns" with the completed structure in the retina. This antigen can thus be regarded as a marker for determination of the maturity of the retina.

Immunofluorescence (data not presented). Anti-human-$alpha_1$ and anti-human-rho sera reacted predominantly with the photoreceptor cell layer and outer synaptic layer, respectively. The same pattern was observed with bovine eyes. No other ocular tissues stained with neither anti-$alpha_1$ nor anti-rho sera.

Properties of The Human Retina-Specific Antigens

Several properties of the human retina-specific antigens are summarized in Table 1.

TABLE 1

COMPARISON OF PROPERTIES OF THE HUMAN RETINA-SPECIFIC ANTIGENS

Property	$Alpha_1$-Ag	Beta-Ag	Rho-Ag
Number of epitopes	2	not deter-mined	1
Molecular weight	220,000	135,000	40,000
Isoelectric point (pI)	5.7	not deter-mined	not deter-mined
Carbohydrate	no	no	no
Sialic acid	no	no	no
Lipid	no	no	no
DNA	no	no	no
RNA	no	no	no

The molecular weight determined by SDS-PAGE with known markers was 220,000 daltons for $alpha_1$-antigen, 135,000 - for beta-, and 40,000 - for rho-antigen. No carbohydrates, sialic acid, lipids, DNA or RNA were identified in neither of these antigens.

Immunochemistry of Broad and Narrow Interorgan Specificity Retinal Antigens

Along with the retina-specific $alpha_1$-, beta- and rho-antigens, several interorgan specificity antigens were found in human and bovine retinas (Fig. 1). There are two categories of such antigens in the retina, broad specificity antigens occurred in most of the body tissues and narrow specificity antigens restricted to retina and nervous tissue (brain predominantly) only. At least, 20 antigens of different specificities could be betected in human and mammals' retina using a panel of the anti-retina polyspecific and oligospecific sera. The retina as itself can thus be regarded as a very complex antigenic natural system containing broad and narrow interorgan specificity antigens as well as organ-specific antigens confined to the retina only.

DISCUSSION

We have investigated the antigenic structure of human and some mammals' retina using a panel of conventional anti-human-retina and anti-bovine-retina immune sera. As it was established, the retina is a very heterogeneous antigenic system which could be regarded as a natural model for study of the evolution of visual proteins (15). We have identified among retinal antigens three novel retina-specific antigens which are different from S-antigen and IRBP, and partly described their properties and distribution in various vertebrate retinas. It is of significance to isolate those antigens from retina and to identify in those antigens uveitopathogenic sites. There is also a need in future studies, to correlate the immunochemical and molecular properties of these highly attractive antigens with their ultrastructural locations in the retina and possible physiological niches.

ACKNOWLEDGEMENTS

We are thankful to Mrs Marina Tretyakh for her secretarial help and technical assistance. We thank Dr Barbara Wiggert and Dr Igal Gery, Bethesda, USA, for providing us with anti-S and anti-IRBP sera. This study was supported by the USSR Ministry of Health.

REFERENCES

1. Shinohara T, Donoso L, Tsuda M, Yamaki K, Singh V (1989) In: Osborne N, Chader J (eds) Progress in Retinal Research. Pergamon Press, Oxford, pp. 51-66

2. Chader G (1989) Invest Ophthalmol & Vis Sci 30: 7-22

3. Faure J (1980) Curr Eye Res 2: 215-221

4. Wiggert B, Lee L, Rodriguez M, Hess H, Redmond T, Chader G (1986) Invest Ophthalmol & Vis Sci 27: 1041-1049

5. Donoso L, Yamaki K, Merryman C, Shinohara T, Yue S, Sery T (1988) Curr Eye Res 7: 1077-1085

6. Donoso L, Merryman C, Sery T, Vrabec T, Arbizo V, Fong S (1988) Curr Eye Res 7: 1087-1095

7. Saari J, Bunt-Milam A, Bredberg D, Garwin J (1984) Vision Res 24: 1595-1603

8. Hirose S, Kuwabara T, Nussenblatt R, Wiggert B, Redmond T, Gery I (1986) Arch Ophthalmol 104: 1698-1702

9. Donoso L, Merryman S, Sery T, Sanders R, Vrabec T, Fong S (1989) J Immunol 143: 79-83

10. Singh V, Yamaki K, Donoso L, Shinohara T (1988) Curr Eye Res 7: 87-92

11. Saari J, Teller D, Crabb J, Bredberg D (1985) J Biol Chem 260: 195-201

12. Suchkov S (1989) In: Petrov R, Khaitov R (eds) Proceedings of The First All-Union Immunological Congress. Meditsina (in Russian), Moscow, p. 124

13. Pfeffer B, Wiggert B, Lee L, Zonnenberg B, Newsome D, Chader G (1983) J Cell Physiol 117: 333-341

14. Lowry O, Rosebrough H, Farr A, Randall R (1951) J Biol Chem 193: 265-275

15. McKechnie N, Alexander R, Sura G, Grierson I (1988) Acta Ophthalmol 66: 514-521

© 1990 Elsevier Science Publishers (Biomedical Division)
Ocular Immunology Today. M. Usui, S. Ohno and K. Aoki, editors.

CHARACTERIZATION OF T CELL SUBSETS IN PATIENTS WITH UVEITIS

SATOSHI MIKI, YOSHIHITO TANOUCHI, TOMOKO OTANI, KEIKO YAMAGUCHI
and YASUO MIMURA

Dept. of Ophthalmology, Tokushima University School of Medicine
3-18-15 Kuramoto-cho Tokushima 770 Japan

INTRODUCTION

The distribution of lymphocyte subsets and their functions have
been investigated in uveitis using single-color flow cytometry.
However, pathophysiology of uveitis is still unclear.

By two-color flow cytometry techniques, T lymphocyte subsets can
be distinguished more clearly. These techniques were used in the
present study to assess T lymphocyte subsets in uveitis.

SUBJECTS AND METHODS

Subjects

Twenty four patients had Behcet's disease with ocular symptoms,
fourteen had Vogt-Koyanagi-Harada disease (VKH disease) and six
had Sarcoidosis. A group of thirty healthy volunteers served as
the controls.

Methods

Peripheral blood samples were obtained from all patients and
controls, and cerebrospinal fluid samples from newly diagnosed six
patients with VKH disease were obtained. Lymphocytes were stained
by fluorescein isothiocyanate (FITC) labelled anti Leu2a (CD8),
Leu8, Leu7 and Leu4 (CD3) antibody and phycoerythrin (PE) labelled
anti Leu15 (CD11), Leu3a (CD4), Leu11 (CD16) and HLA-DR antibody.

Two-color analysis by fluorescein activated cell sorter (FACS)
was conducted.

Data analysis were conducted by the Student's t-test.

RESULTS

The percentages of $CD4^+Leu8^-$ cells (helper T cells) significantly
decreased in the peripheral blood of patients with VKH disease
($p<0.05$) compared with normal controls. Those of $CD8^+CD11^+$ cells
(suppressor T cells) significantly increased in the peripheral blood
of patients with Behcet's disease ($p<0.05$) and Sarcoidosis ($p<0.01$)
compared with the normal controls. $CD4^+Leu8^-/CD8^+CD11^+$ (herper
T cells/suppressor T cells) significantly diminished in the

peripheral blood of patients with Behcet's disease (p<0.05) and Sarcoidosis (p<0.01) compared with the normal controls due to increased $CD8^+CD11^+$ cells (TABLE 1).

The percentages of $CD4^+Leu8^-$ cells (suppression inducer T cells) significantly increased in the peripheral blood of patients with VKH disease (p<0.01) compared with the normal controls. A significant (p<0.05) decrease in the activity of Natural Killer (NK) cells was noted in the peripheral blood of patients with Behcet's disease compated with the normal controls. The percentages of $CD8^-CD11^+$ cells and $CD3^+HLA-DR^+$ cells were essentially the same in uveitis patients and the controls (TABLE 2).

TABLE 1
Two-color flow cytometric analysis in patients with uveitis (No.1)

	$CD4^+Leu8^-$(%)	$CD8^+CD11^+$(%)	$CD4^+Leu8^-/CD8^+CD11^+$
Behcet's Disease	19.0±6.8	7.2±3.7#	3.2±1.7$
VKH Disease	18.0±5.4*	6.0±3.7	4.1±2.8
Sarcoidosis	17.7±5.0	9.0±4.1##	2.3±2.0$$
Unclassified Uveitis	18.5±5.6**	7.5±3.8###	3.9±4.9
Controls	22.1±5.9*,**	5.1±2.6#,##,###	5.4±2.8$,$$

*,**,#,$:p<0.05   ##,###,$$:p<0.01   (mean±SD)

TABLE 2
Two-color flow cytometric analysis in patients with uveitis (No.2)

	$CD4^+Leu8^+$(%)	$CD8^+CD11^-$(%)	NK activity(%)	$CD3^+HLA-DR^+$(%)
Behcet's Disease	15.7±5.4	20.3±5.8	33.4±11.0#	5.7±5.1
VKH Disease	24.2±8.7*	22.5±6.7	38.0±17.2	5.6±4.1
Sarcoidosis	15.8±4.3	18.8±5.0	38.2±12.5	9.2±7.2
Unclassified Uveitis	19.5±7.0**	17.9±7.5	39.4±13.6	6.8±4.5
Controls	14.9±5.6*,**	21.2±6.0	40.6±10.4#	6.6±2.9

*,**:P<0.01   #:P<0.05   (mean±SD)

This comparison was made for the attack and remission stages in the peripheral blood of patients with Behcet's disease and no statistically significant differences could be found (TABLE 3).

TABLE 3

Two-color flow cytometric analysis in patients
with Behcet's disease

	Attack(n=9)	Remission(n=14)
CD4⁺Leu8⁻	18.4 ± 7.4(%)	19.3 ± 6.7(%)
CD8⁺CD11⁺	7.8 ± 3.4(%)	6.7 ± 3.9(%)
CD4⁺Leu8⁺	16.2 ± 6.6(%)	15.4 ± 4.6(%)
CD8⁺CD11⁻	20.5 ± 7.8(%)	20.2 ± 4.4(%)
CD4⁺Leu8⁻/CD8⁺CD11⁺	2.6 ± 1.4	3.6 ± 1.9
NK activity	31.2 ± 6.4(%)	34.9 ± 13.2(%)
CD3⁺HLA-DR⁺	6.4 ± 7.0(%)	5.2 ± 3.6(%)

(mean±SD)

TABLE 4

Two-color flow cytometric analysis in newly diagnosed patients
with VKH disease

	Peripheral blood(n=6)	cerebrospinal fluid(n=6)
CD4⁺Leu8⁻	14.6 ± 2.9*(%)	30.3 ± 12.9*(%)
CD8⁺CD11⁺	6.3 ± 4.4(%)	4.1 ± 2.1(%)
CD4⁺Leu8⁺	25.2 ± 5.5(%)	30.6 ± 18.0(%)
CD8⁺CD11⁻	23.4 ± 7.6(%)	23.0 ± 6.9(%)
CD4⁺Leu8⁻/CD8⁺CD11⁺	3.2 ± 1.9	9.6 ± 6.1
CD3⁺HLA-DR⁺	6.0 ± 5.5(%)	8.8 ± 6.8(%)
T cell	72.1 ± 4.5**(%)	86.2 ± 6.5**(%)
B cell	9.4 ± 6.4(%)	2.3 ± 1.3(%)

*:P<0.05   **:p<0.01   (mean±SD)

A comparison was subsequently made of T-lymphocyte subsets in
the cerebrospinal fluid with those in the peripheral blood of newly
diagnosed six patients with VKH disease. The percentages of CD4⁺
Leu8⁻ cells in the cerebrospinal fluid significantly exceeded those
in the peripheral blood of patients with VKH disease (TABLE 4).

DISCUSSION

Previous reports by our laboratory indicated diminished percentages
of CD4⁺ cells and increased percentages of CD8⁺ cells in the
peripheral blood of patients with Behcet's disease. Increased
percentages of OKIal⁺ cells was noted more frequently in the

peripheral blood of patients with Behcet's disease and VKH disease than in the normal controls as measured by single-color FACS analysis[1]. Two-color flow cytometric analysis was performed in the present study to more clearly determine the distribution of T lymphocyte subsets in patients with uveitis.

Due to variation in the percentages of circulating T lymphocytes in a normal population, an effective means for achieving this purpose is to express findings the ratio of helper T cells to suppressor T cells. No comparison could be made of the true helper T-suppressor T ratio in single-color FACS analysis, but it was possible by two-color flow cytometric analysis[2]. Patients with Behcet's disease and Sarcoidosis diminished $CD4^+Leu8^-CD11^+$ were compared with the normal controls.

Arimori[3] and Kogure[4] reported low activity of NK cells in the peripheral blood of patients with Behcet's disease, as we also did.

There were no significant differences in the peripheral blood of patients with Behcet's disease with respect to attack and remission stages. However, some previous reports indicate high activity of NK cells at the attack stage[5], while others maintain low activity[3,4]. The dynamics of T lymphocytes in patients with Behcet's disease should be elucidated.

The percentages of $CD4^+Leu8^-$ cells in the cerebrospinal fluid exceeded those in the peripheral blood of patients with VKH disease. It would thus appear that local immunoreaction in the first stage of VKH disease is associated with helper T cells[6].

In conclusion, two-color flow cytometric analysis should prove helpful for elucidating the underlying cellular dynamics in uveitis patients.

REFERENCE

1. Mimura Y (1984) Annual Report of Behcet's Disease Research Committee of Japan 206-208
2. Kudo H, Nakano K (1985) Clinical Pathology 12: 1367-1375
3. Arimori S (1983) Annual Report of Behcet's Disease Research Committee of Japan 177-181
4. Kogure M (1987) Annual Report of Behcet's Disease Research Committee of Japan 64-67
5. Mimura Y (1982) Annual Report of Behcet's Disease Research Committee of Japan 224-226
6. Ariga H, Ono S, et al (1988) Acta Soc Ophthalmol Jpn 92: 225-228

© 1990 Elsevier Science Publishers (Biomedical Division)
Ocular Immunology Today. M. Usui, S. Ohno and K. Aoki, editors.

IMMUNOHISTOCHEMICAL ANALYSIS OF VOGT-KOYANAGI-HARADA DISEASE AT THE CLINICALLY CONVALESCENT STAGE

TAIJI SAKAMOTO* ** HAJIME INOMATA*   KATSUO SUEISHI**

Department of Ophthalmology* and Pathology**, Faculty of Medicine, Kyushu University 60, 3-1-1 Maidashi Higashi-ku, Fukuoka 812, Japan

ABSTRACT

The eyes from two autopsy cases of Vogt-Koyanagi-Harada disease (VKH) with sunset sky fundus, the sign of clinically convalescent stage of VKH, were examined by immunohistochemical technique. The first case died at 32 months after the onset and the other at 7 years. Histopathological examination showed lymphocytic infiltrate in the thickened choroid with remarkable disappearance of melanocytes.   Immunohistochemical examination demonstrated both T and B cells including activated ones in the choroid and HLA-DR antigen in the melanocytes. The results indicate that the inflammation of VKH is still active even at the clinically convalescent stage and choroidal melanocytes play some roles in the pathogenesis of VKH.

INTRODUCTION

Vogt-Koyanagi-Harada disease (VKH) is bilateral uveitis of unknown etiology associating extraocular manifestations (cerebrospinal fluid (CSF) pleocytosis, pilosis, alopecia, dysacousia and vitiligo)(1-4). The histopathology of VKH is the granulomatous inflammation throughout the uveal tract. And inflammation tends to subside according as the disappearance of melanocytes showing sunset sky fundus. There are only a few histopathological reports of VKH (4,5), and immunohistochemical report is even limited(6). The aim of this study is to examine whether or not the inflammation of VKH is active at the clinically convalescent stage with sunset sky fundus using immunohistochemical technique.

MATERIAL AND METHODS

Case reports

Case 1 was a 63 year-old Japanese woman with VKH for 32 months

until her death. At the onset of the disease in June 1984, she complained of bilateral visual disturbance. Slit lamp examination revealed cells in the anterior chamber. Ophthalmoscopic examination
found exudative retinal detachment in both eyes. Cells in CSF
numbered 60/mm^3, mostly lymphocytes. She was treated with corticosteroid hormone. After 5 months, the inflammation subsided with
typical sunset sky fundus, but vitiligo and pilosis became manifest.
In February 1987, she died of uterine cancer.

Case 2 was a 68 year-old Japanese man with VKH for 7 years after
the onset. In 1975, he suddenly noticed severe headach and visual
disturbance, and was diagnosed as VKH, and thus treated with
corticosteroid hormone. In August 1982, a typical sunset sky fundus
was observed in both eyes. In December 1982, he died of pulmonary
fibrosis.

Histopathological and immunohistochemical methods

The enucleated eyes, obtained at autopsy, were immediately fixed
in the 6% formaldehyde and embedded in paraffin. The section was
stained with hematoxylin and eosin. The ocular tissue from case 1
was snap frozen and embedded in OCT compound.

Immunohistochemical examination was performed with avidin-biotin-
peroxidase method or alkaline phosphatase anti-alkaline phosphatase
method. The primary antibodies were monoclonal antibodies prepared
against T lymphocytes(UCHL-1, DAKOPATTS), B lymphocytes(MX-Pan B,
KYOWA), HLA-DR (DAKOPATTS), T helper/inducer lymphocytes(CD 4, Beckton Dickinson), T supressor/cytotoxic lymphocytes (CD 8, Beckton
Dickinson), IL-2 receptor (CD25, Immunotech), activated T lymphocytes (CD26, Immunotech) and interferon gamma (Chemicon).

RESULTS

Case 1: The choroid was thickened with lymphocytic infiltration
and the melanocytes remarkably disappeared. No granulomatous inflammation was observed. The retinal pigment epithelium (RPE) was
focally degenerative. Dalen-Fuchs nodules were present in the RPE
(Fig. 1a). Both T and B lymphocytes were present. CD4+ cells were
more numerous than CD8+ cells. CD25+ cells and CD26+ cells were
also noted in the choroid (Fig. 1b). HLA-DR antigen was demonstrated
in the endothelium of choriocapillaris. But interferon gamma was
not apparently exposed.

Case 2: The histopathological features were almost the same as those of case 1. But inflammatory infiltrate was more prominent. There were also T and B lymphocytes in the thickened choroid (Fig. 1c). HLA-DR antigen was present on some infiltrating cells and in some degenerating melanocytes (Fig. 1d).

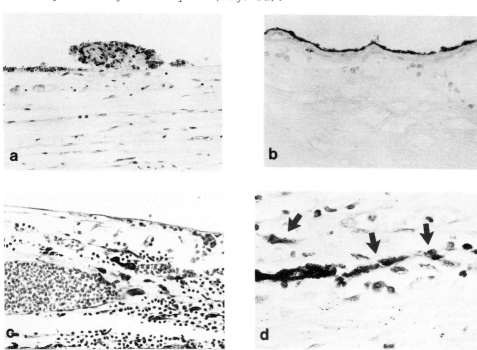

Fig. 1a. Dalen-Fuchs nodule(Case 1). Hematoxylin and eosin (X300).
Fig. 1b. Immunohistochemical staining of anti activated T cell anti-
         body IgG (Avidin-biotin-peroxidase method) (X400)
Fig. 1c. Lymphocytic infiltrate in the choroid(Case 2). Most of the
         melanocytes disappeared. Hematoxylin and eosin (X320)
Fig. 1d. Immunohistochemical staining of anti-HLA-DR antigen anti-
         body (Alkaline phosphatase anti-alkaline phosphatase
         method). Some degenerating melanocytes show positive
         reaction (arrow). (X400)

DISCUSSION

The cases presented herein were clearly diagnosed as VKH from their ocular and extraocular manifestations. Histopathological examination showed lymphocytic infiltrate throughout the uvea without granulomatous inflammation but with remarkable loss of melanocytes. In sympathetic ophthalmia, choroidal melanocytes were destructed and finally disappeared from the choroid (7). Similar mechanism possibly ocurred in our cases so that most of the melanocytes disappeared from the choroid.

In the present cases, the inflammation subsided clinically showing sunset sky fundus. Immunohistochemical studies using monoclonal antibodies demonstrated B and T cells were still present including activated T cell (CD26+) and IL-2 receptor presenting cell (CD25+). Our results indicate that the inflammation is still active even at the clinically convalescent stage. In addition to that findings, HLA-DR antigen, which was not present in the normal melanocytes, was detected in choroidal melanocytes of VKH. The class II major histo-compatibility antigens encoded by genes in the HLA-D region play a key role in the presentation of antigens. And aberrant expression of HLA-DR antigen was present in some autoimmune diseases (8). Our results, therefore, suggest that melanocytes played an important role in the inflammation of VKH, which is possibly induced by auto-immune mechanism (9).

REFERENCES

1. Vogt A (1906) Früzeitings Ergrauen der Zilien und Bemerkungen uber den sogenannten plötzlichen Eintritt dieser Veränderung, Klin Monatsbl augenheilk, 44, 228-242

2. Koyanagi Y (1929) Dysakusis, alopecia und Pilosis bei schwerer Uveitis nicht traumatischen Ursprungs,· Klin Monatsbl Augenheilk, 82, 194-211

3. Harada E (1926) On the acute diffuse choroiditis, Acta Soc Ophthalmol Jpn, 30, 356-378

4. Inomata H, Kato M (1989) In: Vinken P, Bruyn GW, Klawans HL(eds) Handbook of Clinical Neurology, Elsevier, Amsterdam, pp611-626

5. Perry HD, Font RL (1977) Clinical and histopathologic obser-vation in severe Vogt-Koyanagi-Harada syndrome, Am J Ophthalmol 83, 242-254.

6. Chan CC, Palestine AG, Kuwabara T, Nussenblatt RB (1988) Immuno-pathologic study of Vogt-Koyanagi-Harada syndrome. Am J Ophthalmol, 105, 607-611

7. Inomata H (1988) Necrotic changes of melanocytes in sympathetic ophthalmia. Arch Ophthalmol, 106, 239-242

8. Hanafusa T, Pujul-Borrell R, Chivato L, Russel RCG, Doniach D, Bottazo GF (1983): Aberrant expression of HLA-DR antigen on Thyrocytes in Graves′disease:relavance for autoimmunity, Lancet, II:1111-1115

9. Nussenblatt RB, Palestine AG (1989) In: Nussenblatt RB, Palestine AG (eds) Uveitis, fundamental and clinical practice, Year book medical publishers inc., Chicago, pp274-290

© 1990 Elsevier Science Publishers (Biomedical Division)
Ocular Immunology Today. M. Usui, S. Ohno and K. Aoki, editors.

IMMUNOLOGICAL ANALYSIS OF VOGT-KOYANAGI-HARADA DISEASE: IMMUNOSUPPRESSION OF P-36-SPECIFIC CYTOTOXICITY MEDIATED BY HLA-DQ MOLECULES

KAZUMI NOROSE[*], AKIHIKO YANO[**], FUMIE AOSAI[**], ETSUKO ASHIZAWA[*], HIDEMI HASHIZUME[*], KIMIKO KAWAI[*], KENICHI HIRABAYASHI[*] AND KATSUZO SEGAWA[*]

Dept. of Ophthalmol[*]. Shinshu Univ. Sch. of Med., Matsumoto; and Dept. of Med. Zool[**]., Nagasaki Univ. Sch. of Med., Nagasaki, Japan.

INTRODUCTION

 Vogt-Koyanagi-Harada disease (VKH) is thought to be a systemic disorder affecting various organs containing melanocytes (1,2), and it is regarded as an autoimmune attack directed against melanin-bearing cells. As the histopathologic findings of sympathetic ophthalmia with uveal granulomatous inflammation and formation of Dalen-Fuchs nodules (3) resemble those seen in VKH, cellular immune responses to (modified-) self systemic melanocytes, as well as humoral- and lymphocyte-mediated immunities (4), have been suggested to play a key role in determining the immunopathology of VKH. In this work, the leukocytes in the peripheral blood (PBL) of patients with VKH were studied with regard to the cytotoxicity against human melanoma cell line (P-36) and antigen-specific proliferative responses in order to gain more information on the immunological processes taking place during the manifestation of the clinical signs. Here we present the data indicating the existence of the split of the responsiveness against P-36 in patients with acute VKH, and the immune suppression (presumably HLA-DQ-mediated) in a patient with recurrent type of VKH.

MATERIALS AND METHODS

Isolation of PBL

 PBL were isolated from patients with VKH by Ficoll-Conray gradient centrifugation as described in detail previously (5).

Monoclonal antibodies

 Anti-HLA-DR (clone L243) and anti-Leu 10 (reactive with HLA-DQ; clone SK10) monoclonal antibodies (MAb's) were purchased from Becton-Dickinson Co. (USA) (5).

Cytotoxic assay

 Human melanoma cell line (P-36; SK-MEL-28) and the human cervical carcinoma cell line (HeLa-S3) have already been demonstrated (6). Cytotoxicity against P-36 has been described elsewhere (6).

Assay cultures for P-36-specific and PPD-specific proliferative responses

 In order to obtain P-36-specific proliferative responses of PBL, $3 \times 10^4/100$ μl of P-36 cells were added to the responder PBL. P-36 cells were inactivated by the treatment with 100 μl/ml mitomycin C and irradiation (3000 R). Assay cultures were maintained at 37°C in a humidified atmosphere of 5% CO_2 and 95% air for 5 days. Then, [^{3}H] methyl-thymidine (^{3}H-TdR) incorporation was measured. Assay of PPD-specific proliferative responses has been described previously (5). The effect of anti-HLA-DR and -DQ MAb's on proliferative responses has also been described elsewhere (5). To analyze the participation of HLA-DR and -DQ molecules in P-36- and PPD-specific proliferative responses, anti-HLA-DR and -DQ MAb's were added to the culture system in various dilutions.

RESULTS AND DISCUSSION

PBL from all 10 patients with VKH except patient K.K. (18 yr. old, female, HLA: A24,B13,Cw1,Cw3,DR4,DQw3) and patient Y.N. (58 yr. old, male, HLA:A24,A11,Bw61, Cw1,Cw3,DR1,DR4,DQw1,DQw3) showed strong cytotoxicity against P-36, but not against HeLa-S3 (Table I). The specificity of these cytotoxic cells has been revealed to be melanocytes as already reported (6), and HeLa-S3 cells were used as a negative control. It is noted that patients K.K. and Y.N. took an unusual clinical course; patient K.K. suffered from severe iritis with fibrin, in spite of a great dose of corticosteroid therapy, and patient Y.N. showed prominent shallowing of the anterior chamber and dramatic choroidal detachment in the early stage of the disease.

As shown in Table I, PBL from all patients including patients K.K. and Y.N. with VKH showed significant proliferative responses to P-36 as measured by incorporation of ^{3}H-TdR for the antigen-specific proliferative responses. No significant P-36-specific proliferative response was detectable in the PBL from the healthy controls. In sum, P-36-specific proliferative (CD4$^+$) cells were induced in PBL in patients K.K. and Y.N., although P-36-specific cytotoxic T lymphocyte (CD8$^+$ CTL) activity was not significantly observed.

TABLE I

P-36-SPECIFIC CYTOTOXIC ACTIVITY AND PROLIFERATIVE RESPONSES IN PATIENTS WITH UNUSUAL VKH

Patient	Cell Source	% specific ^{51}Cr release				Proliferative responses of PBL to P-36		
		P-36		HeLa-S3				
		10:1	50:1	10:1	50:1	Medium	P-36	cpm
K.K.	PBL	4	5	−1	2	351 cpm	11,062 cpm	10,711
Y.N.	PBL	2	7	5	4	1,126	5,522	4,396
Usual*	PBL	27	46	4	9	838	13,632	12,794
Controls**	PBL	7	8	1	5	772	3,480	2,708

Materials and methods demonstrated previously (5,6).
* :n=10 for % specific ^{51}Cr release and n=6 for proliferative responses.
**:n=6 for % specific ^{51}Cr release and n=6 for proliferative responses.

VKH is classified into two variant clinical types, i.e. Vogt-Koyanagi and Harada's types (1). It is now agreed that the symptoms differ only in their intensity and in the regions of the eye involved (1). Patient K.K. was classified as a typical Vogt-Koyanagi type and patient Y.N. was not classified as either typical Harada's type or typical Vogt-Koyanagi type. The different CTL responses of these patients may be attributed to the intensity of the symptoms and regions of the eye involved. If this is the case, the clinical types of the disease may be influenced by the responses of the P-36-specific cytotoxicity and proliferation to P-36. It is hoped that early diagnosis of the clinical types of the disease will become possible in order to choose the most relevant therapy. It may be possible to improve the criteria for the prognosis of VKH by using these indicators.

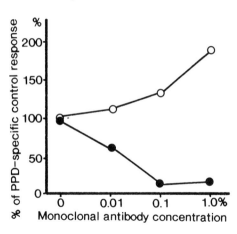

P-36-specific proliferative responses of PBL

PPD-specific proliferative responses of PBL

Fig. 1. Effects of anti-HLA-DR and -DQ monoclonal antibodies on P-36- and PPD-specific proliferative responses of a patient with VKH.

% of blocking= (1-experimental response (cpm)/control response (cpm))x100
○——○ : anti-HLA-DQ,　　●——● : anti-HLA-DR.

Furthermore we examined the involvement of HLA class II molecules in the antigen-specific proliferative responses of the PBL from patient K.K. (Fig.1). The effects of anti-HLA-DR and -DQ MAb's were tested on P-36- and PPD-specific proliferative responses. P-36- and PPD-specific proliferative responses of PBL from patient K.K. were blocked by anti-HLA-DR MAb but not by anti-HLA-DQ MAb. P-36-specific proliferative responses from patient K.K. were significantly inhibited by anti-HLA-DR MAb depending upon the dose of the MAb, while anti-HLA-DQ MAb showed augmenting effects on these antigen-specific responses rather than a blocking effect on the responses. Thus, 2 distinct genetic mechanisms may be involved in controlling antigen-dependent T cell responses of patient K.K. with acute VKH; one is HLA-DR regulation of P-36-specific proliferative (CD4$^+$; helper/inducer) T cell responses, and the other is HLA-DQ regulation of VKH-induced suppressor (CD8$^+$) T cell activity.

In humans, the responses of antigen (such as protein, viral, bacterial and tumor antigens, and so on)-specific T cells are well known to be dependent on HLA-DR molecules of the antigen-presenting cells (APC, macrophages, monocytes, dendritic cells, etc.) (7). There is considerable evidence indicating that immune responses may be depressed by infection with a variety of viruses, intracellular bacteria, protozoa and fungi (8). Thus VKH might be involved in some types (virus) of infection. Recently, Sasazuki et al. (9) elucidated the existence of HLA-linked immune suppression genes (Is genes) in humans that control low or non immune responsiveness through CD4$^-$8$^+$ suppressor T cells, and reached the conclusion that Is genes are mapped within the HLA-DQ subregion and that the HLA-DQ molecule is an Is gene product. In addition, HLA-DQ molecules (probably on the cell surface of APC) may play an important role in the activation of the suppressor T cells (5). In this work, we have also revealed that anti-HLA-DQ MAb released the responsiveness from the suppressive status of patient K.K., who suffered from severe iritis with fibrin in spite of a great dose of corticosteroid therapy and had a bad prognosis. One of the possible mechanisms of the unresponsiveness of antigen-specific cytotoxic T cell responses observed in patient K.K. with acute VKH is HLA-DQ molecules on APC mediated immunosuppression as already reported in another disease (5). If low responsiveness in cytotoxic activity against P-36 affects the bad prognosis of VKH, it is needed to classify the types of HLA-DQ molecules and to analyze their functions. Whether there is a linkage between the prognosis of VKH and HLA-DQ molecules or not is a problem still to be addressed.

REFERENCES

1. Sugiura S (1978) Jpn J Ophthalmol 22:9-35

2. Ohno S, Minakawa R and Matsuda H (1988) Jpn J Ophthalmol 32:334-343

3. Segawa K and Matsuoka N (1971) Jpn J Ophthalmol 15:81-87

4. Ohno S (1981) Trans Ophthalmol Soc UK 101:335-341

5. Yano A, Norose K, Yamashita K, Aosai F et al (1987) J Parasit 73:954-961

6. Norose K, Yano A, Aosai F and Segawa K (1990) Invest Ophthalmol Vis Sci in press

7. Thorsby E, Berle E and Nousiainen H (1982) Immunol Rev 66:39-56

8. Mackowiak PA (1978) N Engl J Med 298:83-87

9. Sasazuki T, Kohno Y, Iwamoto M, Tanimura M et al (1978) Nature 272:359-361

© 1990 Elsevier Science Publishers (Biomedical Division)
Ocular Immunology Today. M. Usui, S. Ohno and K. Aoki, editors.

PRELIMINARY REPORT ON T LYMPHOCYTE SUBSETS IN RECURRENT UVEITIS

ZHENG XIAO-BIN and BAO LI-LING
Research Lab of Immunology, Shanxi Institute of Ophthalmology
No. 92 Fu Dong Jie, 030002, and Department of Ophthalmology,
1st Teaching Hospital of Shanxi Medical College, 030001,
Taiyuan, Shanxi, People's Republic of China

INTRODUCTION

Uveitis has been thought to be associated with immunopathology
for several years[1], and the abnormalities in immunoglobulins,
immune complexes have been found in it. The attention has recently
focused on the changes in the T and B lymphocyte subsets of the
peripheral blood and/or the aqueous or the eye. T cells were found
dominated in the aqueous humour of patients with uveitis[1]. And the
changes of T lymphocyte subsets were found[3,4,5]and not found[6] in the
patients with uveitis. Many uveitises were chronic and recurrent,
for the purpose to see the state of cellular immune in recurrent
uveitis, we conducted this research.

MATERIAL AND METHODS
Collection of Samples

Patients. We selected 12 patients (6 males and 6 females) who
suffered from chronic recurrent uveitis, i.e. the patients had had
uveitis at least several months or several years and recured at
least two or three times. All of them were onset of the disease and
not been treated with hormones systemically (some of them were
treated with Traditional Chinese Medicines) while being examined.
Their average age was 43.2 years.12 age-matched healthy people
(10 males and 2 females) were used as controls. Their average age
was 34.0 years.

Materials

Monoclonal antibodies were offered by Wuhan Institute of Biological
Products. Lymphocytes Seperation Medium was offered by Shanghai
Second Factory of Reagents. Fetal Bovine Serum was offered by Tianjin
Factory of Biochemical Products. And the Fluorescence Microscope
was the type of OLYMPUS BH.

Methods

5ml peripheral blood were taken from each person of both groups
and put in a test tube which contained heparin (1000 unit/ml), then

mixed with equal volume Normal Saline. Mononuclear cells were seperated by the gradient centrifugation method. Wash three times by HBSS (Hanks' Balanced Salty Solution), then suspended them at a concentration of 5×10^{5}--10^{6} in 1ml of HBSS with 20% FBS (Fetal Bovine Serum). Using an ELISA plate, 0.05ml cell suspension were incubated with 0.05ml monoclonal antibodies (CD3, CD4, CD8 and CD25) at 4°C with ice for 30 minutes. Wash three times with HBSS with 2% FBS, then resuspended them to 0.05ml and incubated them with second antibodies which have FITC on them at 4°C with ice for another 30 minutes. Wash three times again and resuspended them. Put the cell suspensions on slides and covered with covering glasses. Lymphocytes were counted under the fluorescence microscope. Counting 100 to 200 cells each. Recken the percentages of CD3, CD4, CD8 and CD25 of the total lymphocytes.

RESULTS

The results are shown in Table 1:

Table 1

RESULTS OF THE TEST

Percentages of CD3, CD4, CD8, CD25 and ratio of CD4/CD8 and the significance between the two groups

	Patients' ($\bar{X} \pm SD$)	Controls' ($\bar{X} \pm SD$)	t-test
CD3	59.12±2.91%	61.90±3.82%	P>0.05
CD4	55.77±5.34%	49.74±2.36%	P<0.002
CD8	51.68±5.01%	31.88±4.77%	P<0.001
CD25	53.88±5.23%	2.97±1.35%	P<0.001
CD4/CD8	1.09±0.18	1.59±0.25	P<0.001

From Table 1 we can see that: CD4 of patients significantly increased than the control, and CD8 also significantly increased than the control. The number of CD8 increased more than that of CD4, so the ratio of CD4/CD8 became lower than the control. But CD3 has no significant change compared with the control. And the increase of CD25 was also very significant than the control.

DISCUSSION

In previous studies of T lymphocyte subsets in uveitis: Nussen-blatt RB et al found that CD8 increased and CD4/CD8 ratio decreased in patients with active posterior uveitis ; in patients with acute untreated uveitis, Abreu MT et al found that CD4 was lower causing the lower ratio of CD4/CD8 in peripheral blood, and the same ratio was found in aqueous humour[4]; but no changes were found in peripheral blood by Murray PI et al[6]; in an interesting study by Usui M et al showed that in rats of experimental S antigen induced uveitis, a rise in CD4 in peripheral blood was found five days after immunization, with the onset of disease CD8 increased, lowing the CD4/CD8 ratio, and as the disease progressed CD4 decreased until they could not been detected in the late stages, this experiment suggests that CD4 initiates the immune response and this is then controls by CD8[7].

Our results showed that both CD4 and CD8 in recurrent uveitis are higher than the normal. Although the high CD8 can be explained to regulate the cellular immune response, the high CD4 perhaps was accumulated by many times of recurrence of the disease. And the lower ratio of CD4/CD8 of the patients suggested that there may be a cellular immune disturbance in such patients.

In our experiment, we detected the CD25 for the first time. CD25 is an antigen of the receptor of interlukin-2 (IL-2). When a lymphocyte is activated, it shows the IL-2 receptors on its surface, so we can see how many lymphocytes are activated by detecting CD25. The very higher percentage of CD25 of the patients showed both the activity of immune and the activity of the disease, and it suggests that systemic cellular immune response is involved in recurrent uveitis.

As for the unchanged percentage of CD3, it needs further investigation.

REFERENCES

1. Spalton DJ (1988) Bri J Ophthalmol 72:81-82
2. Beltort R, Moura NC, Mendes NF (1982) Arch Ophthalmol 100:465-467
3. Nussenblatt RB, Salinas-Carmona MC, Leake W, Scher I (1983) Am J Ophthalmol 95:614-621
4. Abreu MT, Beltort R, Matheus PC, Santos LMB, Sheinberg MA (1984) Am J Ophthalmol 98:62-65
5. Deschenes J, Freeman WR, Char DH, Garovoy MR (1986) Arch Ophthalmol 104:233-236
6. Murray PI, Dinning WJ, Rahi AHS (1984) Bri J Ophthalmol 68:746-749
7. Usui M, Takamar K, Shima Y, Mitsuhashi M, Matsushima T (1986) In: Proceedings of the 4th International Symposium of Immunology and Immunopathology of the Eye

© 1990 Elsevier Science Publishers (Biomedical Division)
Ocular Immunology Today. M. Usui, S. Ohno and K. Aoki, editors.

OCULAR BEHCET'S DISEASE IN THE UNITED STATES:
CLINICAL PRESENTATION AND VISUAL OUTCOME IN 29 PATIENTS

JOHN C. BAER, MD,[1] MICHAEL B. RAIZMAN, MD,[2] C. STEPHEN FOSTER, MD[2]

From the [1]University of Maryland School of Medicine, Department of Ophthalmology, Baltimore, Maryland, U.S.A., and the [2]Hilles Immunology Laboratory, Ocular Immunology Service of the Massachusetts Eye and Ear Infirmary, and Harvard Medical School, Boston, Massachusetts, U.S.A.

INTRODUCTION

Behçet's disease is prevalent in the Mediterranean Basin[1-3], and in the Far East[3,4] but uncommon in the United States. In addition to a difference in incidence, there may be differences in the aggressiveness of the eye disease[3,4], in the sex distribution[3] and HLA antigens[5] in the United States. To address these questions, we retrospectively reviewed a cohort of 29 patients with ocular manifestations from the Massachusetts Eye and Ear Infirmary (21) and the Massachusetts General Hospital (8).

MATERIALS AND METHODS

Twenty-nine patients who satisfied the criteria for Behçet's disease[3] with ocular involvement were identified. Charts were reviewed for date of birth, date of examination, sex, medical history including ocular and systemic symptoms, and family history including ethnic background. For each visit, the visual acuity, external examination, slit lamp examination, intraocular pressure and fundus examination were reviewed and recorded. Treatment, clinical course and visual outcome were recorded for the 21 patients from Massachusetts Eye and Ear Infirmary (MEEI).

RESULTS

Fifteen of the patients were male and 14 were female. Average age at presentation was 33 years (range 11-65 years). The average length of follow-up was 48 months (range 13 - 100). One of the patients was Greek, one was Turkish and four were Italian-surnamed. Three (10%) of the patients were Hispanic. No patients were Oriental, Black or Native American.

Oral mucosal ulceration was present in 26 patients (90%). Sixteen patients (55%) had genital ulcerations, and 15 (52%) had skin involvement. Seventeen patients (59%) had arthralgia or arthritis. Seven patients (24%) had central nervous system involvement.

Twenty-two (76%) patients had typical ocular involvement in both eyes; five (17%) had typical involvement unilaterally. Two patients had scleritis. Manifestations of severe inflammation often appeared only in one eye: 17 eyes of 14 patients developed macular edema, 9 eyes of 11 patients developed hypopyon, and 15 eyes of 12 patients developed papillitis.

HLA antigens were typed in seven Caucasian patients. Three were HLA-B5 positive, one was B27 positive, and three were negative for both antigens.

The subgroup of 21 MEEI patients had a mean presenting age of 33 years. Average follow-up was 45 months. Ten were male and 11 were female. At the end of the study, 16 patients were without inflammation in either eye for a mean of 33 months, three patients continued to have mild ocular attacks which responded to acute management, and two patients were uncontrolled. When presenting visual acuity was compared to final acuity, 9 of 42 eyes showed a decrease in vision. Only four of these lost more than one line. Best visual acuity at any time during the study period was also compared to final acuity. Eleven eyes lost vision, six by more than one line. Twelve eyes of 10 patients had a final acuity of 20/200 or worse, but seven of these presented with vision of 20/200 or worse.

Three of 10 patients treated with cyclosporine (initial dose of 5 mg/kg/d) were controlled. Five of eight patients treated with chlorambucil (8-12 mg/d) were controlled. Three of six treated with oral cyclophosphamide (1 mg/kg/d) and 2 of 2 treated with intravenous cyclophosphamide were controlled. Three of ten patients treated with azathioprine (1.5 mg/kg/d) were controlled. Three patients with mild disease were controlled by colchicine alone. No patients treated achieved long-term control on prednisone.

DISCUSSION

We compared the ocular presentation of Behçet disease in our patients with that reported in the Middle and Far East. The presenting age, and relative frequency of the major manifestations in our patients was typical of that found in other regions[1,4,6,7]. Articular involvement was the most common minor manifestation. Fully 24% of our patients had neuropsychiatric involvement. This is similar to the largest previous American study[6], but contrasts to findings in Japan[4] and the Middle East[1]. The possibility of an ethnic predisposition to neuropsychiatric involvement must not be dismissed.

In contrast to the male predominance described in other areas[1,2,4], we found a nearly equal distribution of males and females. This has also been true of other American studies[6,7]. Male predominance may not be a characteristic of the ocular Behçet's population in the United States[3].

The HLA-B5 antigen is associated with Behçet's disease in Japan[4,5]. Ohno, et al were not able to verify this association for Caucasian patients in the United States[5]. In our cohort, one of the HLA-B5 positive patients was Greek and one Italian-surnamed. Only one of the five non-Mediterranean patients tested was positive.

Ten percent of our patients were Hispanic. Only 3-4% of non-Behçet's patients seen at the MEEI are Hispanic. This supports the suggestion that certain Hispanic sub-populations may have an increased incidence of Behçet's disease[9].

Because of the low incidence of ocular Behçet's disease in the United States, it seems unlikely that prospective data on therapeutic outcome in American patients will become available soon. Large retrospective reviews of patients treated with a *single* therapeutic protocol are equally unlikely. Therefore, we have reviewed the outcome in a subgroup of 21 patients treated with an evolving therapeutic strategy.

The severity of inflammatory signs in our patients was markedly asymmetrical. Asymmetry was also apparent in the visual outcome. Of 10 patients with acuities of 20/200 or worse at the end of the study period, only two had vision worse than 20/200 bilaterally. Of the other eight, the fellow eye saw 20/40 or better in seven. In contrast, studies of natural history from Japan and the Middle East have found that 50% or more of patients will have bilateral acuity of worse than 20/200 after 3 to 6 years of follow-up[2,4]. The asymmetrical presentation and favorable visual outcome may be partially attributable to a less severe prognosis in the United States[3,4], or to a less severe prognosis in female patients[4] who make up a greater percentage of our population, but we suggest that successful management with chemotherapy is more likely to be the explanation. In support of this idea, a recent prospective, controlled, masked study has demonstrated that chemotherapy can halt the progression of eye disease, and protect the fellow eye in patients with unilateral disease[9].

In our hands, no single immunosuppressive agent has been efficacious in all patients. Despite initial enthusiasm about cyclosporine at doses of 10 mg/kg/d, this dose proved renal toxic. Only three of ten patients in our study ultimately remained controlled using 5 mg/kg/d. Currently, our immunosuppressive agent of choice for severe cases is oral chlorambucil or intravenous cyclophosphamide. We use colchicine in mild cases. Prednisone is useful for acute management.

Our study supports previous impressions that male predominance may not be a characteristic of ocular Behçet's patients in the United States, and that, among North American racial groups, Hispanics may be particularly susceptible. American patients with ocular manifestations may also have differences in HLA association, and incidence of neuropsychiatric involvement. Our data also supports the notion that immunosuppressive therapy can alter the course of ocular disease.

ACKNOWLEDGEMENTS
This study was supported in part by the Susan Morse Hilles Immunology Fund.

REFERENCES

1. Mamo JG, Baghdasarian A. Arch Ophthalmol 1964;71:38-48.

2. BenEzra D, Cohen E. Br J Ophthalmol 1986;70:589-92.

3. Michelson JB, Dhisari FV. Surv Ophthalmol 1982;26:190-203

4. Mishima S, Masuda K, Izawa Y, Mochizuki M. Trans Am Ophthalmol Soc 1979;77:225-79.

5. Ohno S, Char DH, Kimura SJ, O'Connor GR. Jpn J Ophthalmol 1978;22:58-61.

6. Colvard DM, Robertson DM, O'Duffy JD. Arch Ophthalmol 1977;95:1813-7.

7. Elliott JH, Ballinger WH. Trans Am Ophthalmol Soc 1984;82:264-81.

8. Lavalle C, Donato AS, Del Giudice-Knippling JA, et al. J Rheumatol 1981;8:325-7.

9. Yazici H, Pazarli H, Barnes C, et al. New Engl J Med 1990;322:281-5.

© 1990 Elsevier Science Publishers (Biomedical Division)
Ocular Immunology Today. M. Usui, S. Ohno and K. Aoki, editors.

STUDIES OF HLA ANTIGENS AND FIBRIN REACTIONS AFTER CATARACT EXTRACTION WITH POSTERIOR INTRAOCULAR LENSE

MAKOTO HIGUCHI* , HIDEO OHTSUKA * , SHIGETO HIROSE**, and SHIGEAKI OHNO **
Ohtsuka Eye Hospital, Sapporo, Japan* and Department of Ophthalmology, Hokkaido University School of Medicine, Sapporo, Japan **

INTRODUCTION

Some patients show fibrin reactions in the anterior chamber after extracapsular cataract extraction (ECCE) with posterior intraocular lense (P-IOL) [1,2] . Many possibilities have been speculated which cause fibrin reaction after ECCE with P-IOL, such as IOL itself, deposit of IOL, ethylene oxide gas, lense material, and so on. However, none of available data could demonstrate a clear interpretation. In our previous study, we examined 400 eyes operated on in our hospital concerning the mechanism underlying the fibrin reaction [3] . Eventually, we suggested that it might be the secondary immune response of type III allergy against lense protein. But, this reaction is not so frequently seen in Caucasians, and even in Japanese, there are 2 groups, one of which does not have this reaction at all. Therefore, some genetic factors are expected to exist in this reaction. In the present study, HLA antigens were tested in these patients in order to investigate whether or not there are genetic factors in the fibrin reactions.

MATERIALS AND METHODS

Fouty patients who had fibrin reactions 4 to 7 days after the operation were the subjects. They were all operated on by the same operator with usual method of ECCE with P-IOL. Seven were males and 33 were females. They were between 46 and 91 years old with an average of 72.2.

Lymphocytes were separated from the heparinized peripheral blood of the patients. Microlymphocytotoxicity test was performed by the NIH standard method. HLA typing was done on HLA-A, B, C and DR antigens and results were evaluated by Fisher's test.

Thirty-eight cases who had had same operations but without fibrin reactions served as controls. Twelve were males and 26 were females. Average age was 71.0 and their ages ranged from 54 to 82 years old.

RESULTS

Among HLA-A antigens, HLA-Aw33 was increased (p=0.30) and A11 was decreased (p=0.30) (TABLE 1). Among HLA-B antigens, HLA-B39 was increased (p=0.13) and B35 and Bw60 were decreased (p=0.19 & 0.07)(TABLE 2). As for HLA-C antigens, HLA-Cw7 was increased(p= 0.41)(TABLE 3). Regarding HLA-DR antigens, HLA-DR1 and DRw52 were increased (p=0.35 & 0.52)(TABLE 4). However, no significant difference was observed between the patients and the controls (Pc>0.05). It was suggested that HLA system did not play an important role in the fibrin reaction after ECCE with P-IOL.

TABLE 1. FREQUENCY OF HLA-A ANTIGENS IN PATIENTS WITH
FIBRIN REACTION AFTER ECCE WITH P-IOL

HLA antigens	Patients(n=40)	Controls(n=38)	
HLA-A 1	1 (3%)	1 (3%)	
A 2	19 (48%)	18 (47%)	
A 3	0 (0)	1 (3%)	
A 24	27 (68%)	23 (61%)	
A 26	5 (13%)	8 (21%)	
A 11	4 (10%)[a]	8 (21%)[a]	
A 31	4 (10%)	3 (8%)	a:p=0.30
Aw33	6 (15%)[b]	2 (5%)[b]	b:p=0.30

TABLE 3. FREQUENCY OF HLA-C ANTIGENS IN PATIENTS WITH
FIBRIN REACTION AFTER ECCE WITH P-IOL

HLA antigens	Patients(n=40)	Controls(n=38)	
HLA-Cw1	13 (33%)	10 (26%)	
Cw3	16 (40%)	17 (45%)	
Cw4	5 (13%)	5 (13%)	
Cw5	0 (0)	1 (3%)	
Cw6	2 (5%)	0 (0)	
Cw7	15 (38%)[a]	10 (26%)[a]	a: p=0.41

DISCUSSION

In our previous study, 400 eyes operated on in our hospital were examinede in order to investigate the mechanism underlying the fibrin reaction after ECCE with P-IOL [3].
And we have got following results.

1. Since there was no fibrin reaction after the operatioin of secondary inplanted P-IOL, this reaction is not caused by IOL.

2. Lens material must be one of the major factors of this reaction, because ECCE without P-IOL is sometimes accompanied by this reaction which had never been seen after intracapsular cataract extraction (ICCE).

TABLE 2. FREQUENCY OF HLA-B ANTIGENS IN PATIENTS WITH
FIBRIN REACTION AFTER ECCE WITH P-IOL

HLA antigens	Patients(n=40)	Controls(n=38)	
HLA-B 51	6 (15%)	5 (13%)	
Bw52	4 (10%)	8 (21%)	
B 7	6 (15%)	3 (8%)	
B 44	7 (18%)	5 (13%)	
B 13	1 (3%)	1 (3%)	
B 15	1 (3%)	0 (0)	
Bw62	4 (10%)	7 (18%)	
B 16	1 (3%)	0 (0)	
B 39	4 (10%)[a]	0 (0)[a]	
B 17	0 (0)	1 (3%)	
B 35	4 (10%)[b]	9 (24%)[b]	
B 37	2 (5%)	1 (3%)	
Bw46	6 (15%)	2 (5%)	
Bw48	3 (8%)	2 (5%)	
Bw54	10 (25%)	7 (18%)	
Bw56	1 (3%)	1 (3%)	
Bw59	1 (3%)	2 (5%)	
Bw60	2 (5%)[c]	8 (21%)[c]	a: p=0.13
Bw61	8 (20%)	5 (13%)	b: p=0.19
Bw67	1 (3%)	2 (5%)	c: p=0.07

3. This reaction was seen much more frequently in the cases with hypermature cataract than those without it ($p<0.001$). Therefore it was thought that lens protein was more important than epithelial cells.

4. This reaction was observed 4-7 days after the operation. There was no difference between 1st and 2nd operated eyes in the patients who underwent operation in both eyes.

These results suggested that this reaction might be the secondary immune response of type III allergy against lens protein. But, this reaction is not so frequently seen in Caucasians [4]. Even in Japanese, not all patients who were in same conditions had this reaction. Some of them did not show it at all. So, we speculated that there might be genetic factors on it and examined HLA antigens. As a result, we could not find any HLA specificities closely related to this reaction. Although certain genetic factors might be involved in the susceptibility of the patients to the fibrin reaction after ECCE with P-IOL, HLA system does not seem to play an important role.

Table 4. FREQUENCY OF HLA-DR ANTIGENS IN PATIENTS WITH
FIBRIN REACTION AFTER ECCE WITH P-IOL

HLA antigens	Patients(n=40)	Controls(n=38)	
HLA-DR 1	7 (18%)[a]	3 (8%)[a]	
DR 2	13 (33%)	15 (39%)	
DR 4	21 (53%)	18 (47%)	
DRw11	1 (3%)	2 (5%)	
DRw12	4 (10%)	2 (5%)	
DRw 6	13 (33%)	9 (24%)	
DRw 8	8 (20%)	8 (21%)	
DRw 9	6 (15%)	9 (24%)	
DRw10	1 (3%)	1 (3%)	
DRw52	26 (65%)[b]	21 (55%)[b]	a: p=0.35
DRw53	27 (68%)	27 (71%)	b: p=0.52

CONCLUSIONS

1. HLA antigens were tested in the patients who had had ECCE with P-IOL, in order to investigate whether or not genetic factors are involved in the fibrin reaction after ECCE with P-IOL.

2. It was shown that HLA-Aw33, B39, Cw7, DR1 and DRw52 were slightly increased, and HLA-A11, B35 and Bw60 were decreased in the patients as compared to controls. However, there was no significance by corrected P-value.

3. These results suggest that HLA system does not play an important role in the fibrin reaction after ECCE with P-IOL.

REFERENCES

1. Nishi,O (1987): Jpn. Clin. Ophthalmol., 41(4);331-336.

2. Sakanishi,Y (1987): Jpn. Clin. Ophthalmol., 41(12);1323-1328.

3. Ohtsuka,H (1989): Ganka Rinshou Ihou, 83(9);1894-1899.

4. Miyake,K (1988): J. Ophthalmic Surgery, 1(1);154-160.

ANTI – LENS CRYSTALLIN ANTIBODIES IN HUMAN SERA AND THE AQUEOUS HUMORS

HITOMI OHGA, TOSHIO KATAYAMA, KUNIAKI EGI, AND HISAKO FUJIWARA
Department of Ophthalmology, Kawasaki Hospital, Kawasaki Medical School
700 2 – 1 – 80 Nakasange Okayama (Japan)

INTRODUCTION

In order for the human crystallin lens to develop independently from fetal circulation during the early embryonic period and, as a result, escape the body's immune tolerance, it is well known that lens antibodies are produced. Crystallin that leaks from the lens causes an autoimmune reaction ; lens – induced endophthalmitis. The authors previously demonstrated that in senile cataracts, even when the capsule is not damaged, crystallin may leak into the aqueous humor[1].

In this study we turned our attention to anti – human crystallin antibodies, investigating them in the aqueous humor and sera using the immune – blotting method and the enzyme – linked immunosorbent assay (ELISA) and studying their clinical significance in cataract patients and postoperative inflammation.

MATERIALS AND METHODS

Senile cataract lenses and aqueous humors obtained during operations and blood obtained from patients with various eye diseases and subjects receiving general check – up were used in this study. Crystallin fractions were determined by column chromatography (Sepharose CL – 6B and Sephadex G – 75), with α, β_H, and γ_H crystallin being obtained. Immune blotting was performed using a Bio – Rad Kit. Human sera and human senile cataract crystallin were used for the primary antigen – antibody reaction and goat anti – rabbit IgG horseradish peroxidase was employed for the secondary reaction.

Anti – human crystallin antibodies were determined by the enzyme – linked immunosorbent assay (ELISA), which was performed using standard procedures. Serum was diluted $1000 \times$. Aqueous humor was diluted $100 \times$ and incubated overnight at 4°C. Absorbancy was determined at 490 nm. Since we were unable to determine IgG in this study, the protein levels in the aqueous humor and sera were ascertained.

RESULTS

1. Immune blotting

Immune blotting pattern is shown in Figure 1. The anti – crystallin antibodies in the serum obtained from a normal 40 – year – old male are shown in Figure 1.

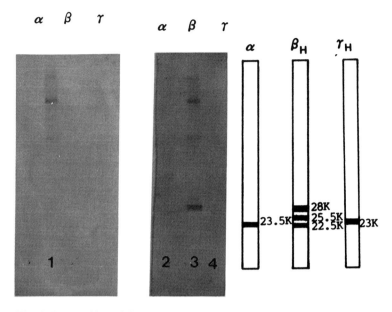

Fig. 1. Immunoblot of human serum. Lane 1 shows standard ; lane 2, α – crystallin antibody ; lane 3, β_H – crystallin antibody ; lane 4, γ_H – crystallin antibody.

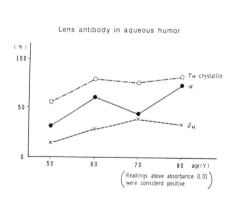

Fig. 2. The anti – crystallin antibodies in aqueous humor based on age. γ_H – crystallin antibody showed the highest level.

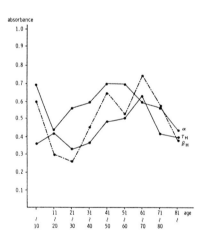

Fig. 3. Anti – crystallin antibodies in serum. A tendency to increase with age was observed.

In the patients with senile cataracts, we were able to observe anti – crystallin antibodies against α, β_H, and γ_H crystallins in the sera.

2. ELISA

As for anti – crystallin antibodies in the aqueous humor, significant differences between subjects of 60 years old or younger and one 70 years old or older were observed at a risk rate below 1 – 2 % with respect to α, β_H, and γ_H crystallins. In the older age group, an increase in the antibody titer was observed.

In judging the antibody titer by ELISA, absorbance of 0.01 or above in the anti – crystallin of the aqueous humor was considered to be positive, and we noted a tendency for the anti – crystallin antibody positive rate in the aqueous humor to increase with age.

With increasing age the antibody positive rate of the various anti – crystallin antibodies tended to increase, the highest rate being that of γ_H crystallin (Fig 2).

No difference was observed in either the anti – crystallin antibody titer or the anti – crystallin antibody positive rate between types of cataracts.

When the relationship between postoperative inflammation and pre – operative anti – crystallin antibodies in the aqueous humor was examined, no tendency for an increase in pre – operative anti – crystallin antibodies in the aqueous humor was observed, even when postoperative inflammation was severe.

With regard to the relationship between the postoperative fibrin reaction and the pre – operative anti – crystallin antibodies in the aqueous humor, only pre – operative γ_H crystallin showed a high level of grade II or above. This indicates, of course, that factors during and after the operation are important.

Next, we studied anti – crystallin antibodies in the serum. Although there were problems with the analysis of individual background factors of the 92 specimens used, generally, higher antibody titers were observed in the order of α, β_H, γ_H crystallins, and the titers tended to increase with increasing age (Fig 3).

As for the relationship between cataracts and the anti – crystallin antibodies in the serum, although there was a difference in mean age between the cataract group (64 years) and the control group (40 years), the anti – crystallin antibody level in the serum was higher in the cataract group, and an increase at a risk rate of 2 % or below was observed for β_H crystallin.

DISCUSSION

Many researchers have conducted studies on anti – human crystallin antibodies[2345]. In recent years, with an increase in the cataract population and an increase in cataract surgery, lens – induced endophalmitis is more often encountered. Also, with the appearance of a rapidly aging society, among the diseases accompanying old age those involving immunity cannot be neglected.

Methods for examining anti – human crystallin antibodies have been improved. In this study, we examined anti – human crystallin antibodies in the aqueous humor and serum using the immune blotting method and ELISA.

In their detailed report on anti – human crystallin antibodies in the peripheral blood, Sunagawa et al[5]. stated that they observed an increase in these antibodies with increasing age and that anti – γ_H crystallin antibodies showed the highest level. In our present results, γ_H crystallin antibodies showed a high level in the aqueous humor and, anti – α crystallin antibodies showed a high level in sera. α – crystallin is an organ – specific protein consisting of two subunits. One of these subunits exists in the tissue but not in the lens, while the other is said to be independent[6]. Many points require further study in evaluating the antibody titers of crystallin in serum and the aqueous humor.

SUMMARY

Human anti – lens crystallin antibodies in sera and the aqueous humor were studied by the immune blotting method and ELISA.

Anti – lens crystallin antibodies in sera, tended to rise with age and higher antibody titer was observed in the order of α, β_H, γ_H crystallin.

The relationship between anti – lens crystallin antibodies and postoperative inflammation is not yet clear.

REFERENCES

1. Fujiwara H (1989) Lens crystallin reactive protein in the aqueous humor of cataract patients. Jpn J Ophthalmol 33 : 418 – 424

2. Hackett E, Thompson A (1965) Natural anti – lens antibody : A non – pathogenic auto – immune system. Proc 10th congr. Int Soc Blood Transf, Stockholm, pp 757 – 758

3. Luntz M H (1968) Anti – uveal and anti – lens antibodies in uveitis and their significance. Exp Eye Res 7 : 561 – 569

4. Nissen S H, Andersen P, Andersen H M K (1981) Antibodies to lens antigens in cataract and after cataract surgery. Brit J Ophthalmol 65 : 63 – 66

5. Sunakawa M, Yoshida H (1986) Anti – lens crystallin antibodies in human sera, 1 Reciprocal change with age. Acta Soc Ophthalmol Jpn 90 : 1361 – 1365

6. Bhat S P, Nagineni C N (1989) α B subunit of lens – specific protein α – crystallin is present in other ocular and non – ocular tissues. Biochem Biophysi Res Commun 158 : 319 – 325

© 1990 Elsevier Science Publishers (Biomedical Division)
Ocular Immunology Today. M. Usui, S. Ohno and K. Aoki, editors.

A NEW PATHOPHYSIOLOGICAL APPROACH TO THE AUTO-IMMUNITY AT THE ORGANISM MOLECULAR LEVEL

L.S. CHABROVA, A.P. RYUMIN, L.F. LINNIK

The IRTC "Eye Microsurgery", Moscow, USSR

INTRODUCTION

Despite a wealth of experience accumulated by clinical immunology, the problem of developing the methods of immunologic diagnostics still retains its topicality. Several laboratories are involved in providing a great number of diagnostic tests whose technical sophistication and difficulties of evaluating the results (1) call for new pathophysiological approaches to study the alterations occured in the immune system. Toxicologists also complain of the fact that reliable and informative immunological criteria are not available at all (2). According to the universal knowledge of today, the status of immunological reactivity is one of the early and sensitive indicators of the harmful effects produced by low-intensity factors, and allergic effects become prominent in concentrations by several orders of magnitude lower than those when general toxic action can be seen. It is essential to reveal these effects when the available materials intended for transplantation are estimated in terms of their toxicity and hygiene.

The development of the immunity theory led to the knowledge that the immune system on the one hand, and endocrine and neurohumoral systems on the other hand, are interconnected, which in its turn provided the rationale for a systemic approach to the homeostasis regulation (3).

In our earlier studies regarding the optical properties of the blood we proceed from an integral approach to the body, viz., that the development of any pathological process, as consistent with current methodology, should be considered primarily in terms of a patient's interaction with the entire aggregate of his or her being (the principle of unity existing between the body and the environment); secondly, it should be considered in terms of interconnection characteristic of local changes of the whole body (the principle of wholeness); and thirdly, in terms of stagewize qualitative development of the disease process proper.

The results of our investigations made it possible to see for the first time how ocular and some other diseases affect the optical properties of the plasm with lysate of autoerythrocytes at different concentrations, i.e. at the molecular level of the body.

R.V. Hoygne (4) proposed a method of toxicological study regarding the body hypersensitivity towards antibiotics, in particular to penicillin. Underlying that method was the provision of dependences of the optical density of mixed blood plasm upon the diagnosticum concentration.

Further on, in order to enhance its diagnostic potentialities, the method had been modified by using, as a diagnosticum, a variety of tissue antigenes, including the lysate of autoerythrocytes (5, 6).

The erythrocytes are known to possess the exceptionally varied antigenic and absorptive properties.

Between the blood plasm and the erythrocytes of the body there is a constant exchange of cholesterine and other lipids. The energy for the body tissues is provided by metabolic process that takes place in blood on the cellular level.

Ioshida et al. obtained the data confirming that the erythrocytes, due to their membrane receptors, are instrumental in the process of elimination of the immune complexes from the body by fixing them on the membrane and by carrying to the cells of reticuloendothelial system where their phagocytosis is taking place. Therefore it is evident that the erythrocytes hemolysate substitutes many biological and chemical reagents employed in the techniques for studying the system of homeostasis by inhancing their standard quality and capability for reproduction.

Keeping in view that the dynamics of the concentration encountered in the course of the Hoygne reaction modified by Klemparskaya, can be caused by the concentration changes in the body occuring in the pathology process, we may conclude that the discovered nodes (7) will reflect, as a model, the dynamics of this pathology. It is owing to the nosological sign providing the difference between the node and the initial selection that the semantic structure of this node is determined. The above structure offers the ground for making diagnosis of a disease throughout the nodes.

In the dynamics of dilutions the nodes form a certain system. This appears to be of importance, since it testifies to the fact that the node systems reflect this or that disease or condition proceeding from the molecular properties of the blood.

MATERIAL AND METHODS

410 in-patients suffering from various ocular diseases underwent our examination.

Having broken the patients down as per sex (200 females and 210 males), we grouped them as per age with the one year interval taking into consideration the nosologic forms. Certain age periods were found to be characteristic of various diseases. To illustrate the case, we took three age groups in women (54-63 years old, 67-73 years, 74-78 years) and two age groups in males (15-25, 67-70 years). Further on, by bringing the dependences of the mixture optical density obtained from the patients of these chosen groups to one initial level (70.0%) we arranged the index of optical density in each age group according to a disease, for each dilution separately.

RESULTS

The results of six dilutions were taken for analysis (1:15360, 1:7680, 1:3840, 1:1920, 1:960, 1:480).

The results of examination were used to prepare a diagnostic Table for women (Table 1) and males (Table 2).

TABLE 1

DEPENDENCE OF THE MIXTURE OPTICAL DENSITY UPON THE DIAGNOSTICUM CONCENTRATION (NODES) IN A VARIETY OF DISEASES, AGE-ORIENTED ASPECT IN FEMALES

Dilution	Level of mixture optical density	Probability of nodes emergence as per disease					
		glaucoma	melanoma	cataract	dacryocystitis	uveitis	retinopathy
1	2	3	4	5	6	7	8
1:15360	680			0.98			
	685			0.90			
	690	0.83			0.70		
	695					0.70	
	700	0.89					
	705			0.90			
	710	0.99					
1:7680	670						0.85
	685			0.99			
	690	0.99		0.95			
	700		0.70				
	705	0.99					
	715			0.83			
	740	0.99					
1:3340	660			0.98			
	670	0.99					
	680	0.98					
	685			0.98	0.90	0.95	
	690	0.97					
	695	0.77					
	700				0.89		
1:3840	705	0.94		0.90			
	710	0.94					
	715			0.90			
	720			0.74			
	745	0.99					
1: 1920	670	0.96					
	685			0.90			0.89
	690			0.72			
	695	0.96	0.95				
	710			0.89			
	720	0.72					
	725	0.89					
	735						0.72

398

TABLE I (continued)

1	2	3	4	5	6	7	8
	680	0.89					
	685			0.82			
	690	0.89					
	695		0.95				
1:960	700	0.98					
	705	0.98					
	710			0.91			
	715	0.98					
	720			0.94			
	750				0.79		
	770	0.99					
	670			0.79			
	675				0.98		
	685			0.95			
1:480	695	0.98		0.79			
	715	0.93					
	745				0.81		
	775	0.98					

TABLE 2

DEPENDENCE OF THE MIXTURE OPTICAL DENSITY UPON THE DIAGNOSTICUM (OF A NODE) IN A VARIETY OF DISEASES, AGE-ORIENTED ASPECT IN MALES

Dilution	Level of mixture optical density	Probability of nodes emergence as per disease					
		glaucoma	cataract	trauma	contusion	myopia	diseases of lacrimal tract
1	2	3	4	5	6	7	8
	690			0.86			
1:15360	700		0.87				
	710		0.72		0.74		
1:7680	700		0.96	0.92			
	705	0.98					
	680	0.98					
1:3840	695		0.98				
	705				0.94		
	685						0.97
1:1920	690			0.88			
	720		0.98				
1:960	690			0.84			
	715		0.81		0.96		

So, the proposed method of autoimmunologic diagnostics involving the determination of dependence of light penetration of the blood plasm mixture and autoerythrocyte diagnosticum upon its concentration as a means of making diagnosis
of ocular diseases -- diminishes the strain on an unhealthy organ (blood properties are studied), enables the diagnostics to be standardized since it refers to
many diseases, reduces economic expenditures for diagnostics due to inexpensive
equipment used for the purpose, and it can be used in clinical setting.

1. Лохов Ф.Ш., Кузьмина Е.Г. и др. Применение нефелометрического
   метода в клинике //Тезисы 1-й респ. научн. конференции молодых
   медиков Грузии. - Бакуриани, 1987. - С.265-266.
2. Виноградов Г.И., Науменко Г.М., Винарская Е.И. и др. Биологичес-
   кая значимость аутоиммунных реакций организма при воздействии
   факторов окружающей среды //Гигиена и санитария. 1987. - № 1. -
   С.55-58.
3. Пантелеев Э.И. Итоги выполнения иммунологической части Гос. про-
   граммы//Иммунология. - 1987.-№2. - С.5-50.
4. Уанье Р.В. //Аллергия к лекарственным веществам. - М., 1962. -
   С.176-186.
5. Варнаган Л.З., Архипов Б.Ф. Унификация и стандартизация методов
   исследования системы гомеостаза с помощью гемолизата эритроцитов
   //Новые методы научных исследований в клинической и эксперимен-
   тальной медицине. - Новосибирск, 1980. - С.10-15.
6. Клемпарская Н.Н. Аутоантитела облучённого организма. - М.: Атом-
   издат, 1972.
7. Путинцева (Чаброва) Л.С., Рюмин А.П. Оптические свойства смеси
   плазмы крови и аутоэритроцитов при некоторых заболеваниях //Вест-
   ник офтальмологии. - 1977. - № 3. - С.23-28.

© 1990 Elsevier Science Publishers (Biomedical Division)
Ocular Immunology Today. M. Usui, S. Ohno and K. Aoki, editors.

A STUDY OF AUTOIMMUNE REACTIONS OF THE ORGANISM IN CASE OF UVEAL
MELANOMA FROM A POSITION OF THE MOLECULAR BIOLOGY

L.F.LINNIK, L.S.CHABROVA, O.N.ZAROBELOVA
The IRTC "Eye Microsurgery",
Beskudnikovsky Blvd.59a, Moscow 127486 (USSR)

INTRODUCTION

A differential diagnosis of uveal melanoma presents considerable
difficulties, because it has a lot of simulating and associating
states.

The traditional methods of preoperative examinations allow one to
determine dimensions and localization of the neoplasm, its ultra-
sound structure, but percentage of diagnostic errors is rather high
(5).

The development of the immunity theory led to a conception of correlation of the immune system with the endocrinic and the neurohumoral one. The last one created a basis to a systemic approach to the
homeostasis regulation. Developing this new pathophysiological
approach to the study of the immune system, in particular the autoimmunity, we obtained that according to the optical properties of
the blood, some eye diseases and their stages can be differentiated
(1,2,3.4).

The purpose of the present investigation was a determination of
optical density for uveal melanoma specific indices in the mixture
of the blood plasma and the set of accumulated concentration of the
lysate of autoerythrocytes, taking into account the stages of the
process and also the sex and age of patients.

MATERIAL AND METHODS

66 patients with the diagnosis of melanoma of uveal tract were
examined. There were the following groups: women aged 25-50 years -
11 patients, 50-75 years - 7 patients; men aged 25-50 years - 9 patients, 50-75 years - 9 patients.

The diagnosis was determined by clinical methods and after the surgery was confirmed by pathohistological methods. Ophthalmoscopy, biomicroscopy, diaphanoscopy, transillumination, ultrasonic A-, B-scan-
ning, radioisotopic diagnosis, fluorescein angiography, computer to-
mography were used for clinical verification of the diagnosis.

In spite of the whole system with many methods for uveal melanoma diagnosis, the difficulties to differentiate it from other states, which are about 40, remained.

By the transvitreal fine-needle aspiration biopsy of the intra-ocular formation or after enucleation the diagnosis was confirmed pathomorphologically.

The optical properties of the blood were studied on the method of microprecipitation with lysate of autoerythrocytes, with the subsequent analysis of data, according to the approach developed by Chabrova L.S. and Ryumin A.P.(1). For this purpose all indices of translucence were referred with a parallel transfer to an equal initial level (70.0%) and further according to the formed groups the specific indices were determined, which were typical for each of these groups on the share method (the Fischer method).

The investigations were performed before and after treatment in different periods (5 days, 10 days, 1 month, 6 months, 1 year). Totally 119 investigations were performed.

RESULTS

The investigations performed in patients with different stages of uveal melanoma showed that each of these groups is characterized with own structure of specificity according to indices of translucence. First, it was obtained that the structure depends on both the disease and sex and age of patients.

TABLE 1

DEPENDENCE OF MIXTURE OPTICAL DENSITY ON THE STAGE OF UVEAL MELANOMA TAKING INTO ACCOUNT SEX AND AGE BEFORE TREATMENT

SEX	AGE	STAGE	Dilution/Translucence
1	2	3	4
MALE	25-50	I-II	4/700
		III-IV	1/420
	50-75	I-II	0
		III-IV	4/730
			6/710
			7/725
			8/730
			9/730
			10/720

1	2	3	4
	25-50	I-II	2/590
		III-IV	3/695
			4/715
			5/740
			6/705
FEMALE			9/750
			10/710
	50-75	I-II	0
		III-IV	1/350
			3/600

Note: in numerator - ordinal number of dilution:

1 - 1:10; 2 - 1:30; 3 - 1:60; 4 - 1:120;

5 - 1:240; 6 - 1:480; 7 - 1:960; 8 - 1:1920;

9 - 1:3840; 10 - 1:7680; 11 - 1:15360.

In denominator - mixture optical density.

Reliability of all presented indices of optical density

0.90   P   0.99

Few of revealed specific indices of optical density with the low titer of diagnosticum dilution (1:240; 1:30) was observed in the 1st-2nd stages of the process, it concerns only the patients aged 25-50 years. In older age neither in men nor in women specific indices were not revealed in these stages of disease.

The specific indices were revealed in all age groups in the 3rd - 4th stages of the process. The intensity of the immune process, which is reflected in these indices, was pronounced in men in the 2nd age group, and in women opposite in the first one. The titer of diagnosticum dilution was similar in men and women and has a wide range (from 1:60 to 1:7680).

A smaller amount of specific indices in low titres was revealed in the first age group of men and in the second group of women. At the III-IV stages of the disease (1:10 to 1:30 and 1:10 to 1:60 correspondingly).

The number of specific indices was found to increase with the increased intensity of the autoimmune state (in healthy people such indices are not detected practically), and this allows one to suppose that in cases of ocular tumors at the III-IV stages of the process, the autoimmunity is in its most tense state in men aged 50 to 75 and in women aged 25 to 50 years.

The obtained data have an undoubted significance in understanding the aging peculiarities of the tumour process which is essential in determining the risk groups and in selecting the tactics of treatment.

It should be noted that the found-out specific indices of translucence were characterized by a very high degree of difference reliability ($0.9 < P < 0.99$) from the initial sample, while in all other translucence indices the reliability was extremely low ($P < 0.2$).

All patients with uveal melanomas underwent treatment corresponding to the process stage: beta therapy was applied at the I - II stages, and enucleation was done at the III - IV stages.

Investigations of the blood optical properties were revealed to reflect efficacy of the beta therapy or surgery (Table 2), and the obvious relationship of the process with non-specific factors can be traced.

TABLE 2

DEPENDENCE OF THE MIXTURE OPTICAL DENSITY ON THE UVEAL MELANOMA STAGES TAKING INTO ACCOUNT SEX AND AGE AFTER TREATMENT

Sex	Age	Stage	Dilution/translucence
MALE	25-50	I - II	11/700
			10/780
			4/660
			3/630
			2/560
		III - IV	5/750
	50-75	I - II	0
		III - IV	0
FEMALE	25-50	I - II	8/730
		III - IV	9/715
			8/715
			6/720
			5/690
			5/715
			2/520
	50-75	I - II	11/730
			10/725
		III - IV	0

Reliability of all presented indices of the optical density:
$$0.90 < P < 0.99$$

Thus, in the beta therapy application, intensification of the autoimmune reactions was noted which manifested itself in the increased amount of specific indices from one (at a dilution of 1:120) to six (at a dilution of 1:30 to 1:15360) in men aged 25 to 50 years and in emergence of two indices (at a dilution of 1:10 to 1:60) in the women of the second age group. But in men of older age (50 to 75 years) at the I - II stages of the process, specific indices were not detected before treatment, and they did not appear after the beta therapy either. If before treatment in the first age group of women only one specific index with low titre was revealed, the only after-treatment changes consisted in the changed value of the specific index (from 590 to 730) and in the increased dilution titre (from 1:30 to 1:1920).

The disappearance of specific indices in other groups of patients observed during six months after the beta therapy evidences the success of the conservative treatment at the I - II stages of uveal melanoma.

Various intensity dynamics of the autoimmune reactions was noted in all patients at the III - IV stages. Thus, in men aged 25 to 50, two specific indices (at a dilution of 1:10 to 1:30) changed to one (at a dilution of 1:240) five days following enucleation, it then disappeared after ten days; in the second age group six specific indices (at a dilution of 1:120 to 1:7680) disappeared after five days and did not appear later. The same tendency is observed in women. But the number of indices in the age group of 25 to 50 years was maintained during five days, although the dilution titre changed (from 2:60 to 1:7680 before surgery and from 1:30 to 1:3840 after it), and one index only with the low titre at a dilution of 1:120) remained after ten days, disappearing after one month in the second age group of women, two specific indices with the low titre (at a dilution of 1:10 to 1:60) disappeared after five days and did not appear later.

Thus, it was for the first time found out that the pronounced degree of the autoimmune response and its intensity depend on the process stage, but the dependence on the patient's sex and age was also noted at all the stages of uveal melanoma.

The data obtained in patients after treatment are found out to be similar in dynamics of specific indices in the groups opposite

in their sex and age, once again indicating an exact correlative relationship between the autoimmune process activity and non-specific
factors.

We obtained that the stages of the tumour process in uveal melanoma are reflected on the optic properties of the autoerythrocyte
lisate and the blood plasma mixture, i.e. on the molecular level of
the organism, as a result of interaction between specific and non-
specific factors.

This reflection allows one to judge of the erythrocytes participation in the pathological process, intensity of the autoimmune reactions in the patient's organism and their specific features depending on the stage of the uveal melanoma, patient's age and sex, it
also presents an opportunity to evaluate the efficacy of the selected treatment.

REFERENCES

1. Putintseva (Chabrova) L.S., Ryumin R.P. Optical properties of a
   blood and erythrocytes mixture in some diseases. - Vestn. Oftal-
   mol., 1977.-No.3.-P.23-28.
2. Chabrova L.S., Ryumin A.P. A pathogenetic function of erythrocytes in glaucoma.//Regulation mechanisms in the blood system. -
   Krasnoyarsk.-USSR Academy of Sciences.-1978.
3. Chabrova L.S., Ryumin A.P. A method of the autoimmunological diagnostics.-Moscow.-1989.-Dep. No. 18330 of 17.08.89
4. Chabrova L.S., Ryumin A.P. A study of diagnostic value of the
   blood optical properties. Dep. No. 18328 of 17.08.89.

IMMUNOTHERAPY

© 1990 Elsevier Science Publishers (Biomedical Division)
Ocular Immunology Today. M. Usui, S. Ohno and K. Aoki, editors.

SYSTEMIC CHEMOTHERAPY FOR OCULAR CICATRICIAL PEMPHIGOID

C. STEPHEN FOSTER, M.D., JOSEPH TAUBER M.D., AND MAITE SAINZ DE LA MAZA, M.D..
From the Immunology Service, Massachusetts Eye and Ear Infirmary, Harvard Medical School, 243 Charles Street, Boston, Massachusetts.

INTRODUCTION

Cicatrical Pemphigoid (CP) is a systemic autoimmune disease characterized by conjunctival cicatrization with subepithelial fibrosis and symblepharon formation with fornix shortening. Untreated, progressive disease inexorably leads to xerosis, corneal opacification, profound visual loss and, in some cases, complete loss of the eye. It is well recognized that topical therapeutic strategies are not effective treatment for this systemic disorder, and that systemic chemotherapy is both safe and effective in halting progressive disease. Review of the literature suggests that cyclophosphamide, azathioprine, methotrexate and dapsone are, in descending order of efficacy, effective agents in the treatment of CP (1-9). Because of limited reports of chemotherapy experience in ocular cicatricial pemphigoid, the most appropriate agent of choice for therapy may be unclear. This study was undertaken to compare efficacies and side effects of chemotherapeutic agents used in a large series of CP patients in the hope of establishing guidelines for the use of systemic chemotherapy in cicatricial pemphigoid affecting the conjunctiva.

PATIENTS, MATERIALS AND METHODS

We reviewed the records of 165 patients with CP followed in the Immunology Service between 1977 and 1988. The study population includes all patients with CP treated for three or more months with any systemic chemotherapy and with adequate followup examination records. One hundred and five patients satisfied these criteria and form the data base for this report. The diagnosis of CP was based on the presence or cicatrizing conjuctivitis with or without symblepharon formation, and the demonstration of immunoreactant deposition at the epithelial basement membrane zone (BMZ) with fluorescence microscopy of conjunctival biopsies. Biopsy technique, tissue processing and criteria for biopsy positivity have been previously published (10). All patients in this study had biopsy proven CP. Staging of CP, performed using the scheme previously reported by Foster (10) and grading of conjunctival inflammatory activity (from 0 to 4+ in steps of 0.5) were performed in all patients by the same physican (CSF) to ensure accurate disease staging and consistent conjunctival inflammation grading. The criteria for institution of systemic chemotherapy, pretreatment patient evaluation, including photographic documentation, and laboratory treating protocols have been described in detail elsewhere (10). Chemotherapies were initiated at 2 mg/kg for diaminodiphinylsulfone (dapsone), cyclophosphamide and azathioprine, but were adjusted for each individual based on clinical judgment, hematologic tolerance and side effects.

Records and ocular photographs were reviewed and disease progression was considered to have occurred if there was clinical or photographic evidence or progressive conjunctival cicatrization within a stage or advancement to a higher stage. Based on previous reports of asymmetry between eyes in CP disease severity (stage) and progression (11) and on our own experience supporting this observation, we chose to report results both in terms of patients and eyes. Data were tabulated and analyzed using customized database software. Statistical analysis was performed using the Student's t test, chi square and linear regression methods.

RESULTS

Thirty-three patients were male (31%) and 72 female (69%). The longitudinal followup of these patients ranged from three to 147 months (mean 35 mos.). All patients had documented disease progression before institution of chemotherapy. The average patient age at the time of diagnosis of OCP was 68 years (range 23 to 95). Extraocular manifestations of cicatricial pemphigoid (skin, mouth, esophagus, trachea, gastrointestinal or genitourinary tract) were present in 50 patients (48%) at the time of initial ocular examination. A history of glaucoma was obtained from 26 patients (25%). A clinical diagnosis of rosacea based on facial skin characteristics was made in 15 patients (14%).

Most patients (90%) were classified at stage III or IV in the worse eye at the time of first examination, accounting for 84% of eyes. Seventy-nine percent of patients had equal disease stages in both eyes. Vision varied considerably at presentation; acuities were 20/40 or better in 32% of eyes, between 20/50 and 20/100 in 33% and 20/200 or worse in 35% of eyes. There was no linear relationship between visual acuity and disease stage at presentation ($R^2 = .12$). Females had significantly more visual loss at presentation, with 63% presenting with acuity of 20/200 or worse in at least one eye, as compared to 36% of males (p<0.03). Two eyes had no light perception at the time or first examination. Most patients (38%) had 2+ conjunctival inflammatory disease activity at first examination.

<u>Outcome - total group</u>. Ninety-two percent of patients were classified at stage III or IV in the worse eye at final examination, as compared with 90% of patients who had disease at these advanced stages at presentation. Over 90% of eyes had 1+ conjunctival inflammatory activity or less at final exanination (compared with 43% at initial examination) while 52% of eyes had no inflammation at all. Vision at final examination was 20/40 or better in 31% of eyes, between 20/50 and 20/100 in 35% and 20/200 or worse in 34% of eyes. Three eyes lost light perception during the study; their initial vision had been 20/100, count fingers and hand motions.

Not all patients had a successful outcome as a result or systemic chemotherapy. Progression of conjunctival cicatrization occurred in 16 eyes (7%) of 14 patients. Because the goal of this study was to evaluate the efficacy of chemotherapy in OCP, all cases of progression in stage were reviewed to ascertain the basis of ocular deterioration. Of the 16 eyes which progressed in stage, one did so before treatment was initiated and one progressed following lamellar keratoplasty in a patient with sicca syndrome and a persistent epithelial defect. Three of the eyes which progressed had presented with corneal perforation and visions of count fingers or worse at stage II or III, but had no active inflammation, and had no progression in the other eye while on chemotherapy. One eye showed progression from stage II to III without loss of acuity, and later had all disease activity halted. Despite progression of cicatriation, these eyes were not felt to represent *therapeutic* failures. The remaining ten eyes on eight patients which had progressed in disease stage had no extenuating circumstances, and were judged treatment failures. The highest incidence of both progression in cicatrization and of therapeutic failure occurred in the patients maintained on azathioprine ($p < 0.01$). For patients in whom conjunctival inflammation was <2+, dapsone was highly effective in halting inflammation and scarring. If conjunctival inflammation was >3+, cyclophosphanide was distinctivly superior in efficacy ($p < 0.01$).

Overall, 42% of patients had their disease brought under control with their initial chemotherapy regimen, including 45% (31/69) begun on dapsone, 40% (10/25) on cyclophosphamide and 33% (3/11) begun on azathioprine. An additional 50% had their disease brought under control with additions or substitutions in their regimens.

DISSCUSSION

Authors dating from as early as von Graefe in 1879, agree that cicatricial pemphigoid affecting the conjunctiva is invariably progressive and that the ultimate prognosis is quite poor (12). Ten to thirty years or more may be required for the disease to run its full course, with bilateral blindness as the end result. The course of the disease is usually slow, but may be punctuated by periods of explosive inflammatory activity with rapid progression of conjunctival cicatrization (13). No topical therapy is effective in stopping the progression of conjunctival scarring in this systemic disease. High doses of systemic prednisone can control the process, and periodic subconjunctival steroid injections can be temporarily ameliorating (10). However, the long-term consequences of the moderate to high doses of systemic steroid required for control of CP and the cataractogenic effects of subconjunctival steroid injections are unacceptable. The collective experience reported in the literature demonstrates unequivocally that cicatricial pemphigoid affecting the conjunctiva is highly amenable to successful abolition of conjunctival inflammation and progressive cicatrization through the use of systemic chemotherapeutic immunosuppressive therapy.

The results of this case control study provides additional insights into the efficacy of various chemotherapeutic regimens and allow recommendations to be made with respect to choice of therapy for patients with cicatricial pemphigoid.

The results of this study show a failure rate, in our hands, of 4% (five eyes in four patients) among those patients successfully maintained on chemotherapy. The failure rate was 9% in our total study population (11 eyes in nine patients), including patients intolerant of treatment. These failure rates are far lower than the high incidence of progression reported as the natural history of untreated cicatricial pemphigoid. In a prospective study with 22 month followup, a 75% incidence of progression has been reported in stage III CP (14).

In the patient with pemphigoid which is of mild to modest inflammatory activity and is not rapidly progressive, dapsone should be the initial drug of choice. It is mandatory to ensure that the patient does not have a history of sulfa allergy and is not glucose-6-phosphate dehydrogenase deficient.

Cyclophosphamide is the better initial drug choice in patients with intense inflammation (3+ or greater conjunctival inflammation) or rapidly progressive disease, with therapeutic failure occurring in one of nine patients (11%), as compared with four failures among 15 patients (27%) treated with dapsone. Prednisone is a reasonable adjunct to induction of therapy, provided there is no contraindication to its use. We typically taper and discontinue the prednisone within two months of its initiation. Azathioprine was effective in achieving disease control when *added* to initially ineffective dapsone.

Cytotoxic chemotherapy should only be used by physicians who are trained and expert in their administration, willing to maintain regular and sometimes frequent followup schedules, maintain constant vigilance for the side effects which may develop, and who are prepared to take responsibility for managing the complications and side effects which might be encountered in these patients.

REFERENCES

1. Dantzig PI (1974) Immunosuppressive and cytotoxic drugs in dermatology. Arch Dermatol 110: 393-406.
2. Lever WF, Schaumberg-Lever G (1977) Immunosupressive and prednisone in pemphigus vulgaris: Therapeutic results obtained in 63 patients between 1961 and 1975. Arch Dermatol 113: 1236-1241.
3. Wolff K (1976) Immunosuppressive therapy. Bull Dermatosem Hautarzt 1: 25.
4. Fellner MJ, Katz JM, McCabe JB (1978) Successful use of cyclophosphamide and prednisone for initial treatment of pemphigus vulgaris Arch Dermatol 114: 889-894.
5. Dave VK, Veckers CFH (1974) Azathioprine in the treatment of muco-cutaneous pemphigoid. Br J Dermatol 90: 183-186.
6. Brody HJ, Piroi DJ (1977) Benign mucous membrane pemphigoid: Response to therapy with cyclophosphamide. Arch Dermatol 113: 1598-1599.
7. Rook A, Waddington E (1953) Pemphigus and pemphigoid. Br J Dermatol 65: 425-431.
8. Person JR, Rogers RS III (1977) Bullous pemphigoid responding to sulfapyridine and the sulfones. 113: 610-615.
9. Rogers RS III, Seehafer JR, Perry HO (1982) Treatment of cicatricial (benign mucous membrane) pemphigoid with dapsone. J Am Acad Dermatol 6: 215-223.
10. Foster CS (1986) Cicatricial pemphigoid. Trans Am Ophth Soc 84: 527-663.
11. Mondino BJ, Brown SI (1983) Immunosuppressive therapy in ocular cicatricial pemphigoid. Am J Ophthalmology 96: 453-459.
12. Duke-Elder S (1965) System of Ophthalmology. St. Louis : C.V. Mosby vol. 8 part 1, p. 502.
13. Mondino BJ, Brown SI, Lampert S, et al (1979) The acute manifestations of ocular cicatricial pemphigoid: diagnosis and treatment. Ophthalomology 86: 543-555.
14. Mondino BJ, Brown SI (1981) Ocular cicatricial pemphigoid. Ophthalmology 88: 95-100.

© 1990 Elsevier Science Publishers (Biomedical Division)
Ocular Immunology Today. M. Usui, S. Ohno and K. Aoki, editors.

NEW IMMUNOSUPPRESSIVE APPROACH TO CORNEAL GRAFT REJECTION :
A CLINICAL AND IMMUNOLOGICAL STUDY IN A RAT PKP-MODEL

CARL P. HERBORT*§, MARC D. de SMET*, FRANCOIS G. ROBERGE*, ROBERT B. NUSSENBLATT*, HAYA LORBERBOUM-GALSKI#, AND IRA PASTAN#.

*Laboratory of Immunology, National Eye Institute; #Laboratory of Molecular Biology, National Cancer Institute. National Institutes of Health, Bethesda, MD 20892. § Department of Ophthalmology, Lausanne University, Lausanne, Switzerland.

INTRODUCTION

Corneal transplantation is achieving astonishingly high success rates when compared to other transplantation procedures. When grafts are placed onto non vascularized corneas, rejection rate does not exceed 5-10% (1). Such a low rejection rate is explained by the immunological privilege the cornea enjoys; although sensitization to the graft occurs through the normal afferent loop, destruction of the graft through the efferent loop is prevented because of the avascular structure of the cornea (2). When grafts are placed onto vascularized corneal beds the immunological privilege is lost and rejection is very frequent despite massive corticosteroid therapy (3). Better immunosuppressive therapy is needed in these situations. Graft rejection is a T lymphocyte mediated process requiring activated T cells (reviewed in 4). Although CD8+ cytotoxic T lymphocytes (CTL) are the primary effector cells in allograft rejection, activation of both CD4+ helper T lymphocytes and CTL cells is necessary. Characteristic features of activated T lymphocytes is dependency on interleukin-2(IL-2), which is also mainly produced by CD4+cells, and expression of high affinity IL-2 receptor (IL-2R). Cyclosporine (CsA) is a very effective immunosuppressive agent but has to be given continuously. It suppresses graft rejection by inhibiting both IL-2R expression and IL-2 production by T lymphocytes. More selective immunosuppressants are presently available. IL-2-PE40 is a recombinant chimeric cytotoxin composed of IL-2, fused to a modified pseudomonas exotoxin. It is extremely toxic to activated T cells which express high affinity IL-2R (5). A more potent and selective effect is therefore expected from this new molecule. We studied the effect of IL-2-PE40 on corneal graft rejection in the rat both clinically and immunologically.

MATERIAL AND METHODS

Animals

Female inbred Lewis and Fisher (F344) rats (Charles River, Raleigh, NC), 8-10 week old, were used. Lewis rats were used as recipients and Fisher rats were used as donors. These strains differ only in their minor and medial transplantation antigens (6).

Experimental protocol

Grafted animals were treated for 12 days with CsA (12mg/kg/day IM, Sandoz A.G., Basle, Switzerland) starting from the day of surgery. On day14, technically successful animals were randomly assigned either to IL-2-PE40 therapy (0.62μg/ g/day IP in 2 divided doses for 10 days) or to PBS treatment. Animals were followed by a clinical scoring method for 8 weeks. Clinical score was based on graft opacity (score 0-4) and graft edema (0-2). With a score > 4.5, a graft was considered rejected. In addition, cytotoxic T cell response in the draining lymph nodes was evaluated in both groups during a period of 2 weeks after the cessation their respective immunosuppressive treatments.

Surgical technique

The surgical method used was penetrating keratoplasty and has been describred previously (7). In brief, 3 mm corneal buttons were taken excentrically to favor rejection and transplanted onto 2.5 mm donor beds by 8 sutures, using 10.0 Nylon monofilament (Alcon Pharmaceuticals Ltd, Fort Worth, TX).

Cytotoxic T cell assay

Cervical lymph nodes were excised in anesthetized recipient (Lewis) rats and cells were cultivated in bulk mixed leukocyte reaction (MLR) in the presence of irradiated donor (stimulator) spleen cells from Fisher rats at the respective concentration of 10^6 cells in a total volume of 30 cc of supplemented RPMI medium. After 5 days cytotoxicity was measured by plating effector and target cells in triplicates in 96-well plates at the effector:target ratios of 50:1, 25:1, 12.5:1 in a standard ^{51}chromium release assay. Con A stimulated donor spleen cells were use as targets.

RESULTS

Clinical evaluation (Figure 1)

Syngeneic grafts had a slightly elevated score during the 2 first weeks because of surgical inflammation. Corneas remained clear during the rest of the observation period. Allogeneic grafts remained clear during the first 2 weeks. Clinical score of the PBS treated group rose sharply from week 3 to reach a maximum on the 4th week. The corneas then gradually cleared due to regeneration of epithelium and endothelium from the recipient side. In contrast, the score of the IL-2-PE40 treated group remained low during the whole observation period. Cumulative rejection rate calculated as the ratio of rejected grafts to total number of grafts per group was 0% in the syngeneic group, 100% in the PBS treated group and 50% in the IL-2-PE40 treated group.

**Fig. 1. EFFECT OF IL-2-PE40 ON CORNEAL GRAFT REJEC-
TION AND CYTOTOXIC RESPONSE IN DRAINING LYMPH NODES**

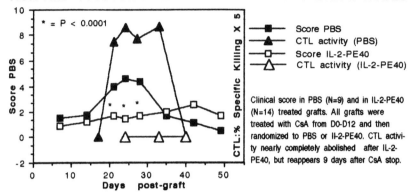

Clinical score in PBS (N=9) and in IL-2-PE40 (N=14) treated grafts. All grafts were treated with CsA from D0-D12 and then randomized to PBS or Il-2-PE40. CTL activity nearly completely abolished after IL-2-PE40, but reappears 9 days after CsA stop.

Legend:
- Score PBS
- CTL activity (PBS)
- Score IL-2-PE40
- CTL activity (IL-2-PE40)

Cytotoxicity assay (Figure 1)

Evaluation of cytotoxicity parallelled our clinical findings. No cytotoxicity in draining lymph nodes was measured 5 days after cessation of CsA in the PBS group but cytotoxic activity was again very strong at 9 days. In the IL-2-PE40 treated 15 days after treatment cessation cytotoxic activity was still unsignificant, indicating very strong immunosuppression.

DISCUSSION

Both CsA and IL-2-PE40 were able to prevent allograft rejection in our model. However rejection occured in all animals in the group that had received only CsA within 2 weeks of treatment cessation. The clinical evaluation was confirmed by the measure of cytotoxic activity in draining lymph nodes which was restored within 9 days after CsA discontinuation. Il-2-PE40 prevented rejection in half of the grafts even after treatment discontinuation, which was also parallelled by an almost absent cytotoxic response in draining lymph nodes. It seems therefore that unlike CsA, IL-2-PE40 conveys tolerance in a certain number of cases. It can be hypothetized that the difference of potency between the 2 immunosuppressants comes from their different mechanism of action : CsA only blocks the activated T lymphocyte whereas IL-2-PE40 is killing the activated cell. IL-2-PE40 appears to be a very efficient agent in T cell mediated diseases because of the association high potency and high selectivity.

ACKNOWLEDGEMENTS

This work was supported in part by the Fondation Suisse de Bourses de Medecine et Biologie (Dr. Carl P. Herbort).

REFERENCES

1. Pollack FM (1985-86) Cornea 4 : 137

2. Coster DJ (1989) Eye 2 : 151

3. Stern GA (1988) Ophthalmology 95 : 842

4. Asher NL, Hanto DW, Simmons RL (1989) In : Flye MW (ed) Principles of Organ Transplantation. W.B. Saunders, Philadelphia, pp 91-104

5. Lorberboum-Galski H, FitzGerald D, Chaudhary V, Adhya S, Pastan I (1988) Proc Natl Acad Sci USA 85 : 1922

6. Gill tJ, Kunz HW, Misra DN, Cortese Hasset AL (1987) Transplant 43 : 773

7. Herbort CP, Matsubara M, Nishi M, Mochizuki M (1989) Jpn J. Ophthalmol 33 : 212

MECHANISM OF PROTECTION FROM HERPES SIMPLEX VIRUS TYPE 1 (HSV-1) RETINITIS IN MICE

S.S. ATHERTON,[*][+] J.U. IGIETSEME,[*] F. MIRANDA,[*] J.W. STREILEIN[*][+]

Departments of [*]Microbiology and Immunology and [+]Ophthalmology, University of Miami School of Medicine, P.O. Box 016960 (R-138), Miami, FL 33101 (USA)

INTRODUCTION

Acute retinal necrosis develops in the uninoculated eye of approximately 90% of BALB/c mice 10 days after uniocular anterior chamber (AC) inoculation of HSV-1 (KOS strain) (1). Recently, we demonstrated that intravenous (IV) injection of in vitro-activated HSV-1 specific immune effector cells (IEC) could protect against contralateral retinitis when these cells were injected IV within 24 hours of virus inoculation into the AC (2). We reported that the incidence of retinitis in mice treated with virus-specific IEC was 10% (4/40) compared with an incidence of 88.1% (37/42) in the untreated mice. If the IEC were transferred later than 24 hours after virus inoculation, there was no protection. Treatment of the IEC prior to adoptive transfer with anti-Thy 1.2 and complement abolished completely the ability of these cells to protect the uninoculated eye. From these results, we proposed that a retinitis-inducing process is established within 24 hours following AC inoculation. Once established, this process is impervious to immune intervention (2). In the experiments reported herein, we studied the mechanism of protection by IEC by (1) examining the ability of various T cell subsets to protect against retinitis and (2) correlating the appearance of virus in the uninoculated eye with the level of protection.

MATERIALS AND METHODS

Animals and Virus

Adult female BALB/c mice (Taconic, Germantown, NY) were used in all experiments and were maintained in accordance with the ARVO Resolution on the Use of Animals in Research. Stocks of the KOS strain of HSV-1 were grown and titered using standard methods (2). Inoculation of virus into the AC was performed by proptosing the eye, removing the aqueous by paracentesis and microinjecting 2×10^4 PFU of virus into the AC (3). Immediately after sacrifice, eyes for virus recovery studies were removed and homogenized. Serial dilutions of the homogenized eyes were plated onto monolayer cultures of Vero cells and overlaid with culture medium containing 0.5% agarose. After 5 days, the plates were fixed and stained; the titer of virus was determined by counting the plaques on duplicate monolayers.

Preparation and Antibody Treatment of Immune Effector Cells

Mononuclear cells IEC were prepared following previously-published methods (2). Within 2 hours of virus inoculation into the AC, groups of mice received an IV inoculation of in vitro-restimulated IEC that had either been depleted of L3T4[+] and Ig[+] cells or that had been depleted of Lyt 2[+] and Ig[+] cells using the appropriate goat anti-mouse antibodies (Becton Dickinson, Mountain View, CA). The two negatively-selected populations were recombined and given to a third group of mice. Using indirect ophthalmoscopy, mice were evaluated on day 10 p.i for retinitis which is characterized by inflammation, hemorrhage and loss of retinal transparency (4).

RESULTS

Role of T cell subsets in Protection Against Retinitis

We were interested in determining which T cell subset was primarily responsible for protection against retinitis. To address this question, we studied the ability of negatively selected (with antibody and complement) subsets of T cells to protect the uninoculated retina following AC inoculation of HSV-1. Table 1 demonstrates that the cell population containing only Lyt 2^+ cells was significantly more efficient at conferring protection than the cell population containing only L3T4$^+$ cells. Four of 11 mice (36.3%) developed retinitis in the former group, compared with 6 of 10 mice (60.0%) with retinitis in the latter group. Neither subset of T cells alone provided the level of protection observed when non-depleted in vitro-activated cells were administered [2 of 21 mice (9.5%) developed retinitis]. Moreover, when the two negatively selected populations were combined and injected together, the level of protection against retinitis approached that observed in mice treated with the unfractionated effectors [2 of 10 mice (20%) developed retinitis]. These results suggest that both the L3T4$^+$ cell and the Lyt 2^+ cell contribute to protection against retinitis and that optimal protection requires both subsets of T cells.

TABLE 1

ROLE OF T CELL SUBSETS IN PROTECTION AGAINST CONTRALATERAL RETINITIS

Group[*]	Type of Transferred Cells	Incidence of Retinitis (%)	
1	None	10/11	(90.9)
2	Unseparated Activated Effectors	2/21	(9.5)[#]
3	Enriched for Lyt 2^+ cells	4/11	(36.4)[#]
4	Enriched for L3T4$^+$ cells	6/10	(60.0)
5	Lyt 2^+ and L3T4$^+$ cells	2/10	(20.0)[#]

*All mice were injected with HSV-1 via the AC route. Adoptively-transferred cells were injected intravenously within 2 hours of virus inoculation.
[#]Significantly different than group 1 at p<0.27 or better (Fisher's Exact Test, 2-tailed)

Activated Immune Effectors Prevent Second Wave Virus from Reaching the Uninoculated Eye

Two distinct waves of virus reach the uninoculated eye following uniocular AC inoculation of HSV-1: an early, low-titered wave within the first 24 hours and a later, higher-titered wave on day 10 p.i. coincident with the development of retinitis (5). To determine whether IV administration of IEC protects by preventing one or both waves of virus dissemination to the uninoculated eye, the amount of virus on days 1, 2, 3 and 10 p.i. in the eyes of HSV-1-infected mice that had been treated with IEC was determined by plaque assay. The amount of virus recovered from treated mice was compared with the amount of virus previously reported from animals inoculated with HSV-1 via the AC route without benefit of exogenous IEC (5). The virus recovery results are shown in Table 2. Administration of IEC had no effect on the replication of virus in the HSV-1-inoculated eye. In this eye, the titer of virus rose to approximately 6.95 Log$_{10}$ PFU/ml by day 2 p.i., a titer comparable to that recovered from the injected eyes of untreated mice infected with HSV-1 via the AC.

In the contralateral eye, the arrival of first wave of virus was delayed by 24 hours in mice that received IEC, although the amount of virus was similar to that recovered from the first wave in control mice (Table 2). The most striking finding in these mice was that the HSV-1 titers on day 10 p.i. were significantly reduced compared to those recovered previously at day 10 p.i. in the contralateral eyes of HSV-1-injected BALB/c mice with retinitis (6). Since the average titer of virus recovered at day 10 p.i. from mice with retinitis was 5.57 Log_{10} PFU/ml (6), we conclude that the low titer of virus recovered at day 10 p.i. from the contralateral eyes of mice treated with IEC is consistent with the observation that treated animals did not develop retinitis. This result supports the hypothesis that activated IEC protect against retinitis by limiting quantitatively the spread of and/or replication of second wave virus.

TABLE 2

VIRUS RECOVERY FROM INJECTED AND UNINJECTED EYES OF MICE TREATED WITH IEC

	HSV-1 TITER (Average Log_{10} PFU/ml $\pm$ SEM)[*]			
	Day 1	Day 2	Day 3	Day 10
Injected Eye	5.37 ± 0.26	6.95 ± 0.01	5.63 ± 0.78	3.44 ± 0.64
Uninjected Eye	$<0.7^+$	2.30 ± 0.66	2.23 ± 0.38	2.12 ± 0.54

[*]Mice were inoculated with HSV-1 via the AC route, and IEC were injected IV within 2 hours of virus inoculation. At each time, 3-7 mice were sacrificed. Both eyes were removed and assayed for HSV-1 as described in Materials and Methods.
[+]Lower limit of virus detection

DISCUSSION

We demonstrated previously that protection from retinitis was mediated by the T cells in the adoptively-transferred activated immune effector population (2). The results of experiments using populations of IEC enriched for either Lyt 2^+ or L3T4$^+$ cells suggest that Lyt 2 cells contribute most of the protective ability in the transferred IEC, since there was a significant difference in the incidence of retinitis between untreated virus-infected mice and virus-infected mice injected with Lyt 2 cells. This finding is consistent with observations of other investigators that transferred HSV-1-specific Lyt 2 cells could protect the majority of mice against fatal herpes virus infections (7,8). In our experiments, transfer of Lyt 2 cells alone reduced the incidence of retinitis from 90.9% in untreated mice to 36.4%, a significant reduction but one which is higher than the 9.5% incidence in the mice treated with unselected activated IEC. Treatment of mice with L3T4 cells alone reduced the incidence of retinitis slightly (60%), a result which suggests that the L3T4 cells in the population of HSV-1-specific IEC also contribute to retinal protection. Further support for a contribution from L3T4 cells is provided by the finding that when both the Lyt 2 cells and L3T4 cells were combined, the incidence of retinitis was reduced to 20%, a rate approximating that observed in HSV-1 infected mice treated with unseparated IEC (10%). In vivo, the L3T4 cells in the transferred IEC may provide help which allows virus-specific cytotoxic cell precursors to differentiate to fully functional effector cells and, in so doing, increase the level of protection over that afforded by the Lyt 2 cells alone.

It is important to identify the anatomic location at which the transferred IEC act to prevent retinitis in the uninoculated eye. We examined the early (day 1, 2, 3 p.i) and late (day 10 p.i.) virus titers in both the inoculated and the uninoculated eye to determine if IV transfer of IEC affected virus titers. After AC inoculation of HSV-1, virus replicates to high titer (approx. 6.0 Log_{10} PFU/ml) in the inoculated eyes of mice within 24 hours of infection, and the titer of virus reaches a peak on day 3 p.i. (5). In these experiments, the early titers of virus in the inoculated eyes of mice treated IV with IEC were not significantly reduced from the titers of virus in the inoculated eyes of untreated HSV-1-infected mice. Since virus replication in the inoculated eye was not affected by treatment with virus-specific IEC, these results suggest that IEC do not protect against retinitis by preventing virus replication in the inoculated eye.

After uniocular AC inoculation of HSV-1, virus spreads from the injected eye through the central nervous system (CNS) to the uninoculated eye (5,9). In uninoculated eyes of IEC-treated mice, only low titers of virus were recovered on day 10 p.i., the day on which the maximum titer of virus was recovered from uninjected eyes of untreated mice with retinitis (5). This result suggests that transferred IEC prevent replication of the virus comprising the second wave which, in turn, reduces the amount of virus in the uninoculated eye on day 10 p.i. below the threshold needed for retinitis. Thus, transferred IEC must protect by limiting virus replication and/or spread within the CNS - either by direct killing of virus-infected cells or by elaboration of cytokines such as gamma interferon which would limit the replication and/or spread of the virus. Studies are in progress to determine the location in the CNS where the interaction of virus and adoptively-transferred IEC occurs.

ACKNOWLEDGEMENTS

This work was supported in part by NIH grants AI 23285 (SSA, JWS), EY 06012 (SSA) and EY 05678 (JWS).

REFERENCES

1.   Whittum JA, McCulley JP, Niederkorn JY, Streilein JW (1984) Invest Ophthalmol Vis Sci 25:1065-1073
2.   Igietseme JU, Calzada PJ, Gonzalez AR, Streilein JW, Atherton SS (1989) J Virol 63:4808-4813
3.   Niederkorn JY, Streilein JW, Shadduck JA (1981) Invest Ophthalmol Vis Sci 20:355-363
4.   Kielty D, Cousins SW, Atherton SS (1987) Invest Ophthalmol Vis Sci 28:1994-1999
5.   Atherton SS, Streilein JW (1987) Invest Ophthalmol Vis Sci 28:571-579
6.   Cousins SW, Gonzalez AR, Atherton SS (1989) Invest Ophthalmol Vis Sci 30:1485-1494
7.   Larsen HS, Russell RG, Rouse BT (1983) Infect Immun 41:197-204
8.   Sethi KK, Omata Y, Schneweis KE (1983) J Gen Virol 64:443-447
9.   Olson RM, Holland GM, Goss SJ, Bowers WD, Meyers-Elliot RH (1987) Curr Eye Res 6:59-62

© 1990 Elsevier Science Publishers (Biomedical Division)
Ocular Immunology Today. M. Usui, S. Ohno and K. Aoki, editors.

ANTI-IDIOTYPIC ANTIBODIES (INTERNAL IMAGE) MODULATE AUTOIMMUNE UVEORETINITIS INDUCED BY S-ANTIGEN

Y. DE KOZAK[1], M. MIRSHAHI[1], C. BOUCHEIX[2] AND J.P. FAURE[1].
[1] INSERM U86, Immunopathologie de l'Oeil, Centre des Cordeliers, Paris, France.
[2] INSERM U268, Villejuif, France.

INTRODUCTION

According to the network theory of Jerne (1), idiotypic interactions occur during immune responses to external or self antigens at humoral and cellular levels and can modulate these reactions. The regulation of the response to self antigens has been called the "autoimmune network" by Zanetti et al.(2).

The injection of an antigen induces the production of a first set of antibodies (Ab1 or idiotype) which stimulate a second cascade of antibodies (Ab2, anti-idiotypic (anti-Id) antibodies). Ab2 beta, called "internal image" are able to mimic the antigen structure of an epitope of the antigen and induce an immune response (Ab3) that is anti-antigen.

Experimental autoimmune uveoretinitis is an ocular inflammatory disease induced in laboratory animals by a single injection of a purified protein from the retina: S-Antigen (S-Ag) leading to the destruction of the visual cells of the retina. We have previously reported the suppression of the disease by injecting monoclonal antibodies (mAbs) against the autoantigen (3) given either simultaneously (4) or prior (5) to the S-Ag challenge. Anti-idiotypic (anti-Id) antibodies were detected in the sera of mAb-injected rats (5). The suppression of EAU was adoptively transferred by using cells from donors immunized with the mAb S2D2 to naive recipients, prior to immunization with S-Ag in CFA (6). MAb S2D2 (IgG 2b) was found particularly effective in disease suppression. It is directed against an epitope located in the N-terminal region of the S-Ag molecule in the amino acid sequence 40-50 (R. Stiemer et al., article in preparation). This sequence (peptide S2) is distant from the region containing the presently known uveitogenic sites (241-320).

The aim of the present study was to determine the role of anti-Id-S2D2 antibodies, internal image of the epitope recognized by the mAb S2D2, in the regulation of the immune response to S-Ag.

MATERIAL AND METHODS

Anti-Id S2D2 antibodies preparation

Antibodies against the idiotype S2D2 were raised in heterozygous rnu/+ rats by 3 injections of 100 µg of protein A purified mAb S2D2 with adjuvant, one injection every two weeks. Control antibodies were prepared using antibodies against monoclonal antibody PM1 of the same isotype IgG2b as S2D2 but with an unrelated specificity (directed against a human leukocyte differentiation antigen).

Anti-Id S2D2 antibodies (internal image) were purified by immunoaffinity chromatography on PM1 bound Sepharose 4B followed by immunoaffinity chromatography on S2D2-bound Sepharose 4B. The removal of antibodies directed against constant-region determinant on mouse immunoglobulin was monitored in ELISA by the progressive failure of the rat sera to bind to wells coated with the control mAb.

Induction of EAU

Rats were preimmunized with 3 subcutaneous injections on the back of the purified rat polyclonal anti-Id S2D2 antibody in adjuvant. Seven days after the last mAb injection, rats were challenged in the foot pads with 50 or 100 µg of purified bovine S-Ag in 0.1 ml of saline mixed with 0.1 ml of complete Freund's adjuvant containing 150 µg of M. tuberculosis H37 Ra.

Histological assessment of EAU

Animals were sacrificed 30 days after S-Ag immunization. Disease severity was graded from 0 to 4 according to the extent of the destruction of the outer layers of the retina (6).

Lymphocyte proliferation assay

Draining lymph node cells were collected 7 days after the last injection of anti-Id S2D2 antibody and tested for specific responses to anti-S2D2 antibody (20 µg/ml) and S-Ag (20 or 100 µg/ml) by an in vitro proliferation assay. The stimulation was measured by thymidine uptake and expressed as stimulation index values (SI=mean cpm/min in cultures with antigen/mean cpm/min in cultures without antigen).

Titration of anti-S-Ag antibodies

Anti-S-Ag antibodies were detected in rat sera by ELISA (4) using
a peroxidase-labeled mouse anti-rat kappa chain mAb (MARK,
Immunotech, Luminy, Marseille, France).

RESULTS
Inhibitory effect of anti-S2D2 antibody immunization on EAU

Histological examination showed that almost all rats (18/20 eyes)
preimmunized with anti-S2D2 antibodies in adjuvant before S-Ag were
protected while most of the controls preimmunized with 3 injections
of IgG directed at the control mAb PM1 before S-Ag challenge
developed an ocular inflammation (Fig.1).

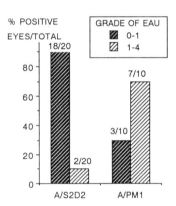

Fig.1. Inhibitory effect
(histological examination) of
preimmunization with 3 injections
of anti-S2D2 antibodies
on EAU induced by 1 injection of
S-Ag in adjuvant.

In vitro proliferative response of cells from rats immunized with anti-S2D2 antibodies

All the 6 rats immunized with anti-S2D2 antibodies presented a
lymphocyte stimulation to anti-S2D2, and cells from the 4 rats
presenting the highest stimulation to anti-S2D2, were stimulated by
S-Ag. Rats injected with the control anti-PM1 antibodies were not
stimulated by any of the 2 stimulants tested. (Fig.2).
So these cells respond to both anti-S2D2 and the S-Ag molecule,
indicating that anti-S2D2 antibodies act as an internal image for
the antigen at the T-cell level.
Antibodies against S-Ag in rats injected with anti-S2D2 antibodies

Injection of anti-S2D2 antibodies induced the production of
antibodies directed at S-Ag (Ab3, equivalent to S2D2). They are
specific for S-Ag, as an incubation with S-Ag, allowed to decrease

the serum S-Ag reactivity on S-Ag coated plates (Fig.3).

These results confirm that anti-Id S2D2 antibodies act as an internal image, inducing the formation of Ab3 antibodies, equivalent to S2D2.

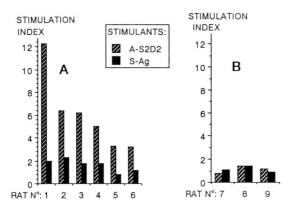

Fig.2. Proliferative response of draining lymph node cells to anti-S2D2 antibodies or to S-Ag in rats immunized with 3 injections of anti-S2D2 antibodies (A) or with antibodies directed at the control mAb PM1 (B).

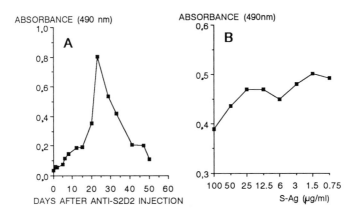

Fig.3. A : Evolution of anti-S-Ag antibodies of sequential sera from a rat immunized with one injection of 200 µg of purified anti-S2D2 antibodies in adjuvants. Anti-S-Ag antibodies appear from the 6th day after immunization, to peak on the 23th day, and decrease thereafter.(plates coated with 5 µg/ml of S-Ag were incubated with sera diluted 1:80 then with MARK/PO diluted 1:1000 for detection of anti-S-Ag rat antibodies). B : inhibition of S-Ag reactivity of rat serum,(taken on the 23th day after immunization with anti-S2D2 antibody), diluted 1:80 and incubated with serial dilutions of S-Ag, before testing on S-Ag coated plates.

CONCLUSION

Immunization of rats with purified rat polyclonal anti-S2D2 antibodies allows to inhibit EAU induced by S-Ag challenge. It has been shown in other systems that the immunization with anti-Id antibodies can induce specific antibody and/or T-cell responses to a given antigen (7,8,9). Rats immunized with anti-Id-S2D2 present a cellular response to both S-Ag and anti-Id S2D2, and develop Ab3 antibodies (equivalent to S2D2). So, the inhibitory effect of anti-S2D2 injections on EAU is related to the presence, at the time of S-Ag immunization, of anti-S2D2 cells and S2D2 equivalent antibodies. These results suggest that the suppression of EAU can be produced through an activation of the idiotypic network. Internal image of selected epitopes used as surrogate antigen could be of value to therapy of autoimmune diseases

ACKNOWLEDGEMENTS
The authors would like to thank J. Cozette, B. Thillaye, M. Barral for their collaboration in this work.

REFERENCES
1. Jerne NK (1984) Immunol Rev 79:5-24
2. Zanetti M (1986) Crit Rev Immunol 6:151-183
3. Faure JP, Mirshahi M, Dorey C, Thillaye B, de Kozak Y, Boucheix C (1984) Curr Eye Res 3:867-872
4. de Kozak Y, Mirshahi M, Boucheix C, Faure JP (1985) Eur J Immunol 15:1107-1111
5. de Kozak Y, Mirshahi M, Boucheix C, Faure JP (1987) Eur J Immunol 17:541-547
6. de Kozak Y, Mirshahi M, Boucheix C,, Faure JP (1990) Regional Immunol in press
7. Eichmann K, Rajewski K (1975) Eur J Immunol 5:661-666
8. Gaulton GN, Sharpe AH, Chang DW, Fields BN, Greene MI (1986) J Immunol 137:2930-2936
9. Singhai R, Levy JG (1987) Proc Natl Acad Sci USA 84:3836-3840

© 1990 Elsevier Science Publishers (Biomedical Division)
Ocular Immunology Today. M. Usui, S. Ohno and K. Aoki, editors.

THE INDUCTION OF SPECIFIC TOLERANCE TO THE RETINAL S-ANTIGEN VIA FEEDING

ROBERT NUSSENBLATT, STEPHAN THURAU, RACHEL CASPI, AND
HOWARD WEINER*

Laboratory of Immunology, NIH, Bldg 10, Rm 10N-202, Bethesda MD
20892, (USA), and *Center for Neurologic Disease, Brigham and
Women's Hospital, Boston, MA, 02115 (USA).

INTRODUCTION

The development of specific therapies for human disorders of putative autoimmune cause is a goal for those in many specialties where there is sole organ disease. Therapy for severe sight threatening intraocular inflammatory disease (or uveitis) is today dependent on medications that are non-specific in their mode of action. While still non-specific, cyclosporine begins to approach this therapeutic goal, with its mode of action more specific than other medications presently available since its primary effect is limited to T-cells (1). Newer methods by which such antigen and organ specific immunosuppression can be acheived seems now to be a reasonable goal. One such an approach is presented here, with the use of feeding of ocular antigen capable of inducing specific suppression of experimental autoimmune uveitis. Additionally, we will show that this suppression can be transferred to naïve animals, with prevention of disease expression in these animals as well.

MATERIAL AND METHODS

Animals. Female adult Lewis rats weighing 180-200 gms were used for all the experiments.

Feeding protocol. Animals were fed with either the whole S-antigen molecule, or the two fragments that have been shown to date to induce uveitis in rats. Animals were fed with 1 mg of S-antigen on days -7, -5, and -2 (2). For active challenge,immunization was performed as described below.

Immunization. Animals were challenged with 30 μg of retinal S-antigen emulsified with complete Freund's adjuvant, given in 0.1 ml of the mixture in one hindpad injection. No pertussis was given.

In vitro suppression of proliferative response to T-cell lines. Two T cell lines prepared as described elsewhere (3) were used as responder cells. The first cell, designated as TH S, is S-antigen specific and has the capacity to induce EAU in naïve recipients. The second T-cell line, designated as TH P, responds in vitro to stimulation with the purified protein derivative (PPD). These cells were mixed in co-culture with modulator cells obtained from the spleens of animals fed with S-antigen or not fed.

Adoptive transfer of protection. Lewis rats were fed with 1 mg of S-antigen on day -17, -15, -13, -10, and day -7. On day -2, the animals were sacrificed and the spleens placed in culture and stimulated with concanavalin A. After 48 hours in cultures (i.e. day 0), the cells were collected, washed and a total of .4 to 1 x 10^8 cells were transferred to each naïve host, who was then immunized with the retinal S-antigen (30 µg) in complete Freund's adjuvant. The experiment was then terminated on day 21.

RESULTS

Effects of feeding S-antigen on active immunization. Feeding animals with the complete molecule of S-antigen was capable of protecting animals subsequently immunized with either the S-antigen or the uveitogenic fragments of the S-antigen, N and M. However, feeding with these fragments in quantities several times the amount found in the S-antigen molecule, either separately or together, was not capable of protecting animals from the expression of uveitis after immunization with the S-antigen.

In vitro mixing experiments. In order to determine whether cellular elements were being induced by feeding with the S-antigen, mixing experiments with antigen specific T-cell lines were performed. An example of such a mixing experiment can be seen in Figure 1. As can be seen in the experiment labeled as TH S/S-AG, the response of this antigen specific T cell line, when stimulated with the retinal S-antigen not in the presence of spleen modulator cells from S-antigen fed animals (1:0) gives a strong proliferative response, with a stimulation index of about 75. However, with the addition of these modulator cells the proliferative response precipitously drops to almost zero at the 1:5 mixing combination. These results are in marked contradistinction to the responses seen when the responder cell is the T-cell specific to PPD. Here the addition of the splenic derived modulator cells induced essentially no change in the proliferative response. A similar response can be seen in the series of experiments labeled TH S/NONE. Here the modulator cells originated from animals that were not fed antigen. In the presence of these cells, no significant change in the proliferative response can be noted.

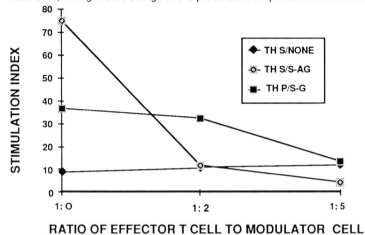

Fig. 1. Mixing of splenic modulator cells with antigen specific T-cells.

Adoptive transfer of suppression to naïve hosts. Figure 2 shows the ability to adoptively transfer this protection. The initial line shows the lack of protection when animals actively immunized are fed an unrelated antigen, such as KLH or BSA. The second line shows the lack of protection obtained when the animals that donated cells were fed a similar unrelated antigen. Line three demonstrates the excellent protection obtained when animals actively immunized with the S-antigen are fed the same antigen. The final line demonstrates the protection achieved when cells from S-antigen fed animals are transferred intra-peritoneally to animals then actively immunized with the same antigen.

434

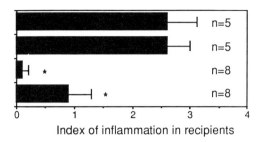

Animals directly fed with unrelated antigen   n=5

Donor fed with unrelated antigen   n=5

Animals directly fed with S-Ag   n=8 *

Donor fed with S-Ag   n=8 *

Index of inflammation in recipients

Fig. 2. S-Ag induced inflammation in recipients of spleen cells from antigen fed donors

DISCUSSION

We have been able to demonstrate that feeding uveitogenic antigens is a viable approach by which effective suppression of EAU can be achieved. Further, the cellular basis of this protection can be demonstrated by the adoptive transfer of splenic-derived modulator cells. This approach to therapy has now been demonstrated in at least two animal models for autoimmune disease (2,4). We feel that this approach is a practical one to be considered for the treatment of human disease. Such a project has begun at the National Eye Institute, with the hope that immunomodulation will be achieved for the first time without the use of an exogenous medication, but rather an autoantigen.

ACKNOWLEDGEMENTS

We wish to thank Mr. Rashid Mahdi for his excellent technical help. SRT received a scholarship from the German Research Council (DFG)

REFERENCES

1.   Nussenblatt RB, Palestine AG (1986)   Surv Ophthalmol 31:159-169

2.   Nussenblatt RB, Caspi RR, R Mahdi, CC Chan, F Roberge, O Lider, HL Weiner (1990)   J Immunol (in press)

3.   Caspi RR, Roberge FG, McAllister CG, El-Saied M, Kuwabara T, Gery I, Hanna E, Nussenblatt B (1986) J Immunol 136:928-933

4.   Lider O, LMB Santos, CSY Lee, PJ Higgins, HL Weiner (1989) J Immunol   142:748-752.

© 1990 Elsevier Science Publishers (Biomedical Division)
Ocular Immunology Today. M. Usui, S. Ohno and K. Aoki, editors.

MODULATION OF EXPERIMENTAL ALLERGIC UVEITIS BY PERTUSSIN TOXIN

GEORGE E. MARAK, JR., D. S. GREGERSON, L. ATTLA, N. A. RAO
Georgetown University, Washington, D. C.; University of
Minneapolis and University of California, Los Angeles (U.S.A.)

Pertussin Toxin (PT) is frequently employed as an adjuvant in
the introduction of experimental allergic uveitis (EAU). Unfortunately, the immunomodulatory effects of PT are highly variable and
not well understood. PT appears to be immunostimulatory when
given at the time of sensitization[1] but immunosuppressive when
introduced at the onset of the effector response.[2] PT is a
profound inhibitor of inflammatory cell activation.[3]

Lewis rats sensitized to 50 μg of retinal 's' antigen given 1 μg
PT intraperitoneally at the time of sensitization had enhanced
inflammation compared to controls. The animals receiving PT on
days 10-14 after sensitization were completely clear of inflammation. A second group of Lewis rats were sensitized to lens protein
according to a protocol which produces a severe Arthus reaction
in nearly all animals within 24 hours of lens injury.[4] Only a
small antiphlogistic effect was observed with PT treatment.

One component of the antiphlogistic activity of PT is attributed
to inhibition of stimulus-response coupling in inflammatory cells.
After binding of the B-oligomer of PT to the cell surface, the
A-protomer penetrates the cell membrane where it catalyses the
ADP ribosylation of G-proteins. This results in loss of the
activity of the G-protein and interference in signal transduction.[5,6] PT has been demonstrated to inhibit a variety of phlogsitic
activities of several types of inflammatory cells.[7,8]

The observed complete inhibition of EAU and the minimal effect
of PT treatment in lens induced uveitis suggest that other
antiphlogistic mechanisims may be more important than the effect
on G-proteins.

Another significant antiphlogistic activity of PT is interference
in lymphocyte migration and homing to sites of inflammation.
Lymphocytes exit the circulation at specialized post-capillary
venules termed high endothelial venules (HEV) by virtue of their
tall cuboidal endothelium, by differences in metabolic activity
and the character of the surrounding inflammation.[9]

Specialized receptors or ligands found on inflammatory cells and HEV are important for adhesion of cells to vessels in inflammatory foci.[10] There appears to be some regional specialization of adhesion mechanisms since MEL-14 does not block adhesion to inflammed synovium.[11]

Two systems of adhesion molecules have been studied in detail, the system defined by the monoclonal antibody MEL-14 (the human counterpart CD44) and the CD11/CD18 complex of integrins (LFA-1, MAC-1, p150, 95). Additional adhesion molecules include MHC-II antigens and soluble components of lymphocyte adhesion molecules termed HEBF's.[12] Ia antigens are important for the binding of CD4+ lymphocytes and it is known that there is increased expression of Ia antigens on vascular endothelium in uveitis.[13]

Additional endothelial cell receptors or ligends have been described including ICAM-1 which is the ligand for LFA-1, ELAM-1, MECA-325, etc. Specific adhesion sites on vascular endothelial cells have been termed addressins.[10]

There appear to be differences in the adhesion molecules on various inflammatory cell types. Lactose-1-phosphate inhibits macrophage adhesion but has little effect on lymphocyte adhesion. Mannose-6-phosphate inhibits lymphocyte adhesion but not monocyte binding. Under comparable conditions (HUVEC monolayers, 37°, 15 min) TS1-22 a monoclonal antibody to CD11a (LFA-1) has no effect on the binding of lymphocytes but inhibits neutrophil binding to vascular endothelium. Although TS1-22 does not inhibit lymphocyte adhesion it does inhibit migration across endothelial cell monolayers.[15, 16]

Pertussis toxin does not interface with lymphocyte adhesion but appears to block lymphocyte migration to foci of inflammation in the absence of any effect on proliferative or cytotoxic responses (since the local injection as opposed to intravenous injection of PT treated lymphocytes produces a normal inflammatory response).[8] PT has also been reported to interfere with macrophage, neutrophil and lymphocyte chemotaxis. The antiphogistic effects of PT in EAU are hypothesized to be related to the inhibiting effects of PT on the migration of lymphocytes to the uvea and retina possibly through effects on the CD11/CD18 complex or alterations in adenate cyclase activity.

Pertussis vaccine contains a variety of immunomodulating
agents. One of these agents PT has a variety of immunomodulating
activities. Since many studies of EAU employ PT as an adjavant
investigators should be aware of the many ill understood and
poorly controlled immunomodulatory variables that use of PT involves.

REFERENCES

1. de Kozak Y, Tillaye B, Reynard G, Faure JP (1978)
   Graefe's Arch Exp Ophthalmol 208:135-142

2. Spangrude GV, Aranco BP, Daynes RA (1985) J. Immunol 134:2900-
   2907

3. Jakeway JP, DeFranco Al (1986) Science 234:734-735

4. Marak GE, Font RL, Alepa FP (1977) Ophthalmic Res 9:162-170

5. Ui M (1984) Trends Pharmacol Sci 5:222-279

6. Okajima F, Ui M (1984) J. Biol Chem 259:13863-13871

7. Meade BO, Kind PD, Manclark CR (1985) Develop Biol Standard
   61:63-78

8. Spangrude GJ, Sacchi F, Hill HR, VanEpps DE, Daynes RN (1985)
   J. Immunol 135:4135-4134

9. Yednock TA, Rosen SO 1989 in Dixon FJ (ed) Advances in
   Immunology Vol. 44 Academic Press, New York pp 313-378

10. Jalkanen S, Reichert R, Gallatin WMG, Bargatze RF, Weissman IL,
    Butcher EC (1986) Immunol Rev 91, pp 39-60

11. Jalkanen S, Steere AC, Fox RI, Butcher EL, Science 233: 556-559

12. Chin YH, Cary GO, Woodruff JJ (1983) J.Immunol 131:1368-1374

13. Fujikawa LS, Chan CC, McAllister C, Gery I, Hooks JJ, Detrick B,
    Nussenblatt RB 1989 in Secchi A, Fregona IA (eds) Modern Trends
    in Immunology and Immunopathology of the Eye, Masson, Milan
    pp 69-75

14. DiCorletto PC and de la Molte CA (1989) J. Immunol
    143:3666-3672

15. Van Epps DE, Potter J, Vachula M, Smith CW, Anderson C
    (1989) J. Immunol 143:3207-3210

16. Lo SK, Van Seventer S, Levin M, Wright SD (1989)
    J. Immunol 143:3325-3329

© 1990 Elsevier Science Publishers (Biomedical Division)
Ocular Immunology Today. M. Usui, S. Ohno and K. Aoki, editors.

PROLACTIN IN HUMAN AQUEOUS HUMOR OF UVEITIS AND NONUVEITIS CATARACT PATIENTS

*U. Pleyer, *E.G. Weidle, *M. Zierhut, *W. Lisch, *H.-J. Thiel
**D. Gupta

*   University Eye Hospital, Dept. of General Ophthalmology
**   University Children´s Hospital
Dept. of Diagnostic Endocrinology, Tübingen (R. F. Germany)

INTRODUCTION

Cumulative data suggest that the immune response as a homeostatic system is subject to neuroendocrine control (1). Especially polypeptide hormones of pituitary origin are involved in immune modulation. Among these, prolactin (Prl) furnishes the clearest evidence of having regulatory effects on both, humoral and cell mediated immune response. Hypophysectomy or treatment with Prl-release inhibitor bromocriptine (Brc) suppresses antibody formation and development of delayed type hypersensitivity, while exogenous Prl reconstitutes physiological immune response in rodent models (2,3). Diminished inflammatory response in different autoimmune models including Experimental Autoimmune Uveitis (EAU) by lowering circulating Prl levels with Brc treatment, suggest a possible role in these diseases (4,5,6). A basis for this immunomodulatory effects has been established by the finding of specific Prl receptors on peripheral T- and B- lymphocytes (7). Based upon these observations and the presumed immune mediated pathogenesis of idiopathic anterior uveitis (IAU), we measured Prl concentrations in patients with and without history of this disease.

PATIENTS AND METHODS

Prl concentrations in aqueous humor and serum were analysed in 28 cataract patients, 13 women and 15 men between 18 and 85 years of age. Group A consisted of 14 subjects (mean age: 53 +/- 22 a) with a previous history of IAU subsided for at least 3 months at the time of surgery. Five of these patients have been HLA B 27 positive. 14 cataract patients (mean age : 55 +/- 14.6 a) without any history of intraocular inflammation volunteered as controls. All except two operations were done with re-trobulbar anesthesia containing an mixture of xylocaine 1% along with epinephrine (1:100 000). Paracentesis was performed under microscopic control with a tuberculin syringe before opening the anterior chamber allowing about 50-150 ul of aqueous humor to be aspirated. At the same time 5 ml venous blood was withdrawn. To avoid major circardial variations of Prl levels, only samples taken between 8.oo to 14.oo hours were accepted.

Prolactin concentrations were measured by radioimmunoassay (IBL Hamburg, F.R.G.) in large series at the end of the protocol to avoid variations between assays.

Statistic analysis

Students t-test was used to evaluate the significance of differences between both groups. Values are expressed as means +/- SE. All p-values were two-sided.

RESULTS

Prl was detected in each sample. Serum concentrations varied in a wide range from 3.6 - 44.6 ng/ml (mean 13.6 +/- 8.3), aqueous humor levels from 0.1 - 3.4 ng/ml (mean 1.25 +/- 1.05). No correlation between serum and aqueous humor concentration was found in either group (fig.1a/b). Wheras serum levels failed to show significant difference between both groups (p< 0.11), intraocular hormone concentrations were significantly higher in uveitis patients (1.9 +/- 0.9 ng/ml) than in controls (0.53 +/- 0.47 ng/ml , p < 0.001, fig. 2).

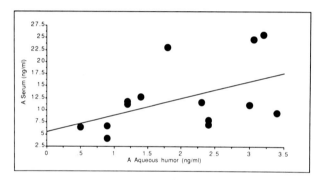

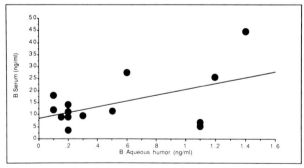

Fig.1a/b.:   Regression analysis. No correlation between aqueous humor and serum prolactin levels has been found in IAU/nonuveitis patients.

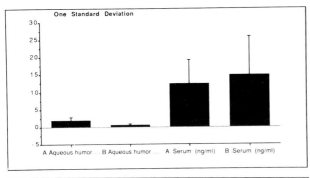

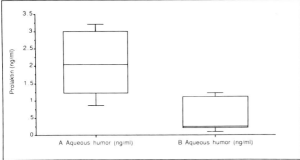

Fig 2: Prolactin concentrations in aqueous humor. Significant difference (p<0.001) has been observed in patients with a positive history of idiopathic anterior uveitis (A n=14) to a control group (B n=14). Values are represented as Mean +/- SEM. Statistical analysis were based on 2-tailed Student's t-test.

DISCUSSION

Prolactin has been observed in blood, milk, cerebrospinal fluid and tears, but we found no reports of PRL levels in aqueous humor (8,9). Since numerous data suggest an immunomodulatory role of the hormone, we evaluated its concentration in uveitis and nonuveitis patients. The significantly increased intraocular Prl level raises the questions of access of the polypeptide (MG 26 000-60 000) into aqueous humor and the relevance of increased concentrations to intraocular inflammation. Because de-stabilisation of the blood-aqueous humor barrier after paracentesis has been similar in both groups, it should not have played a major role. It is more likely that Prl concentrations in uveitis patients may represent a secondary aqueous humor in the postinflammatory state of the disease. Of interest are observations that among all other polypeptide hormones, Prl has an unique cerebrospinal accessibility (10). Radioautografic studies indicate that Prl is transported by a specific receptor mediated

442

mechanism at the choroid plexus (11). Since the aqueous producing ciliary epithelium and the choroid plexus are embryogenically similar , their transport mechanism may be identical too.

In attempting to explain how elevated intraocular Prl levels occur, a particular attention has to be focused on its impact on uveitis. Since the pathogenesis of IAU is presumed to be immune mediated, modulation of neuroendocrine origin may have importance. It has been demonstrated that elevated levels of Prl were consistently associated with decreased suppressor cell functions and production of interleukin-2 in man (12). Of further interest are findings that lymphocytes themselves synthesize mRNA for Prl (13). In addition, data of Hiestand and Mekler suggest that T-cell response to antigen is dependend on pituitary derived Prl, and these activated lymphocytes produce a secondary signal in form of a Prl related polypeptide, which amplify immune response (13). Whether local Prl levels in the eye are of immune stimulatory importance still remains speculative. No inflammatory signs were present in our patients in spite of elevated intraocular hormone levels. It is possible, however, that we had observed the waning of a high prolactin level during the peak period of the disease. The question whether the rise of PRL in aqueous humor is primarily related to uveitis or indirectly associated with it, remains to be elucidated.

REFERENCES

1. Besedovsky, H., A. Del Rey, E. Sorkin (1983) In: Fabris, Garaci, Hadden (eds.) Immunoregulation Plenum Press, New York, pp 315-339
2. Berczi, I., E. Nagy, S. Asa and K. Kovacs (1983) Allergy 38: 325-330
3. Nagy, E., Berczi I., Friesen H. (1983) Acta endocrinol. 102: 351-357
4. Berczi, I., E. Nagy, S. Asa , K. Kovacs (1983) Arthritis Rheum. 27: 682-688
5. Nagy, E., I. Berzci, G.Wren, S. Asa, K. Kovacs (1983) Immunopharmacol. 6: 231-243
6. Palestine A.G., G. Mullenberg-Coulombre, M. Kim, M. Gelato, R. B. Nussenblatt (1987) J. Clin. Invest. 79: 1078-1081
7. Russell, D., R. Kibler, L. Matrisian, D. Lason, B. Poulos and B. Magun (1985) J. Immunol. 134: 3027-3031
8. Nicoll,C. (1974) In: Knobil. Sawyer, Handbook of Physiology sect 7, Vol. 2 part 2, pp 253-293
9. Frey, W., J. Nelson, M.Frick, R. Elde (1986) In: Holly F. Preocular tear film pp 798 -806
10. Login, I. and R. Mac Leod (1977) Brain research 132: 477-48o
11. Walsh, R. J., F. Slaby and B. Posner (1987) Endocrinology 120: 1846-1850
12. Vidaller A., L. Lorente., F. Larrea, J. Mendez., J. Alcocer-Varela., D. Alarcon-Segovia (1986) J. Clin. Immunol. 38: 337-343
13. Hiestand P.C., P. Mekler (1986) Prog. Allergy 38: 239-246

© 1990 Elsevier Science Publishers (Biomedical Division)
Ocular Immunology Today. M. Usui, S. Ohno and K. Aoki, editors.

IMMUNOSUPPRESSIVE THERAPY OF UVEITIS: MID- AND LONG-TERM FOLLOW-UP AFTER CLASSICAL
CYTOSTATIC TREATMENT

ANNE-CATHERINE MARTENET
Eye Clinic, University Hospital, CH-8091 Zurich

Immunosuppression has been one of the most important therapeutic modalities in
chronic severe uveitis for many years. The first assays with the cytostatic drug
nitrogen mustard were published in 1951 (1) and 1952 (2) by Roda-Perez, almost
before the era of steroids. If since, these last compounds have become the most
utilized, the cytostatics have also kept an important place in the treatment
of uveitis, and recently, the promising non cytotoxic drug cyclosporine A has
been added to our therapeutic arsenal.

Up to now there has been almost no report on very late results of all these
therapies. We would like to present here patients who had cytostatic treatment
for uveitis and were followed 1 to 20 years after therapy.

MATERIAL AND METHODS

Between 1968 and 1989, we treated 268 uveitis patients with cytostatic drugs,
principally cyclophosphamide, combined in most adults with the antimitotic drug
procarbazine (3). Only a few patients were treated with azathioprine or chlorambucil, none with cyclosporine A. Of 64 patients with Behçet'disease, the 45 followed for more than one year were presented in 1988 (4). Among the 204 patients
with other forms of uveitis, 73 could not be included in the present study, because the follow-up remained under one year, or the records were insufficiently
documented or lost. We therefore present 131 patients followed 1-4 years, and
81 of them followed 5-20 years. The evaluation of the results is based on the
visual acuity before treatment and at the end of the follow-up, a parameter also
chosen by Nussenblatt et al (5) or BenEzra et al (6).

RESULTS (Fig. 1-5)

We consider the effect of the therapy to be a success if the inflammation is
stopped and the function improved, half a success if the inflammation is stopped
without improvement of the function, and a failure if the treatment had no effect
on inflammation. The classification into these three categories was done shortly
after the end of therapy, but has been reconsidered now if late complications
caused a marked late visual loss. We classified such cases as failures, even
if the inflammation was definitively stopped. But we retained in the groups of
success or half success the cases where a cataract or a discrete macular edema
without inflammatory signs caused a slight decrease of visual acuity.

444

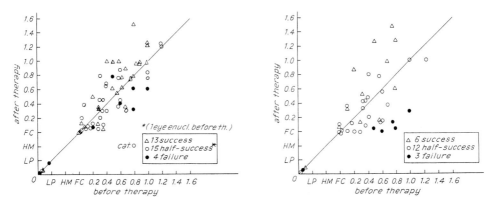

Fig. 1. Immunosuppressive therapy of intermediate uveitis in adults
Visual acuity 1-4 years (left) and 5-12 years (right) after therapy

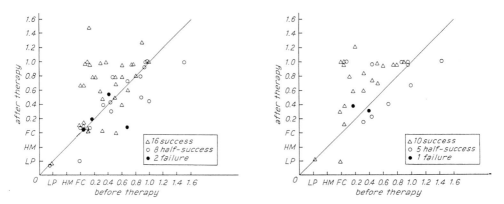

Fig. 2. Immunosuppressive therapy of intermediate uveitis in Children
Visual acuity 1-4 years (left) and 5-16 years (right) after therapy

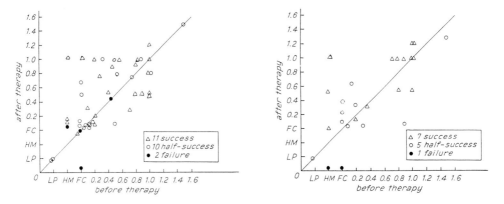

Fig. 3. Immunosuppressive therapy of anterior uveitis in children (JRA)
Visual acuity 1-4 years (left) and 5-17 years (right) after therapy

In *intermediate uveitis in adults*, Fig 1 shows that, 1-4 years after therapy, about 2/3 of the eyes had a visual acuity identical or better to the pretherapeutical value. However, after a longer follow-up, almost half of the eyes had a slightly decreased visual acuity, mostly due to lens opacities or macular edema. The same remarks can be done for the *intermediate uveitis in children* (Fig. 2). In *anterior uveitis in children with JRA* (Fig 3), the late decrease of vision is mostly due to a secondary glaucoma, or, in the milder cases, to lens opacities.

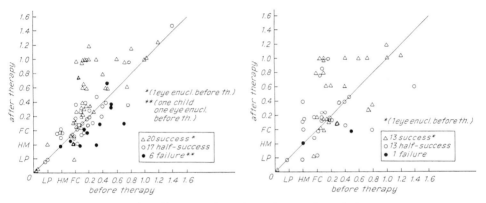

Fig. 4. Immunosuppressive therapy of various forms of uveitis
Visual acuity 1-4 years (left) and 5-20 (right) after therapy

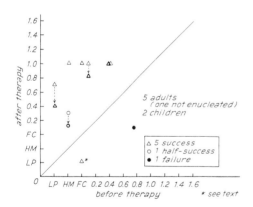

Fig. 5. Immunosuppressive therapy of sympathetic ophthalmia. Visual acuity 1-4 years (thin signs) and 5-13 years (thick signs) after therapy (* see text)

In the *various forms of uveitis* (Fig 4), which include chronic anterior uveitis, chronic panuveitis and rare cases of VKH and ARN, we have some failures with rather good visual acuity, but still a discrete inflammatory activity, at least in the first post-therapeutic period. Later on, the results appear quite satisfactory. In *sympathetic ophthalmia* (Fig 5), the slight visual decrease in very late stages is due to a beginning cataract (of the senile type in a 67 year old patient). The eye recorded as a success* despite visual decrease is the sympathizing eye which was not enucleated and was finally lost by secondary glaucoma due to angle synechiae, while the inflammatory process was absolutely healed.

Only in a few cases, a post-cure with the same cytostatic drugs was necessary after the primary treatment: 3 in intermediate uveitis in adults, 2 in the same in children, 1 in anterior uveitis in JRA, and 5 in the various forms of uveitis. Some more patients, however, had steroids for some period during the follow-up. Post-cure was never necessary in sympathetic ophthalmia, and 5 of these 7 patients had the drugs only 5-8 months.

DISCUSSION

The main observation in this series is a slight decrease of visual acuity through the years, even in successful cases. Several factors contribute to this point. First, the slow post-inflammatory (or sometimes age-related) development of lens opacities, then, especially in intermediate uveitis, the occurrence of a late post-inflammatory macular edema, and, finally, in anterior uveitis associated with JRA, the development of a severe secondary glaucoma, often in aphakic eyes. On the other side, there were not many cases with persistent inflammatory signs, i.e. late failures. We finally note that no systemic or haematologic important complication of the treatment was ever observed, except for a few cases of azoospermia.

In conclusion, we think that immunosuppressive treatment by classical cytostatic drugs remains a valuable alternative in severe uveitis and has long-lasting, satisfactory effect on visual acuity. However, we feel that similar studies should be undertaken after cyclosporin A or steroid therapy.

ACKNOWLEDGMENTS

We are grateful to Ivan Glitsch for drawing the figures and to Phillip Hendrickson for proofreading the manuscript.

REFERENCES

1. Roda-Perez E (1951) Sobre un caso de uveitis de etiologia ignota tratado con mostaza nitrogenada. Revista clinica espanola, 40: 265-267

2. Roda-Perez E (1952) El tratamiento de las uveitis de etiologia ignota con mostaza nitrogenada. Arch Soc oftal hisp-amer 12: 131-151

3. Martenet AC, Verrey F, Witmer R (1969) Importance d'un nouveau cytostatique (dérivé de la méthylhydrazine) sur l'uvéite expérimentale du lapin. Ophthalmologica, 150: 97-106

4. Martenet AC, Paccolat F (1989) Traitement immunodépresseur du syndrome de Behçet: résultats à long terme. Ophtalmologie 3: 40-42

5. Nussenblatt RB, Palestine AG, Chan CC (1985) Cyclosporine therapy for uveitis: long-term follow-up. J ocular Pharmacol 1: 369-382

6. BenEzra D, Nussenblatt RB, Timonen P (1988) Optimal use of Sandimmun in endogenous uveitis. Springer, Berlin, Heidelberg, New York, London, Paris, Tokyo, pp 1-22

© 1990 Elsevier Science Publishers (Biomedical Division)
Ocular Immunology Today. M. Usui, S. Ohno and K. Aoki, editors.

THE EFFECT OF TOPICAL ANTI-Ia ANTIBODIES ON OCULAR SURFACE LANGERHANS CELLS AND THY-1 LYMPHOCYTES

YOSHITSUGU TAGAWA, FUMIHIKO KITAGAWA AND HIDEHIKO MATSUDA

Department of Ophthalmology, Hokkaido University School of Medicine, Sapporo, JAPAN

INTRODUCTION

We have previously demonstrated that Langerhans cells and Thy-1 lymphocytes were predominant populations of immunocompetent cells resident in the murine ocular surface epithelium, and these cells may play an important role in the ocular surface immune system. (1~2)   We also described that topical application of corticosteroids to normal eyes reduced the number of those immunocompetent cells in the ocular surface, and therefore, it is postulated that the anti-inflammatory action of topical corticosteroids in ocular surface may be through the drug's action to alter those cells. (3~4)   Recently, it became obvious that Ia antigens of MHC class II antigens on Langerhans cells and macrophage-monocyte lineage cells play a critical role in the process of antigen recognitions by T cells and in the regulation of immune responses, and it was shown that in vivo treatment of mice with anti-Ia antibody leads to a temporary loss of all Ia molecules from Ia-bearing spleen cells through modulation. This loss was accompanied by a loss of the immunologic functions of spleen cells from these animals. (5)

In this study we attempted to clarify the effect of topical application of anti-Ia antibodies on those immunocompetent cells in the ocular surface epithelium in normal and pathological eyes, in comparison with those of corticosteroids.

METHODS

Mice : C3H/He mice 4 through 8 weeks of age were used throughout the experiments. Prior to use, all eyes were carefully screened clinically to rule out preexisting disease.

Immunofluorescence : EDTA-separated epithelial sheets were stained by immunofluorescence as previouly reported. (1)

Antisera : anti-I-A^k and anti-Thy-1•2 (Cedarlane Lab.: CL8705, CL8600) were used for the cell surface marker for Langerhans cells and Thy-1 lymphocytes, respectively.

Topical application : anti-I-A^k antibody or 0.1 % betamethasone were instilled topically on mouse eyes five times per day for four days.
Corneal sutures : Corneal sutures of 10-0 nylon were put in the center of the cornea to make pathological conditions in the cornea. Two weeks later, the above eye drops were instilled in mice eyes.

RESULTS

In normal eyes the density of Langerhans cells and Thy-1 cells remained normal four days after treatment with anti-Ia antibodies, whereas betamethasone eye drops markedly reduced the number of Langerhans cells and Thy-1 cells. In sutured eyes Langerhans cells and Thy-1 cells increased in number in the conjunctiva, and migrated into the cornea two weeks after suturing. Anti-Ia antibodies did not affect the density of Langerhans cells and Thy-1 cells in sutured eyes, whereas betamethasone eye drops markedly reduced the number of Langerhans cells and Thy-1 cells in the same fashion as in normal eyes.

DISCUSSION

The above findings suggest that topical anti-Ia treatment on Langerhans cells in the ocular surface epithelium is not effective in reducing or suppressing Ia antigens on ocular surface Langerhans cells, and therefore it does not seem to affect their function as antigen presenting cells (APC). These results are consistent with the results on epidermal Langerhans cells, namely, that in vivo anti-Ia antibodies do not modulate Ia expression by epidermal Langerhans cells, but are in contrast with the report that in vivo treatment of mice with anti-Ia antibodies leads to a temporary loss of all Ia molecules from Ia-bearing spleen cells. (5)

Our results also confirm our previous findings that topical glucocorticoids reduce the number of Ia positive Langerhans cells in either normal or pathological eyes, induced by 10-0 nylon sutures in the cornea. (3~4) Thus, steroids applied topically induce a strong suppression on Ia molecules of ocular surface Langerhans cells. The effect on ocular surface Langerhans cells seemed to be stronger than on Langerhans cells in the epidermis. (6)

We conclude from these findings that topical application of anti-Ia antibodies may not be useful to suppress the local immune response or immune-mediated inflammation of the ocular surface.

REFERENCES

1. Tagawa Y, et al (1985) In: O'Connor GR, Chandler JW(eds) Advances in Immunology and Immunopathology of the Eye. Masson Publishing, New York, pp 203-207

2. Tagawa Y, et al (1985) Acta Soc Ophthalmol Jpn 89:832-837

3. Tagawa Y, et al (1983) Acta Soc Ophthalmol Jpn 87:927-934

4. Tagawa Y, et al (1985) Invest Ophthalmol (suppl) 26:236

5. Aberer W, et al (1986) J Immunol 136:830-836

6. Belsito DV, et al (1982) J Exp Med 155:291-302

© 1990 Elsevier Science Publishers (Biomedical Division)
Ocular Immunology Today. M. Usui, S. Ohno and K. Aoki, editors.

THYMIC INSUFFICIENCY AND ITS CORRECTION IN PATIENTS WITH RECURRENT OCULAR HERPES

Yu F MAICHUK, S G MIKULI

Department of Viral and Allergic Eye Diseases,
Helmholtz Institute of Eye Diseases, 103064 Moscow USSR

INTRODUCTION

The latest research data show that development of severe and chronic diseases should mainly be attributed to a pathologic condition of one's immune system (1,2). There are several studies into ocular herpetic infection which indicate qualitative and functional deficiency of T-lymphocytes in patients with recurrent ocular herpes (3-5). Until recently, however, ophthalmologists seem to have underestimated a possible pathogenic correlation between ocular herpes and functional state of the thymus gland – the central organ of the immune system which controls immunity with its active hormones.

MATERIALS AND METHODS
Methods

To know the functional capacity of the thymus gland, even indirectly, we studied its activity in the blood serum using the method of the sensitivity restoration to azathioprin in the rosette-formative cells of the rats' spleen after thymectomy. This technique was described by Bach et al in 1976 (6). The titre of the thymic activity in the blood serum was considered such a maximal delution of the serum that ensured restoration of lymphocytes to azathioprin by 50%. The final result was expressed as binary logarithms of the titre.

Patients

The level of the thymic avtivity was studied in two groups of patients. The first group enrolled 25 patients with newly diagnosed ocular herper, the other group included 29 patients with recurrent attacks of the infection (at least three attack per current year). A control group enrolled 26 clinically healthy people.

RESULTS

As literary data indicate a drop in the titre of the thymic activity with age, all participants of the study were divided into two age groups: 20-40 and 41-60 years of age.

In patients under 40 years of age with initial herpetic infection of the eye, the mean thymic activity was found to be significantly lower than that in the healthy volunteers of the same age. In patents over 40 years of age, index of the thymic activity was almost similar to that in the control group.

In patients suffering from frequent recurrences of ocular herpes, the level of the thymic avtivity in serum was decreased in both age groups. In patients within 20-40 years of age, the thymic activity appeared to be four times lower in comparison with the control group, and in patients older 40 years of age its level was 2.4 times lower than that in the healthy volunteers. No statistically significant difference in the thymic activity was found in patients with recurrent herpes from different age groups(Table).

TABLE

SERUM THYMIC ACTIVITY IN PATIENTS WITH OCULAR HERPES (STA)

Groups	Age(yr)	M+m Log_2 STA titre	P_1	P_2
Patients with primary attack	20-40	3.46+0.006	<0.001	<0.05
	41-60	2.10+0.001	>0.05	
Patients with frequent recurrences	20-40	1.12+0.005	<0.001	>0.05
	41-60	1.00+0.001	<0.001	
Healthy volunteers	20-40	4.78+0.01		<0.001
	41-60	2.58+0.25		

Note: P_1 - significant difference between patients and healthy people of the same age; P_2- significant difference between patients of different age within a group under study

Interestingly, patients from both age groups with frequent attacks of ocular herpes had lower thymic activity in serum as against those with primary infection. This finding indicates a deeper disturbance in the thymic function induced by recurrent herpetic process.

Thus our results show that in patients with ocular herpes and, especially in those with its frequent attacks, the function of the thumus gland is insufficient. Several publications also indicate qualitative and quantitative deficiency of T-lymphocytes in the peripheric blood in patients with ocular herpes. All that serve as a strong argument in favour of using factors of thymus as natural immune modulators for ocular herpes in humans. For such a modulator we have been using Tactivin manufactured in the Soviet Union (7). This drug has already been used to treat 500 patients with severe ocular herpes. Tactivin has been part of a complex treatment which also includes IDU, zovirax, interferon, bonafton, etc. Tactivin is injected subcutaneously once a day each other day. A single dose makes up 25 mkg, a total dose being 150-250 mkg depending on the clinical and immunologic status of a patient. Patients treated with levamisol serve as a control group. Our results are as follows: by the day 7-8 patients treated with Tactivin demonstrate an increase of the initial low level of the thymic activity irrespective of the age. In patients within 41-60 years, the thymic activity increases more than twicely remaining, however below the normal age limits. Improved thymic activity is accompanied with expressed clinical improvement of the condition. In severe intractable cases Tactivin was found to arrest the process and increase the final visual acuity. In addition, the period of treatment shortened from conventional 48 days to 23 days.

Serial testings of the peripheric blood over the period of six months after the treatment showed that the thymic serum activity steadily went down, and 6-12 months later the treatment a new attack might develop. To stabilize clinical and immune indexes, 3-6 months after the first course of treatment we indicate a repeated course.

In the control group of patients treated with levamisol we did not find a statistically significant change in the thymic serum activity throughout the whole course of study.

In conclusion, a five-year period of observation of patients treated with Tactivin indicates its strong antirecurrent properties: the number of severe herpetic recurrences has reduced by 3-4 times. We believe our research data demonstrate a pathogenic correlation between severe recurrent ocular herpes and functioning of the thymic gland. Its dysfunction can be improved with active factors of thymus. One of them proves to be Tactivin.

REFERENCES

1. Lopukhin YM, Petrov RV, Makhonova LA et al (1986) Immunologia (Moscow) 2:50-53

2. Petrov RV (1982) Immunologia. Nauka, Moscow

3. Maichuk YF, Mikuli SG (1983) Oftalmologicheskii zhurnal (Odessa) 4:217-219

4. Russel RG, Nosisse MP, Larsen HS et al (1984) Invest. Ophthalmol 25:938-944

5. Kita M, Yoshida H, Sunakawa M et al (1987) Acta Soc. Ophthalmol. Jpn 91:240-245

6. Bach JF, Karnaud C (1976) Progress in Allergy 21: 342-408

7. Arion VYa (1987) Zhurnal Microbiologii, Epidemiologii i Immunologii 4:98-104

© 1990 Elsevier Science Publishers (Biomedical Division)
Ocular Immunology Today. M. Usui, S. Ohno and K. Aoki, editors.

VALUE OF SCLERAL HOMOGRAFTING IN NECROTIZING SCLERITIS MANAGEMENT

MAITE SAINZ DE LA MAZA, C. STEPHEN FOSTER AND J. TAUBER

Immunology Service, Massachusetts Eye and Ear Infirmary, Harvard Medical School, Boston, Massachusetts, USA

INTRODUCTION

Necrotizing scleritis is a rare but devastating consequence of certain connective tissue disorders, including rheumatoid arthritis (1), Wegener´s granulomatosis (2), polyarteritis nodosa (3), systemic lupus erythematosus (1) and relapsing polychondritis. While systemic chemotherapy is effective in halting progressive necrotizing scleritis, the onset of its action may be too slow (typically 4-8 weeks after initiation) to prevent profound scleral thinning and/or traumatic or spontaneous perforation. Scleral grafting can be a useful temporizing procedure for maintaining the integrity of the globe during the time before the effects of systemic chemotherapy become manifest. Variable results have been reported with the use of auricular cartilage (4), fascia lata (5), aortic tissue (6) and homologous sclera (7) as donor material. We report our experience with donor sclera homografts used in association with systemic immunosuppressive therapy in severe necrotizing scleritis.

MATERIAL AND METHODS

We reviewed the records of patients with necrotizing scleritis seen in the Immunology Service of the Massachusetts Eye and Ear Infirmary in Boston, MA, between 1978 and 1988 in whom scleral homografting had been performed. All patients had been treated elsewhere with topical and systemic steroidal and/or non steroidal antiinflammatory drugs. Necrotizing scleritis was defined as progressively destructive scleral melting with more than 85% of scleral wall thinning and wxposure of underlying choroid, eith or without uveal bulging and/or perforation. Historical review, clinical exam and laboratory results were recorded for each patient. Scleral and conjunctival biopsies for light and immunofluorescence microscopy were obtained during surgical grafting not only for diagnostic purposes but also as a therapeutic procedure for removing necrotic and inflammed tissue. The presence of vasculitis, perivasculitis, granulomas, eosinophils, masts cells and polymorphonuclear or lymphocytic infiltrate was evaluated. Details of tissue handling, processing and staining have been previously reported (8).

Under local anesthesia and operating microscope control, as much as possible of the necrotic and inflammed conjunctival and scleral tissues were carefully resected without perforation of the globe. Next, a template was made from plastic surgical drape to approximate the area of resected sclera. Frozen or gly- cerine preserved full thickness human donor sclera was cut to match template size and shape and secured with 10-0 nylon sutures to the edges of the resection site. Conjunctiva was pulled down over the graft whenever possible and secured with 8-0 Vicryl sutures. In cases with uveal prolapse with or without vitreous loss, uveal excision and/or anterior vitrectomy were performed, followed by application of cryotherapy over the scleral graft.

Patients with necrotizing scleritis associated with a specific systemic vasculitic disease received systemic immunosuppressive therapy, either during the early post-operative period or later in the course. Doses of chemotherapeutic agents and guidelines for patient follow-up have been reported elsewhere (9).

RESULTS

Twelve patients (15 grafts in 12 eyes) form the basis of this report, including eight females and four males, with a mean age of 63 years (range:45-87 years) and a mean follow-up period of 11 months. In addition to necrotizing scleritis, peripheral ulcerative keratitis was present concomitantly in three eyes. Uveal bulging with perforation of the necrotic scleral area occurred in two patients. Six patients had histories of prior ocular surgical procedures (five cataract extractions with or without IOL and one scleral buckle) within a period of 5 to 24 months (mean 13 months) before the necrotizing scleritis was diagnosed.

Underlying systemic autoimmune diseases were present in 10 of the 12 patients, all of them with evidence of vasculitis in the biopsied ocular tissue. Diagnosis included rheumatoid arthritis (3 patients), suspected Wegener´s granulomatosis (incomplete syndrome, 4 patients), definite Wegener´s granulomatosis (complete syndrome, 1 patient), relapsing polychondritis (1 patient) and ulcerative colitis (1 patient). Necrotizing scleritis occurred in one patient with Romberg´s hemi- facial atrophy, and no specific etiology was identified in one case. Neither of these patients had vasculitis demonstrated on biopsy.

Preoperative and final visual acuities, the timing of use of immunosuppressive chemotherapy (initial or subsequent) and scleral graft outcome are recorded in Table 1. Chemotheapy was begun before or immediately following surgery in eight of the 12 patients. The scleral grafts in these patients remained stable long term (mean F/U: 12 months) in all cases except two. Patient 4 had a microbial keratitis with subsequent endophthalmitis, which, in spite of aggressive medical and surgical therapies, required enucleation. Patient 3 had a stable scleral graft for one year after which time the chemotherapy was discontinued; complete melting of the scleral graft ensued within 10 months. Resumption of chemotherapy and repeat scleral grafting resulted in ocular stability (F/U: 35 months).

TABLE 1

SCLERAL GRAFT OUTCOME AND CHEMOTHERAPY

Pt	Preop VA	Chemo begun early	Early outcome post-sg	Sub-sequent chemo?	Late outcome	Final VA
1	HM	Yes	Stable	No	Stable sg late rd	HM
2	20/40	Yes	Stable	No	Stable	20/20
3	20/100	Yes	Stable early Melt on d/c	Yes	Stable	20/100
4	20/50	Yes	Endoph-thalmitis	No	Enucleation	-
5	CF	Yes	Stable	No	Stable	HM
6	CF	Yes	Stable	No	Stable	CF
7	20/400	Yes	Stable	No	Stable	CF
8	CF	Yes	Stable	No	Stable	20/400
9	CF	No	Melted	Yes	Stable	CF
10	20/70	No	Melted	Yes	Stable	20/40
11	20/70	No	Stable	No	Stable	20/30
12	20/25	No	Stable	No	Stable	20/25

VA: visual acuity   rd: retinal detachment   CF: counting fingers
HM: Hand motions   sg: scleral graft   d/c: discontinuation of chemotherapy

Two of the four patients not treated initially with chemotherapy (patient 9 and 10) experienced early graft melting, within 45 and 14 days respectively (mean 4 weeks). Both had evidence of active vasculitis on biopsy. The subsequent institution of immunosuppressive chemotherapy (and regrafting in patient 10) arrested the necrotizing process (F/U: 13 months).

Two patients (patients 11 and 12) were not treated initially with chemotherapy since neither showed evidence of active vasculitis on biopsy. Both remained stable (F/U: 7 months) with secure scleral grafts.

Two of the 12 patients in this study suffered significant complications. One patient with prior history of retinal detachment and scleral buckle had a recurrent postoperative detachment. One patient developed Staph. aureus keratitis one month following grafting, which progressed to endophthalmitis and eventual enucleation.

Nine patients had improved (mean of one Snellen line, (range 0-3) or unchanged final vision compared with preoperative acuity. Three patients had final acuity less than preoperative vision; one of these was the patient requiring enucleation.

DISCUSSION

Necrotizing scleritis is the most severe and destructive form of scleritis. The general implications of this problem are underrecognized. Watson and Hayreh reported that 29% of their patients with this problem died within five years of the onset of the disease; 67% of these deaths may have resulted from extraocular vasculitic lesions (1). Clearly, the presence of necrotizing scleritis may be the first sign of a systemic vasculitic disease, representing an unequivocal worsening of prognosis for survival. Progression of the necrotizing process may occur with astonishing rapidity (within two to four weeks) leaving the tissue behind the advancing edge very thin or perforated. Systemic immunosuppressive chemotherapy has been shown to be highly efficacious in arresting the vasculitic process (10), but the time required for the effects of orally administered chemotherapeutic agents to become manifest (4-8 weeks) may be too long to avoid complications such as spontaneous or traumatic perforation. Scleral grafting, as a temporizing procedure, can supply a collagen framework for support and maintenance of the integrity of the globe. Because the active cellular components of connective tissue (fibroblasts, macrophages, mast cells and plasma cells) are not needed, preserved scleral tissue meets all requirements for an appropiate donor material.

The experience summarized in this report indicates that in patients with active vasculitis, without systemic immunosuppression, scleral grafting is at best a temporizing procedure. When used as an adjunctive procedure to the institution of chemotherapy, scleral grafting is a safe and efficaceous technique, both as a treatment for or as prevention of ocular perforation due to progressively destructive necrotizing scleritis.

REFERENCES
1. Watson PG, Hayreh SS (1976) Brit J Ophthalmol 60:163-191
2. Cogan DG (1956) Trans Am Acad Ophthalmol Soc 53:321-44
3. Straatsma BR (1957) Am J Ophthalmol 44:789-99
4. Renard G, Lelievre P, Mazel J (1953) Bull Soc Ophtal France 66:243-249
5. Armstrong K, McGovern VJ (1955) Trans Ophthalmol Soc Australia 15:110-21
6. Merz EH (1964) Am J Ophthalmol 57:766-770
7. Paufique L, Moreau PG (1953) Ann Oculist 186:1065-1076
8. Foster CS, Fong LP, Azar D, Kenyon K (1988) Ophthalmology 95:453-462
9. Foster CS (1983) Int Ophthalmol 23 (1):183-196
10. Foster CS (1980) Ophthalmology 87:140-149

© 1990 Elsevier Science Publishers (Biomedical Division)
Ocular Immunology Today. M. Usui, S. Ohno and K. Aoki, editors.

Cyclosporine Treatment of Uveitis/Scleritis and Effects on Class II MHC Antigen Expression

Leslie S. Fujikawa, M.D.

Cyclosporine (cyclosporin A, CsA) is a potent immunosuppressive agent which has been very effective in the treatment of a variety of immune disorders, including vision-threatening posterior uveitis. It is a drug which suppresses T helper cell function, and thus, it has the potential for more effective treatment of T cell-mediated diseases (1,2).

The mechanisms by which CsA acts to treat ocular immune diseases are unclear at present. CsA is a potent inhibitor of antigen-driven lymphokine production, including interleukin-2 (IL-2) and interferon-γ (IFN-γ) production, and it blocks the lymphokine-induced expression of class II major histocompatibility complex antigens *in vivo* and *in vitro* (1). Furthermore, recent work in our laboratory indicates that during both experimental autoimmune uveoretinitis and human uveitis, as well as *in vitro* upon the addition of IFN-γ, the retinal vascular endothelium presents an immunologically active surface to circulating lymphocytes, expressing class II antigens, and that this may be very important in generating the local ocular immune response (3-5). Based upon these findings, a possible site of action of CsA is prevention of induction of class II antigens on vascular endothelium.

Ocular Immunology Laboratory, Smith-Kettlewell Eye Research Institute, San Francisco, CA

In this study, we undertook a clinical trial to assess the effectiveness of oral CsA in treating severe autoimmune uveitis and scleritis, and we examined the immunopathology of conjunctival biopsies from these patients before and during CsA treatment in order to characterize CsA's direct ocular effects.

Materials & Methods

Patient population. Ten patients with previously refractory non-infectious posterior uveitis and/or scleritis were treated with oral CsA (initial dose = 6 mg/kg/day) for a period ranging from 3 to 15 months (Table I). Conjunctival biopsies from 6 patients were obtained and processed as previously reported (6) before and during treatment with CsA.

Monoclonal antibodies. Primary antibodies obtained from Becton-Dickinson (Mountainview, CA) were directed against a panel of inflammatory cell markers, including those for T helper/inducer cells (T_H) (Leu-3a), T suppressor/cytotoxic cells (T_S) (Leu-2a), B cells (Leu-14), monocytes (Leu-M1), Langerhans' cells (Leu-6), the IL-2 receptor (Tac antigen), and the class II antigens (HLA-DR and HLA-DQ).

Tissue specimens. Tissues were frozen in OCT compound and 4 μm frozen sections were studied using an immunoperoxidase

Table I.
Uveitis/Scleritis Cases

Case	Age	Diagnosis	Improvement with CsA	Biopsy on Rx	Follow-up
1	54	Panuveitis, scleritis	2+	3 months	8 months
2	27	Retinal vasculitis	4+	6 weeks	3 months
3	51	Scleritis, posterior	4+	4 months	8 months
4	61	Birdshot retinochoroidopathy	2+	9 weeks	6 months
5	72	Uveitis, scleritis, rheumatoid	3+ → 1+	9 weeks	5 months
6	27	Vogt-Koyanagi-Harada syndrome	3+	8 weeks	3 months
7	28	Sympathetic ophthalmia	2+	-	6 months
8	53	Scleritis, anterior	3+	-	6 months
9	66	Anterior scleritis, post surgical	-	-	d/c CsA
10	27	Behcet's syndrome	4+	-	15 months

technique. Tissue sections were incubated with the primary (monoclonal) antibody, followed by biotinylated anti-mouse IgG (heavy & light chain-specific) (Accurate, Westbury, NY), each for 15 minutes at 37° C. After a 15-minute incubation with avidin and biotinylated horseradish peroxidase (Vector Labs, Burlingame, CA), sections were stained with 3,3'-diaminobenzidine (Sigma, St. Louis, MO), nickel sulfate, and hydrogen peroxide. Slides were counterstained with 1% methyl green.

Evaluation of specimens. Sections were evaluated as to the positively stained cells for each antigen. Each slide stained was given a numerical grade on a scale of 0 to 4: "4+" >80% of cells positive; "3+" 60-80% positive; "2+" 40-60% positive; "1+" 20-40% positive; "0.5" 5-20% positive; "0" <5% positive or no staining. Approximate T_H:Ts ratios were calculated from the above and reported as <1.0, 1.0, 1.5, 2.0, 2.5, 3.0, and >3.0.

The degree of class II antigen expression was evaluated: "4+" widespread positive staining of the resident cells, e.g. vascular endothelium, in addition to staining of the inflammatory cells; "3+" focal staining of resident cells; "2+" very limited staining of resident cells; "1+" positive staining limited to inflammatory cells; "0" no staining.

Results

Clinical response to CsA. Significant clinical response was noted with CsA treatment (Table I). If there was both uveitis and scleritis, the response to CsA was similar externally and intraocularly. In one case (case #5) the improvement was temporary due to a lack of compliance with the medication.

Immunopathology of conjunctival biopsies. There was a dramatic reduction of T_H cells with CsA treatment in all cases studied (Figures 1a, 1b, and 2a). Ts cells were much less affected by CsA, decreasing only slightly or even increasing focally in the biopsies. These results were reflected in the T_H:Ts ratios in the biopsies before and during CsA. Before therapy T_H:Ts ratios were ≥ 2.0: 2.5 ± 0.45 (normal in peripheral blood=2.0); during therapy, T_H:Ts ratios of cases 1-4 were ≤ 1.5: 1.25 ± 0.29. The exception to this was case #5 in which lack of compliance was reflected in the clinical response to CsA and T_H:Ts ratio which was 2.5 during treatment.

The results for the class II antigens HLA-DR and HLA-DQ showed a similar response to CsA treatment. Both inflammatory cell and vascular endothelial class II antigen expression was affected in the conjunctival biopsies. The results shown

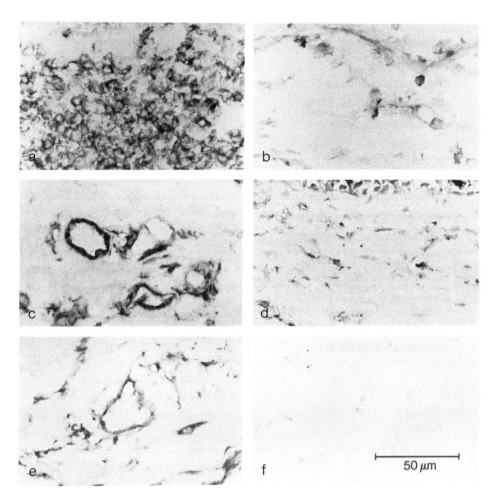

Figure 1. Immunopathology. (a) Many T helper cells prior to CsA treatment. (b) Greatly diminished T helper cells during treatment (Case 3, anti-Leu-3a). (c) Vascular endothelium was positive for class II antigen HLA-DR prior to treatment, and (d) negative during treatment (Case 2, anti-HLA-DR). (e) and (f): The separate class II antigen HLA-DQ showed similar results to that for HLA-DR, (e) prior to treatment and (f) during cyclosporine treatment (Case 1, anti-HLA-DQ).

focus upon the vascular endothelium. HLA-DR and -DQ class II antigens were both positive on the vascular endothelium prior to treatment with CsA and negative during treatment (Figures 1c-f, 2b and 2c).

Discussion

Cyclosporine was a very effective alter-native in the treatment of autoimmune uveitis or scleritis, both for the relief of severe pain and improvement of inflammation and visual acuity.

Our immunopathologic studies show that there was a coordinate decrease in expression of class II antigens HLA-DR and -DQ, particularly on the vascular endothelium, as well as decreased TH cells upon CsA treatment. This decrease in class II anti-

462

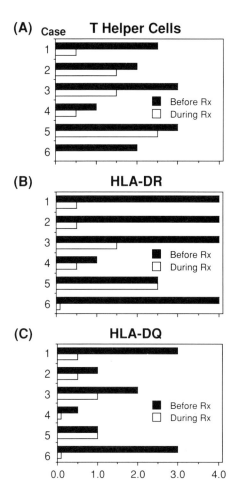

(A) Case **T Helper Cells**

Before Rx
During Rx

(B) **HLA-DR**

Before Rx
During Rx

(C) **HLA-DQ**

Before Rx
During Rx

Figure 2. Summary of Results for Conjunctival Biopsies. (a) Reduction of T helper cells with CsA in all cases studied (anti-Leu-3a). (b) Class II antigen HLA-DR and (c) HLA-DQ were positive on the vascular endothelium prior to and greatly diminished during therapy.

gens correlated positively with the clinical response to CsA.

These studies thus indicate that class II antigens on vascular endothelial cells *in vivo* are not a constant property of these cells, but rather might be dependent upon effects of immunomodulatory mediators, such as IFN-γ, secreted by resident inflammatory cells in the tissues, and which is known to be diminished by CsA.

The results of our study indicate potent ocular actions of CsA, and they are consistent with the hypothesis that prevention of induction of class II antigens on the vascular endothelium is an important mechanism by which CsA exerts its immunosuppressive effect. Since quantitative variation in class II antigen expression has a direct effect on the efficiency of T cell activation (7), the changes induced by CsA would be expected to reduce the efficiency of antigen recognition during a T cell response. Our previous results indicate that class II positive retinal vascular endothelium may be a significant determinant of the immune response by functioning as antigen-presenting cells during uveitis (8). Therefore, it is likely that the present findings involving class II antigens apply also to the retinal vascular endothelium, and that this may be a very important mechanism by which CsA successfully treats local retinal inflammation in many forms of uveitis and retinal vasculitis.

Acknowledgements
Supported by NIH grant EY06948, Research to Prevent Blindness, NY, Smith-Kettlewell Eye Research Institute, and Pacific Presbyterian Medical Center, San Francisco, California.

References

1. Shevach EM (1985) *Ann Rev Immunol* **3**:399
2. Nussenblatt RB and Scher I (1985) *Invest Ophthalmol Vis Sci* **26**:10
3. Fujikawa LS et al (1989) *Invest Ophthalmol Vis Sci* **30**:66
4. Fujikawa LS and Haugen J-P (1987) *Ophthalmology* **94**:136
5. Fujikawa LS et al (1990) *In*: Proc 5th Int Symp Immunol Immunopathol of the Eye. Elsevier Sci Publ, Amsterdam, in press.
6. Fujikawa LS et al (1985) *In*: O'Connor GR, Chandler JW (eds), Adv Immunol and Immunopathol of the Eye. Masson Publ USA, Inc, New York, pp 43-47
7. Janeway CA et al (1984) *Immunol Today* **5**:99
8. Fujikawa LS (1989) *Ophthalmology* **96**:1115

© 1990 Elsevier Science Publishers (Biomedical Division)
Ocular Immunology Today. M. Usui, S. Ohno and K. Aoki, editors.   463

CHRONIC ANTERIOR UVEITIS TREATED WITH BROMOCRIPTINE

MANFRED ZIERHUT, UWE PLEYER, RICHARD WAETJEN, HANS-JUERGEN THIEL,
EGON G. WEIDLE
University Eye Hospital, Schleichstr. 12, 7400 Tuebingen, West-Germany

INTRODUCTION
    The pituitary gland seems to play an important role in the neuroendocrine
immunoregulatory system. One of the most potent hormones seems to be
prolactin. Hypophysectomy leads to antibody-depression (1), and prolactin
replacement normalizes antibody levels (2). Prolactin receptors have been
demonstrated on T and B-lymphocytes (3), and activated lymphocytes can
synthesize mRNA for prolactin leading to secretion of prolactin (4). In
addition thymus hormones can also stimulate the pituitary gland for release
of prolactin (5).
    Bromocriptine, a dopamine- and prolactin antagonist, can inhibit the
immunologic effect of prolactin in in vivo and in vitro animal models (6).
Bromocriptine had been used in the therapy of Parkinson's disease,
prolactinomas and for prevention of lactation.
    In such patients Hedner and Bynke (7) could demonstrate a remission of an
accompanying uveitis in 4 patients.
    After positive results in our own patients suffering from different forms of
uveitis (8) we started a placebo-controlled double blind study in patients
with anterior uveitis.

METHODS
    Only patients with at least 3 or more recurrences of anterior uveitis during
the previous year were included in this study. Therapy was initiated
gradually during a symptom-free interval and eventually reached a dosage of
2.5 mg of Bromocriptine twice daily. This treatment was considered to be
ineffective in patients who had two recurrences during the study. Local
corticosteroid treatment at the beginning of the study was tapered off in the
first two weeks. The study was undertaken in a double blind placebo
controlled manner. All recurrences in the course of the study were treated
with locally applied prednisolone-acetate and scopolamine. Ophthalmological
and laboratory controls were performed after 1 week, 1, 3, 6, 9 and 12
months. The study period was 1 year but was stoped when relevant side
effects were found or at request of the patient.

RESULTS
    15 patients have been participated in the study. Seven patients had
bromocriptine and six placebo. Two patients were excluded because of lack of
compliance. Table 1 demonstrates age, sex, duration of the disease and
etiology of the anterior uveitis in our patients.
    Figure 1a and 1b represent the results of the study. In the bromocriptine
group 2 patients had no recurrences during the study (29%). Two patients

PATIENTS IN THE BROMOCRIPTINE STUDY

N	SEX/AGE	DURATION OF DISEASE (YEARS)	ETIOLOGY
1	f/78	2	unknown
2	f/40	5	seronegative arthritis
3	f/75	25	unknown
4	f/38	3	ankylosing spondylitis
5	m/28	8	unknown
6	m/21	2	seronegative arthritis
7	f/24	1	unknown
8	f/75	1	unknown
9	m/35	13	ankylosing spondylitis
10	m/48	5	ankylosing spondylitis
11	f/18	1	seronegative arthritis
12	m/28	1	unknown
13	f/28	2	unknown

Table 1

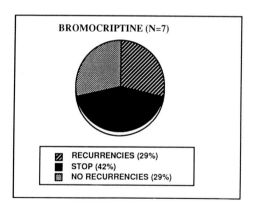

Figure 1a

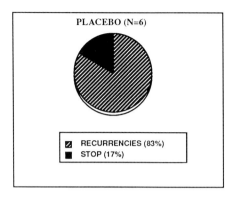

Figure 1b

had to stop because of two recurrences. These, however, were much milder than previous ones. In earlier recurrences they were treated with systemic corticosteroids and in our study the recurrences resolved in a few days with local corticosteroids. Three patients (two without recurrences, one with one recurrence) (42%) were released from the study due to side effects (arterial hypotension, nausea, arthritic complains) (table 2).

Treatment was terminated in five of six patients in the placebo group due to two recurrences and stopped in the remaining patient when she believed she was experiencing a bromocriptine side-effect (mammary atrophy).

SIDE EFFECTS
OF THE THERAPY WITH BROMOCRIPTINE

*   arterial hypotension (5 patients)

*   nausea (1 patient)

*   arthritic complains (?) (1 patient)

Table 2

466

DISCUSSION

Bromocriptine appears to have a prophylactic effect for chronic anterior uveitis recurrences in this study group. This is in contrast to the study of Palestine and Nussenblatt (9), who could not find a clear clinical improvement in 11 patients with bromocriptine treatment.

The patients in this study had taken 4 x 2.5 mg daily but surprisingly there is no report of any side effects in spite of twice the dosage of our patients. The finding of lowering of antiribonuclear antibodies in bromocriptine patients has been interpreted as an immunosuppressive effect by these authors. In our study side effects were frequent but mild compared to common immunosuppressives. Well known is the arterial hypotension which nearly always exists at the beginning of therapy possibly caused by sudden change in serum level of this dopamine-antagonist. Nausea seems to be caused by the alpha-1-adrenergic effect of bromocriptine. It is unclear if the arthritic complains of one of our patients are related to the therapy. Whyte and Williams (10) described a suppression of arthritis by bromocriptine in an animal study.

In summary all the patients receiving bromocriptine had better results (no recurrence or recurrences which were more easily treatable) than in the year prior to the study.

REFERENCES

1. Berczi I, Nagy E, Kovacs K et al (1981) Regulation of humoral immunity in rats by pituitary hormones. Acta endocr. (Copenh.) 98:506
2. Nagy E, Berczi I, Friesen HG (1983) Regulation of immunity in rats by lactogenic and growth hormones. Acta endocr. (Copenh.) 102:351
3. Russell DH, Kibler R, Matrisian L et al (1985) Prolactin receptors on human T and B lymphocytes. J Immunol 134:3027
4. Hiestand PC, Mekler P, Nordmann R et al (1986) Prolactin as a modulator of lymphocyte responsiveness provides a possible mechanism of action for cyclosporine. Proc Natl Acad Sci USA 83:2599
5. Spangelo BL, Hall NR, Dunn AJ et al (1987) Thymosin fraction 5 stimulates the release of prolactin from cultured GH3 cells. Life Sci 40:283
6. Berczi I, Nagy E (1982) A possible role of prolactin in adjuvant arthritis. Arthritis Rheum 25:591
7. Hedner LP, Bynke G (1985) Endogenous iridocyclitis relieved during treatment with bromocriptine, Am J Ophthalmol 100:618
8. Zierhut M, Pleyer U, Waetjen R et al (1989) Bromocriptine in the treatment of uveitis. Proceedings of the Int Uveitis congress Guaruja, Brasil (in print)
9. Palestine AG, Nussenblatt RB (1988) The effect of bromocriptine on anterior uveitis. Am J Ophthalmol 106:488
10. Whyte A, Williams RO (1988) Bromocriptine suppresses postpartum exacerbation of collagen-induced arthritis. Arthritis rheum 31:927

© 1990 Elsevier Science Publishers (Biomedical Division)
Ocular Immunology Today. M. Usui, S. Ohno and K. Aoki, editors.467

ANTIFLAMMINS: INHIBITION OF ENDOTOXIN - INDUCED UVEITIS IN LEWIS RATS

CHI-CHAO CHAN, MING NI, LUCIO MIELE*, ELEONORA CORDELLA-MIELE*, ANIL B.
MUKHERJEE*, AND ROBERT B. NUSSENBLATT

Laboratory of Immunology, National Eye Institute and *Section on Developmental Genetics, Human
Genetics Branch, NICHD, NIH, Bethesda, Maryland, 20892 USA

INTRODUCTION

Antiflammins are phospholipase A2 (PLA$_2$) -inhibitory, anti-inflammatory peptides derived from the region of highest local similarity between uteroglobulin and lipocortin I[1]. Two nonapeptides, MQMKKVLDS and HDMNKVLDL (P1 and P2, or antiflammin 1 and 2 respectively) have shown potent PLA$_2$ inhibitory activity in vitro and striking counter action on carrageenan-induced rat footpad inflammation and edema in vivo[1]. Both synthesized oligopeptides, antiflammin 1 and 2, are water soluble and without the known side effects of corticosteriods.

Endotoxin induced uveitis (EIU) is an experimental model for anterior uveitis of the eye by footpad injection of endotoxin, the lipopolysaccharide (LPS) components of Gram-negative bacterial cell wall.[2] It has been suggested to be induced through PLA$_2$ activation, not from a direct action of endotoxin into the eye.[3,4] EIU usually peaks at 16-20 hours and subsides at 48 hours after endotoxin injection.[2-4] Here, we report the effects of antiflammins on EIU as measured by inflammatory cell count and protein concentration in the anterior chamber, as well as the histopathological study of the treated eyes. We also examined and compared different dosages, schedules, and delivery routes of antiflammins as therapeutic agents for EIU.

MATERIALS AND METHODS

Induction of EIU

Female Lewis rats (Charles River, Raleigh, NC), 8 to 10 weeks old, weighing approximately 200 grams were used in this study. Each animal was injected into one hind footpad with 100 ug *Salmonella typhimurium* endotoxin (Difco Lab, Detroit, MI) diluted in 100 ul sterile pyrogen-free saline (American Quinine, Shirley, NY).

Treatment with antiflammins

Antiflammin 1 and 2 were dissolved in Dacriose sterile ophthalmic irrigating solution (Cooper Vision Pharmaceuticals Inc., Puerto Rico, USA). They were administered topically or in combination with intramuscular injection. For evaluation of the topically administered antiflammins, the animal's left eye (O.S.) was treated with antiflammin whereas its right eye (O.D.) was given Dacriose alone as a control. Animals receiving systemic medication were given bilateral topical treatment as well. The dosage of the antiflammins were as follows: 0.2 mg for intramuscular injection; 0.25, 1.25, or 2.5 mg/ml for topical application. Each rat received two eye-drops in each eye every five hours.

Disease evaluation

The animals were sacrificed 20 hours after endotoxin injection. Immediate aspiration of aqueous humor was performed under a dissecting microscope. 2 ul of aqueous humor was placed on a gelatinized slide, air dried, and stained with Wright's stain. The inflammatory cells on each slide were counted under light microscopic examination. Another 4 ul of aqueous humor were measured for protein concentration by Lowry method. Aqueous humor obtained from four normal rats was studied in a similar manner for the cell count and protein concentration.

Histopathology

For some animals, enucleation was performed immediately after sacrifice. The enucleated eye was processed for histopathological studies by fixation in 4% gluteraldehyde and 10% formalin. After it was sectioned through its vertical plane, the eye was embedded in methyl methacrylate, and 3 um-thick sections were stained with hematoxylin-eosin. The presence of ocular inflammation was determined by quantitation of cellular inflitrate and exudates.

RESULTS

Systemic treatment

Twenty hours after EIU induction, the eyes of animals treated with Dacriose developed profound inflammation as measured by large numbers of inflammatory cells and increased amount of protein in their anterior chambers (Fig 1). Histopathological examination revealed moderate to marked cellular infiltration consisting of polymorphonuclear cells and mononuclear cells in the anterior and posterior chambers and in the vitreous surrounding the ciliary body. Proteinaceous material was present in the anterior chamber. In contrast, the rats treated with antiflammin 1 and 2 developed milder ocular inflammation. Both inflammatory cells count and protein content in their anterior chambers were lower (For P1, cell count: $p<0.05$; protein concentration: $p<0.05$. For P2, cell count: $p<0.05$; protein concentration: $p>0.05$) (Fig.1). Histopathological examination of the eyes from the rats treated with antiflammins also disclosed milder cellular infiltration. However, by histology the amount of proteinaceous material in the anterior chamber was not significantly less than that in the control rats. All evaluated parameters between two eyes in the same rat, treated or untreated, were similar ($p>0.05$).

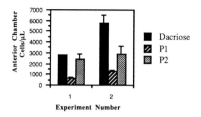

Figure 1a. Inflammatory cell counts in the anterior chamber of EIU rats

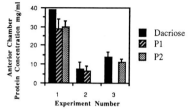

Figure 1b. Protein concentration in the anterior chamber of EIU rats

Topical treatment

In the normal rat, there were no inflammatory cells and no statistical difference in the anterior chamber protein concentration between O.S. and O.D. (p>0.05). No significant difference was found between the two eyes of the untreated EIU rat with respect to inflammatory cell count, protein concentration, and histopathology (Fig.1). There were, however, significant elevations of inflammatory cell count and protein concentration in the anterior chamber of the untreated eye compared to the treated eye of the same animal (For P1, cell count: p<0.05 at the dosages of 2.5 and 1.25mg/ml, p>0.05 at the dosage of 0.25mg/ml; protein concentration: p<0.01 at the dosage of 2.5mg/ml, p>0.05 at the dosages of 1.25 and 0.25mg/ml. For P2, cell count: p<0.05 and protein concentration: p>0.05 for a dosage of 2.5 mg/ml) (Fig 2 and 3). In general, by histopathological examination O.S. demonstrated a lesser degree of ocular inflammation as compared to O.D. of the same rat. The inhibition of inflammatory cellular infiltration was more effective than inhibition of protein leakage into the anterior chamber. No toxicity was observed in the animals treated with antiflammins.

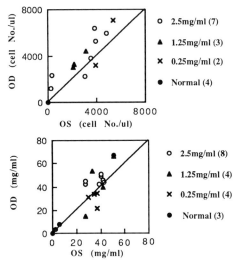

Figure 2. Above- cell counts of EIU animals after treatment with P1 OS. Below- protein concentration of aqueous in same animals

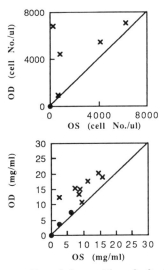

Figure 3. Same as Figure 2. after treatment with P2 OS

DISCUSSION

The present study shows that both antiflammin 1 and 2 can inhibit EIU in rats as measured by inflammatory cell count and protein concentration in the anterior chamber and ocular histopathology. Antiflammin 1 is a synthetic peptide derived from a portion of uteroglobin based on local similarity with lipocortin I (a family of glucocorticoid-induced proteins with anti-inflammatory effects in vivo)[1]. Uteroglobulin also is a steroid-induced secretory protein with PLA_2 inhibitory and anti-inflammatory activity.[5] Antiflammin 2 is a synthetic peptide derived from lipocortin I residues 246-254[1]. These peptides are anti-chemotactic and anti-thrombotic as well.

PLA_2 controls the release of arachidonic acid from phospholipids, residing mainly in cell membranes. Once arachidonic acid is released, the arachidonate cascade involving cyclooxygenase and lipoxygenase pathways proceeds producing numerous inflammatory mediators such as prostaglandins and leukotrienes[7]. Therefore, a PLA_2 inhibitor may produce the same effects as inhibiting both cyclooxygenase and lipoxygenase enzymes. This inhibition would diminish the production of proinflammatory eicosanoids (i.e. prostaglandins and leukotrienes).

The ocular inflammation in EIU is characterized by alteration in vascular permeability with protein leakage and inflammatory cells escape into the iris, ciliary body, and anterior and posterior chambers[2-4]. Various inflammatory mediators such as arachidonic acid metabolites and substance P have been measured and shown to have positive correlation with the severity of the ocular inflammation. It has been suggested that EIU may be elicited by PLA_2 activation [4]. Recently, a PLA_2 inhibitor, EPC, was reported to be a potent anti-inflammatory agent in EIU[8]. However, EPC, a water insoluble drug, is required to be administered systemically two hours before and at the time of LPS challenge in order to achieve its therapeutic action[8]. In contrast, antiflammins are water-soluble and can be administered topically starting from the time of LPS injection. The in vivo pharmacological properties of PLA_2 inhibitory antiflammins make these peptides better therapeutic agents with potential for clinical applications in humans.

REFERENCES

1. Miele L, Cordella-Miele E, Facchiano A, and Mukherjee AB: Nature. 335: 726-730, 1988.

2. Rosenbaum JT, McDevitt HO, Guss RB and Egbert PR: Nature. 286:611-613, 1980.

3. Rosenbaum JT, Hendricks PA, Shively JE, and McDougall IR: J. Nucl. Med. 24:29-33, 1983.

4. Herbort CP, Okumura A, and Mochizuki M: Albrecht Von Graefe's Arch. Klin. Exp. Ophthalmol. 226:553-558, 1988.

5. Miele L, Cordella-Miele E, and Mukherjee AB: Endocrine Rev. 8:474-490, 1987.

6. Flower RJ: Adv. Inflamm. Res. 8:1-34, 1984.

7. Salmon JA: in Prostaglandin (ed. Herman AG et al) Raven Press, N.Y. 1982,. pp 7-22.

8. Herbort CP, Okumura A, and Mochizuki M: Exp. Eye Res. 48:693-705, 1989.

© 1990 Elsevier Science Publishers (Biomedical Division)
Ocular Immunology Today. M. Usui, S. Ohno and K. Aoki, editors.

SUPPRESSION OF MURINE EXPERIMENTAL AUTOIMMUNE UVEITIS WITH ANTI-I-A MONOCLONAL ANTIBODY

H. GOTO, L. R. ATALLA, M. LINKER-ISRAELI, N. A. RAO
Doheny Eye Institute and the University of Southern California
Los Angeles, California (USA)

INTRODUCTION

Corticosteroids and cytotoxic agents have been the mainstay in the management of uveitis. However, as these agents control uveitis by nonspecific immune suppression, they frequently lead to serious side effects.

Major histocompatibility complex (MHC) class II antigens on the surface of antigen-presenting cells have been known to play a role in the immune response, and antibody against class II antigens have been found to selectively block this interaction.

In the study described herein, we showed that in vivo administration of monoclonal anti-I-A antibody suppresses the experimental autoimmune uveoretinitis induced by interphotoreceptor retinoid binding protein (IRBP) in mice.

MATERIALS AND METHODS

EAU induction

Eau was induced in female B10A mice, 8 weeks of age, by repeated injection of IRBP. Fifty μg of IRBP in a 1:1 (v/v) emulsion with complete Freund's adjuvant containing 2.5 mg/ml of Mycobacterium tuberculosis was injected in the foot-pad and intramuscularly.[1] Two days prior to immunization, the mice were treated intraperitoneally with 20 mg/kg cyclophosphamide. Pertussis toxin was injected intraperitoneally with the first immunization and again three days later. Groups of animals were treated with either the monoclonal anti-I-A or IgG. Other animals were sacrificed for in vitro studies on the effect of anti-I-A antibody.

Administration of monoclonal antibody

Animals were divided into two groups. The first group was treated with the monoclonal 10 - 3.6 anti-I-A^K in a dose of 500 μg/injection; the other group, which served as control, was

treated with IgG in a dose of 500 μg/injection. These agents
were injected intraperitoneally, 1 day prior to, and on days
1,2,5,8 and 11 after immunization.

Histopathologic evaluation

Treated animals were sacrificed on day 24 after primary IRBP
injection. Globes were enucleated, fixed in 10% formalin and
prepared for H & E staining. Animals used for in vitro studies
were killed on days 10 and 15 after primary immunization with
the antigen.

In vitro studies

To determine in vitro effects of anti-I-A antibody,
mononuclear spleen cells from animals sacrificed on days 10 and
15 after antigen immunization were cultured with the antigen
and mitogen in the presence or absence of the monoclonal anti-
I-A antibody.

Monoclonal antibody

Hybridoma cell lines producing the monoclonal 10 - 3.6 anti-
I-A^K were a gift from Dr. L. Steinman, Stanford University.
Upon receipt, the cultures were split every other day. After a
large volume had been obtained, the contents of the flasks were
centrifuged, resuspended in serum-free medium, and incubated
for 48 hours. Supernatants containing the monoclonal
antibodies were then collected and concentrated by
ultrafiltration. Protein concentration of the supernatants was
measured using the BioRad assay. Dialysis was performed
through membrane tubing; molecular weight cut off was 12-14 kd.
Immunoglobulins were sterilized with 0.22 μm filters,
aliquoted, and stored at -70°C prior to injection.

Detection of antibody to IRBP

Blood samples were collected and analyzed by enzyme-linked
immunosorbent assay (ELISA). 96-well polyvinylchloride plates
were coated with IRBP (50 ng/well). After 1 hour incubation at
37°C, plates were washed with phosphate buffered saline (PBS)
conaining 0.05% Tween 20. The wells were then incubated with
PBS-Tween at room temperature for 30 minutes. Diluted serum
samples (100 μl) were added after the wells were washed again.
Following incubataion for 1 hour at 37°C, plates were washed
with PBS-Tween. 100 μl of peroxidase-conjugated anti-mouse IgG
in a dilution of 1:1000 was then added to each well, followed

by incubation at room temperature for one hour. After washing the plates, 100 μl of the substrate O-phenylendiamine in citrate buffer using 3% H_2O_2 was added to the wells. The reaction product developed in 15 minutes and was measured by absorbance at 490 nm. Antibody level was expressed as the absorbance value at 1:400 dilution of each sample.

Lymphocyte proliferation assay

Mouse mononuclear cells were obtained by Ficoll-Paque centrifugation of dissociated spleen preparations. Proliferation assays were performed with RPMI-1640, 10% fetal calf serum, and 5 x 10^{-5} M 2-mercaptoethanel in 96-well plates. One hundred microliters of mononuclear cell suspension (10^5 cells) was dispensed into each well, followed by 100 μl of appropriately diluted antigen (IRBP) of mitogen (Con A). Cultures were incubated for 4 days at 37°C in 5% CO_2. At the end of the culture periods, 1.0 μCi of ^{3}H-thymidine was added to each well, the cultures harvested, and incorporation counts assessed. Thymidine uptake, in counts per min (CPM), was expressed as stimultion index:

$$\text{Stimulation index} = \frac{\text{CPM with IRBP (or Con A}}{\text{CPM with medium}}$$

RESULTS

Histologically there was a total suppression of EAU in 80% of the animals treated by I.P. injection of the anti-I-A monoclonal antibody. Uvea and retina were protected by this treatment and did not show evidence of any vascular changes or cellular infiltration. In the remaining 20%, variable degrees of inflammation were noted, but vasculitis, cellular infiltration and/or destruction of different retinal layers were usually minimal. All control animals treated with IgG showed uveoretinitis, retinal perivasculitis and vasculitis. Lymphocyte transformation assay showed a decrease in the lymphocyte proliferation index in the treated group as compared with the controls. Anti-IRBP antibodies were also marakedly diminished in the treated group. In vitro, spleen cells cultured with antigen in the presence of anti-I-A antibody showed suppression of proliferation.

DISCUSSION

It is known that the antigen is processed and presented to lymphocytes via the MHC class II antigens. In lymphocytes this antigen triggers several reactions that result in the release of lymphokines and mediators that are necessary for eliciting the inflammatory immune response. In a previous study, blocking the I-A determinant of the MHC (Ia) class II antigen with anti-I-A antibodies resulted in suppression of uveitis induced by retinal S-antigen in Lewis rats.[2] In the present murine model of uveitis induced by IRBP, we were able to suppress the development of uveoretinitis in 80% of the animals. Total inhibition was not achieved, probably because of the use of an inappropriate antibody isotype, or due to processing of the antigen through the I-E molecule of the Ia region on the suface of macrophages in uveitis.

CONCLUSIONS

1. Monoclonal antibodies to MHC class II antigens, if applied properly, could lead to suppression of EAU development.

2. It appears at least in mice, that the IA subregion of the Ia molecule plays a role in antigen presentation.

REFERENCES

1. Caspi RR, Roberge FG, Chan CC, Wiggert B, Chader GJ, Rozenszjan CL, Lando Z and Nussenblatt RB. A new model of autoimmune disease. Experimental autoimmune uveoretinitis induced in mice with two different retinal antigens. J Immunol (1988) 140:1490-1495.

2. Rao NA, Atalla L, Linker-Israeli M, Chen FY, George FW IV, Martin WJ, and Steinman L. Suppression of experimental uveitis in rats by anti-I-A antibodies. Invest Ophthalmol Vis Sci (1989) 30:2348-2355.

© 1990 Elsevier Science Publishers (Biomedical Division)
Ocular Immunology Today. M. Usui, S. Ohno and K. Aoki, editors.

IMMUNOTHERAPY OF MURINE AUTOIMMUNE UVEITIS BY ANTI-L3T4 ANTIBODY

L. R. ATALLA, M. LINKER-ISRAELI, N. A. RAO

Doheny Eye Institute and the University of Southern California
Los Angeles, California (USA)

INTRODUCTION

Murine T-cells recognize antigens in the context of class II
MHC molecules. Cytolysis, proliferation and release of
lymphokines by T-cells are tightly coupled to the specific
recognition of antigen. L3T4 is a determinant that is expressed
on the surface of T-cells and correlates primarily with class II
MHC antigen-reactivity. Monoclonal antibody (mAb) GK 1.5
directed to L3T4 molecule blocks antigen specific functions of
antigen-reactive T-cell clones. Administration of mAb GK 1.5 has
been reported to inhibit autoimmune diseases such as experimental
allergic encephalomyelitis and rheumatoid arthritis. Using this
monoclonal antibody, we were able to prevent the development of
experimental autoimmune uveitis in mice.

MATERIALS AND METHODS

Female B10A mice, 8 weeks of age were immunized with interphotoreceptor retinoid binding protein (IRBP). Cyclophosphamide,
20 mg/kg was injected prior to immunization. Immunization was
accomplished by two injections of IRBP, one week apart.[1]
Pertussis toxin was given with the primary immunization, and
again 3 days later. The animals were divided into 6 groups, each
with 6 animals. Groups 1 and 2 were injected with the monoclonal
antibody GK 1.5 and IgG, respectively in a dose of 125
ug/injection. The I.P. injections began on day 7 after primary
immunization and were repeated on days 10, 13, 16 and 19. In
groups 3 and 4, where the antibody used for immunotherapy animals
were injected with the same agents, respectively. GK 1.5 was
administered in a dose of 300 μg/injection followed by 2 doses 24
hours apart, each of 150 μg. The last two groups did not receive
any treatment and were used for in vitro studies. Groups 1 and 2
were sacrificed on day 23, groups 3 and 4 on day 16 and the last
two groups on days 10 and 15 after primary immunization. In
groups 1 and 2, the eyes were submitted for histologic
examination; spleens were used for lymphocyte transformation

assay and sera for ELISA. In groups 3 and 4, the eyes were processed for histological studies. Spleens from the last 2 groups were cultured with IRBP or Con A, with and without GK 1.5, and the stimulation indices under different conditions were estimated. The monoclonal antibodies were a kind gift from Dr. L. Steinman, Stanford University.

Lymphocyte Proliferation Assay

Spleen mononuclear cells (10^5 cells/well) in RPMI-1640 were incubated with the antigen (4 μg/well) and the mitogen (Con A) (2 μg/well). After 4 days incubation at 37°C in 5% CO_2, cultures were pulsed with 1.0 μci of ^{3}H-thymidine/well, harvested and counted. Stimulation indices were calculated.

ELISA

Anti-IRBP antibodies were measured using the method described before.[2] Briefly, ELISA plates were coated with the antigen (50 ng/well). After incubation, the plates were washed and serum samples in the proper dilutions were added. Plates were washed and incubated with peroxidase conjugated goat-anti-mouse IgG. To develop the color reaction, the substrate o-phenylendianine in citrate buffer with 3% H_2O_2 was used and absorbance was measured at 490.

RESULTS

Histologically, inhibition of uveitis was found in 100% of the animals in group 1, in which GK 1.5 was administered beginning on day 7 after primary immunization. In this same group, stimulation indices and anti-IRPB antibody titers were markedly diminished as compared with those in controls.

In group 3, when GK 1.5 was administered beginning on day 16 after antigen sensitization, this immunotherapy prevented disease in 80% of the animals; the remaining 20% showed mild uveoretinitis. In the control groups 2 and 4, all animals exhibited inflammatory reactions with vasculitis, cellular infiltration, and retinal damage. In the last 2 groups where spleen cells were used for in vitro proliferation assays, inhibition of the proliferation was noted in cultures incubated with GK 1.5.

DISCUSSION

Administration of monoclonal antibodies directed against T-cell subset markers might constitute an effective treatment of autoimmune disorders. Such therapy was proven successful in different animal models.[3] Treatment with antibody to the L3T4 markers selectively reduced the number of L3T4[+] T-cells. The dramatic effect of monoclonal antibody GK 1.5 on the development of EAU in the present study may be attributed to this same mechanism, or may be due to blocking of T-cell activation. Both effects could result in the production of a dominant suppressor population.[4] Further studies are needed to clarify the role of specific lymphocyte subsets in the induction of tolerance by anti-L3T4.

Inhibition of T-cell activation is accompanied by inhibition of T-cell binding to antigen-presenting cell, indicating that anti-L3T4 may block the interaction of L3T4 on T-cell with MHA II on antigen-presenting cells.[5]

This treatment with Mab to L3T4 could alter immune responses by blocking the interaction between T-cells and antigen presenting cells, by directly inhibiting T-cell function, by depleting L3T4[+] cells or by stimulating the development of suppressor T-cells.

CONCLUSIONS

1. It can be concluded that immunotherapy is an effective means of preventing the development of EAU, at least in this model.
2. Further studies are required to detect beneficial effects of such therapy in the treatment of other forms of uveitis.
3. Studies are in progress to delineate the mechanism of beneficial effects noted with the monoclonal antibody therapy.

REFERENCES

1. Caspi RR, Roberge FG, Chan CC, Wiggert B, Chader GJ, Rozenszajn CL, Lando Z, Nusenblatt RB: Experimental autoimmune uveoretinitis induced in mice with two different retinal antigens. J of Immunol (1988) 140:1490-95.

2. Mochizuki M, Kuwabara T, McAllister C, Nussenblatt RB, and Gery I: Adoptive transfer of experimental autoimmune uveoretinitis in rats: Immunopathogenic mechanisms and histologic features. Invest Opthalmol Vis Sci (1985) 26:1.

478

3. Waldor MK, Sriram S, Hardy R, Lanier L, and Lim M: Reversal of experimental allergic encephalomyelitis with monoclonal antibody to a T-cell subset marker. Science (1985) 227:415.

4. Dialynas DP, Wilde DB, Marvack P et al.: Characterization of the murine antigenic determinant, designated L3T4Á, recognized by monoclonal antibody GK 1.5. Immunological Rev (1983) 74:29.

5. Wilde DB, Marvack P, Kappler J, Dialynas DP, and Fitch FW. Evidence implicating L3T4 in class II MHC antigen reactivity: monoclonal antibody GK 1.5 (anti-L3T4a) blocks class II MHC antigen-specific proliferation, release of lymphokines, and bindings by cloned murine helper T lymphocyte lines. J Immunol (1983) 131:278.

© 1990 Elsevier Science Publishers (Biomedical Division)
Ocular Immunology Today. M. Usui, S. Ohno and K. Aoki, editors.

479

COMBINATION TREATMENT WITH CYCLOSPORINE AND BROMOCRIPTINE IN
BEHCET'S DISEASE

TAKASHI HARADA, KYOKO MURAKAMI, MIKA NIWA, SHINOBU AWAYA
Department of Ophthalmology, Nagoya University School of
medicine, Nagoya (Japan)

INTRODUCTION

In recent years, a potency to modulate immuno-competence
has been ascribed to prolactin, pituitary anterior lobe hormone (1).   Administration of bromocriptine, dopamine agonist
of prolactin, induced reduction of host versus graft reaction
in mice (2).   Combination of bromocriptine with low-dose
cyclosporine in experimentally induced auto-immune uveitis in
rats produced effects equivalent to those with high-dose cyclosporine therapy (3).   The efficacy of the combined treatment
in man has been reported in three articles (4,5,6).
We report the results of combination treatment in 10 cases of
Behçet's disease with cyclosporine associated with bromocriptine.

MATERIAL AND METHODS

20 eyes in 10 cases with Behçet's disease who underwent
cyclosporine-bromocriptine combination treatment because of
failure to respond favorably to other modalities of therapy
were admitted for study.   Combination treatment was achieved
with (1) cyclosporine with an initial dose of 5 mg/Kg/day,
usually adjusted according to a severity of the disease or a
reaction of the patients to a given dose of cyclosporine, and
with (2) bromocriptine with an initial dose of 1,25 mg which
was elevated to 7,5mg finally in 3 cases.   The therapy was
continued throughout the period varying from 10 to 19 months
with an average of 15 months.   Blood cyclosporine levels and
serum prolactin ones were monitored usually once per month; in
3 cases blood cyclosporine levels could be determined in 3
days following initiation of bromocriptine medication.
Visual acuity prior to and following the treatment was recorded
from medical charts; in this context, visual acuity at conva-
rescent stage and not at attack stage was adopted.   Number
of acute attacks prior to and following the treatment was also
enumerated for comparison.

480

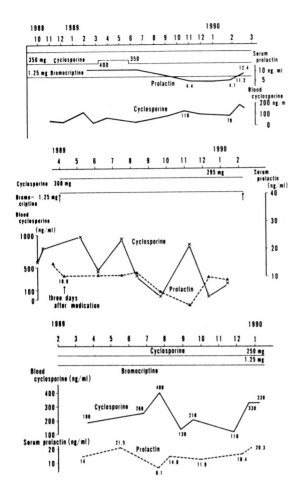

Fig.1 Blood cyclosporine levels and serum prolactin levels in 3 representative cases.

RESULTS

Fig.1 illustrates blood cyclosporine levels and serum prolactin ones in 3 representative cases with Behçet's disease
wherein an overall stabilization of ocular conditions dominated
their clinical course, and cyclosporine dosage did undergo
only a slight change, bromocriptine dosage being fixed to 1,25
mg. The confrontation of blood cyclosporine values and of
serum prolactin ones disclosed that there exists some sort of
reciprocal relationship between the two, that is, as blood
cyclosporine augmented, on the contrary, serum prolactin
lowered, and vice versa.

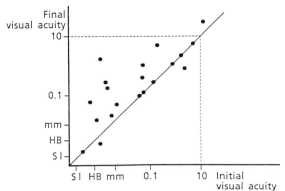

Fig. 2.   Visual acuity prior to and following treatment

An unrestricted rise in blood cyclosporine did not result
in our series as the period of medication proceeded. In 7 cases
out of our series wherein occasional changes of dosage in cyclosporine and bromocriptine rendered the evaluation of interrelationship between blood cyclosporine and serum prolactin less
pronounced,
there were nevertheless an overall tendency to an increase in
blood cyclosporine levels as the period of combination therapy
proceeded, with or without augmentation of dosage of bromocriptine.
With respect to visual acuity prior to and following treatment,
it was ameliorated in 9 eyes(45%),, stabilized in 9 eyes (45 %),
and deteriorated in 2 eyes (10 %). Table 1. demonstrates
significant decrease in acute episode in as much as 85 % of our
series.

TABLE 1.   **Influence of treatment upon attacks**

Attacks	No. eyes
augmented	2 ·········· 10 %
stabilized	1 ··········· 5
reduced	17 ·········· 85
Total	20

DISCUSSION

Results of our study exhibited a reciprocal relationship existing between blood cyclosporine levels and serum prolactin ones and confirmed, like results of other studies (4,5), that medication of bromocriptine with a dose of 1,25 mg or more, exerting suppressing influence on serum prolactin levels, led to raised blood cyclosporine levels.

However, medication of bromocriptine did not develop unrestricted rise in blood cyclosporine levels; when blood cyclosporine increased to attain a given value, it presently sustained gradual decrease, being autoregulated in all likelihood by intervening immunomodulatory systems, and it restored its original level.

Adjunct of bromocriptine to the regimen consisted solely of cyclosporine did not produce adverse effects all the more, as compared with this regimen.   Results of our combined treatment corroborated marked efficacy in reducing acute episode in virtually as many as 85 % of cases and sustaining visual function to a sufficiently acceptable degree, judging from natural course that patients with Behçet's disease usually assume.

Consequently we are convinced that the combination therapy with cyclosporine and bromocriptine is justified in the treatment of this disease.

REFERENCES

1. Nagi EI,Berczi,I, Friesen,HG (1983) Acta Endocrinol 102: 351-357
2. Hiestand,PC,Mekler,P.,Nordmann,R., Grieder,A,Permmongkol,C (1986) Proc.Natl.Acad.Sci,USA, 83:2599-2603
3. Patestine,AG, Muellenberg-Coulobre,CG, Kim,MK,Gelato,MC, Nussenblatt,RB (1987) J clinical Invest., 79:1078-1081
4. Minakawa R, Ohno,S, Ariga H, Tanaka,K, Hirano T (1988) Jpn J Clin Ophthalmol 42:1161-1166
5. Fukuyado K,Banto Y,Tanouchi Y,Fujita Y,Mimura Y (1988) Combination treatment of cyclosporine and bromocriptine in Behçet's disease, 16th Group discussion Uveitis, 23 September, Tokyo
6. Zierhut M,Pleyer U,Waetjen R,Thiek HJ,Weidle G (1989) Klin Mbl Augenheilk 195:221-225

© 1990 Elsevier Science Publishers (Biomedical Division)
Ocular Immunology Today. M. Usui, S. Ohno and K. Aoki, editors.

INTRAVITREAL INJECTION OF ANTI-PSEUDOMONAS GLOBULIN AGAINST PSEUDOMONAS ENDOPHTHALMITIS IN RABBITS

HIROSHI HATANO, MD AND YUTAKA ISOBE, MD
Department of ophthalmology, Yokohama City University School of Medicine, Yokohama, Japan

INTRODUCTION

Bacterial endophthalmitis belongs to devastating eye diseases threatening visual function. Pseudomonas aeruginosa is the causative agent which is most frequently isolated among gram-negative bacteria in endophthalmitis. Pseudomonas tends to become resistant to various antibiotics and systemic use of effective antibiotics are very limited for their side effects. Therefore, antibiotics can not be all mighty in the treatment of pseudomonas infections. In general, pseudomonas aeruginosa hardly be pathogenic in healthy persons because of the naturally aquired humoral immunity against this organism[1]. However, vitreous body of the eye is very far from reach of serum because of absence of blood supply, which can be said a very special part in human body isolated from immunity. It has been reported that intracorneal injection of immunoglobulin on corneal ulcers in horses experimentally infected with pseudomonas aeruginosa has a therapeutic effect[2]. The current experiment was designed to examine and evaluate the efficacy of intravitreal application of antibody alone to pseudomonas endophthalmitis in rabbits, as a possible supplementary treatment in addition to antibiotics.

MATERIALS

30 adult white rabbits and Pseudomonas aeruginosa ; strain 75 and strain Itoh were used. The former strain is virulent to the intraocular tissue producing both protease and elastase, while, the latter is avirulent to it producing neither enzyme[3]. Globulin used for intravitreal injection is human anti-pseudomonas globulin (Pyocyanbulin-I ® , Midorijuji, Osaka, Japan) containing antibodies anti-original endotoxin protein (OEP) x80, anti-protease x8, anti-elastase x8, and anti-exotoxin x32 (PHA: passive hemagglutinin). Human albumin (purity 99%) was used as a control to globulin. Pseudomonas aeruginosa cell suspension 10^2 CFU/ml saline abbreviated as (Ps), human anti-pseudomonas gamma globulin 200mg/ml saline (Glb), and human albumin 200mg/ml saline (Alb) were prepared as materials for intravitreal injection.

METHODS

This experiment was separately done in two series. The first series includes observation and evaluation of clinical courses and the second series does viable cell count in eyes of the rabbits tested. And, each series was conduced for and with respect to each of two different strains of pseudomonas aeruginosa.

Experiment 1. (clinical courses) : Six rabbits were used here. After anesthesia with intravenous injection of pentobarbital sodium, 0.1 to 0.2 ml aqueous humor was aspirated using a syringe with a 30 gauge needle from both eyes of the six rabbits to be injected. Followingly, the right vitreous cavity was injected with 0.1 ml of a mixture of eaqual volume of Ps and Glb preparations mentioned above. On the contrary, the left eyes were injected with 0.1 ml of the mixture of eaqual volume of Ps and Alb preparations which served as a control. And then, the clinical courses of the eyes were followed with a slit-lamp biomicroscope for five days after injection. We evaluated the severity of clinical findings of each rabbit using two keys consisting of exudates volume 0 to 4 in the anterior chamber and transillumination 0 to 2 to get integrated clinical scores 0 through 6.

Experiment 2 (viable cell count) : Another nine rabbits were used here for investigation of the dynamics of viable cell number in whole vitreous cavity of each eye. Three rabbits were sacrificed at each time of 6, 24, and 48 hours after injection using intravenous anesthesia. We removed the cornea, iris and lens out of each eye tested and then took the whole vitreous to homogenize and count the total viable pseudomonas cell number in each eye by step dilution of the supernatant and culture plate method.

RESULTS (figures 1,2,3,4)

Experiment 1 (clinical courses)

1) strain Itoh (figure 1): All of six right eyes which received the mixture of Ps and Glb showed no clinical findings at all. On the other hand, all of six left eyes which received the mixture of Ps and Alb suffered from endophthalmitis with a variety of severity in clinical scores ranging 1 to 5 at one day, 1.5 to 5 at two days, 1.5 to 4 at three days, 2 to 3.5 at four days, and 2 to 3 at five days after injection.

2) strain 75 (figure 2): All six right eyes which received the mixture of Ps and Glb showed no clinical finding except one eye developing endophthalmitis only since the third day after injection. On the contrary, all six left eyes which received the mixture of Ps and Alb progressed to severe endophthalmitis since second day, having score 6 except one eye.

Experiment 2 (vable cell count)

1) strain Itoh (figure 3): At all three given times, all eyes which received Ps and Glb did not recover any pseudomonas cell at all. On the other hand, from two left eyes (one out of three rabbits was dead) which were injected Ps and Alb, 1.0×10^6 and 6.0×10^6 CFU/eye were recovered at 24 hours. At both of 48 hours and 4 days, no viable cell were isolated from the left eyes.

2) strain 75 (figure 4): At 24 hours after injection, the viable cell numbers

recovered from total vitreous of each of three right eyes which received Ps and Glb were 5.3×10^2, 7.0×10^2 and 4.5×10^3 CFU/eye. Those at 48 hours were 2.0×10^2, 6.9×10^3, and 2.5×10^7 CFU/eye, and those at 4 days were 4.5×10^2, 9.3×10^4, and 3.6×10^5 CFU/eye. On the other hand, the viable cell numbers at 24 hours of the left eyes which were injected with Ps and Alb were 3.0×10^6, 1.3×10^7, and 5.1×10^7. Those at 48 hours were 6.3×10^5, 2.4×10^6, and 6.0×10^6 CFU/eye and those at 4 days were 3.5×10^3, 5.8×10^3, and 9.5×10^4 CFU/eye.

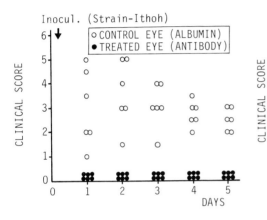

Fig. 1. Clinical course of Pseudomonas endophthalmitis in rabbits (strain Itoh)

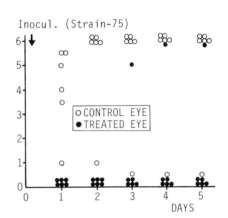

Fig. 2. Clinical course of Pseudomonas endophthalmitis in rabbits (strain 75)

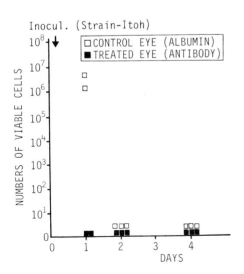

Fig. 3. Viable cells in vitreous cavity of rabbit (strain Itoh)

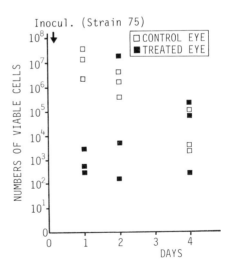

Fig. 4. Viable cells in vitreous cavity of rabbit (strain 75)

486

DISCUSSION

In both strains of pseudomonas aeruginosa, the right eyes which received Ps and Glb invariablby showed lower clinical scores than the left eyes which received Ps and Alb at any given time. Furthermore, the viable cell numbers in the vitreous cavities were much smaller in globulin injected right eyes than albumin injected left eyes in both pseudomonas strains. Therefore, the results in both series of experiments indicates that intravitreal injection of human anti-pseudomonas globulin is effective to suppress the intraocular inflammation of pseudomonas endophthalmitis in rabbits and also the cell growth of pseudomonas aeruginosa in the vitreous cavity.

The possible major mechanism of efficacy of globulin in this experimental model may include an opsonization effect of globulin accelerating adherence of bacteria to the surface of polymorphonuclear leucocytes through Fc receptors and phagocytosis. Another possible cause can be the bacteriolysis by complements activated by globulin.

The biggest problem in clinical application of globulin in endophthalmitis, for whatever therapy or prevention it may be, is the specificity against causative bacteria. The globulin used this time contains the antibody against OEP (original endotoxin protein; OEP). Prior immunization of mice with OEP of pseudomonas aeruginosa has been known to protect mice against infection with any of Fisher's immunotypes and Homma's serotypes of the bacteria. It has been also revealed that OEP is an antigen existing serologically in common in pseudomonas aeruginosa, and can be the common protective antigen in all pseudomonas aeruginosa[4]. Therefore the current experimental findings that infections by two pseudomonas strains were samely suppressed by the globulin, seems to reveal that the most effective fraction of anitbodies in those series of experiments maybe that against OEP, instead those against protease and or elastase.

REFERENCES

1) Doi T, Yoshioka M and Nakajima T: Psedomonas aeruginosa antibodies in human plasama. Jap. J. Exp. Med. 46:149-154, 1976

2) Ueda Y, Sanai Y and Homma JY: The therapeutic effect of intracorneal injection of immunoglobulin on corneal ulcers in horses experimentally infected with Pseudomonas aeruginosa. Japanese Journal of Veterinary Science. 44:301-308, 1982

3) Hatano H: Experimental Pseudomonas Endophthalmitis in Rabbits. Intracameral Inoculation of Two Pseudomonal Strains. Acta Soc. Ophthalmol. Jpn. 86:839-845, 1982

4) Abe C, Shionoya H, Hirano Y, Okada K and Homma JY: Common protective antigen (OEP) of Pseudomonas aeruginosa. Japan J. Exp. Med. 45:355-359, 1975

INDEX OF AUTHORS

488